Praise for Stephen A. Appelbaum's
THE MYSTERY OF HEALING

"I read [*The Mystery of Healing*] on the plane to Los Angeles last week and found myself having a hard time putting it down ... In an era in which expenditures on alternative medicine are rapidly approaching those of conventional treatments, we are sorely in need of a guidebook to help us navigate our way through the murky waters of the healers, hucksters, and hoodwinkers. Stephen Appelbaum has provided us with a thoroughly absorbing and intelligently written volume that cuts to the core of the healing experience. Appelbaum is the ideal guide; both participant and observer, he samples an assortment of alternative treatments with an open-minded skepticism that allows for the fantastic while always looking for plausible alternative explanations. Those who accompany him on this journey will be richly rewarded."

— GLEN GABBARD, M.D., Callaway Distinguished Professor, The Menninger Clinic; author, *Love and Hate in the Analytic Setting*

"This book follows Dr. Stephen A. Appelbaum on a personal voyage through the territory of alternative healing practitioners. These waters are perilous, yet Appelbaum navigates them well, with an attitude both critical and fair-minded. Of the many books on this topic, Appelbaum's is unique in its emphasis on immediate experience; he was a participant-observer in this saga, and the result is an authoritative text that absorbs the reader in its account."

— STANLEY KRIPPNER, PH.D., Professor of Psychology, Saybrook Graduate School; co-author, *The Mythic Path*; co-editor, *Broken Images, Broken Selves*

"Dr. Stephen Appelbaum has provided a valuable contribution in his book *The Mystery of Healing*. He has open-mindedly researched a variety of alternative healing methods, and through his personal participation he helps people be better consumers."

— STEVEN HASSAN, author of the best-seller *Combatting Cult Mind Control*

Praise for Stephen A. Appelbaum's
A Psychoanalyst Explores the Alternative Therapies: Out in Inner Space

"Appelbaum is rigorous in his theoretical thinking and well equipped for studying the many new psychotherapies. I found [this book] not only a vicarious way of learning about unconventional therapies, but an interesting personal experience. It has a unique mixture of honesty and innocence, straightforwardness and exhibitionism, and also humility. I would suggest that it be required reading for any psychotherapist, psychoanalyst, or psychiatrist."

— RALPH R. GREENSON, M.D.

"This book is fun to read ... essential for anyone currently involved with the many aspects of psychotherapy; it compares and contrasts, in a most lucid and interesting manner, several currently debated topics. The book is a powerful argument for informed sensibility and an overcoming of narrowness. It is highly recommended."

— JAMES D. GILL, *The Psychology Bulletin*

"I was particularly impressed with Appelbaum's ability to enter into the different therapies, describe the experience in a vivid way, and then subject them to critical analysis from the standpoint of psychoanalytic theory. I recommend the book to anyone who is interested in learning something about the spectrum of theories flourishing today."

— JEROME D. FRANK, M.D., Professor Emeritus of Psychiatry, Johns Hopkins University

"This book is a thoughtful account of a return from nearby strange, mysterious, and evocative places. It is also an invitation. One cannot come away from the book without being intrigued and challenged. There is simply too much of obvious relevance to modern psychiatry and medicine to ignore."

—JUSTIN SIMON, M.D., *American Journal of Psychiatry*

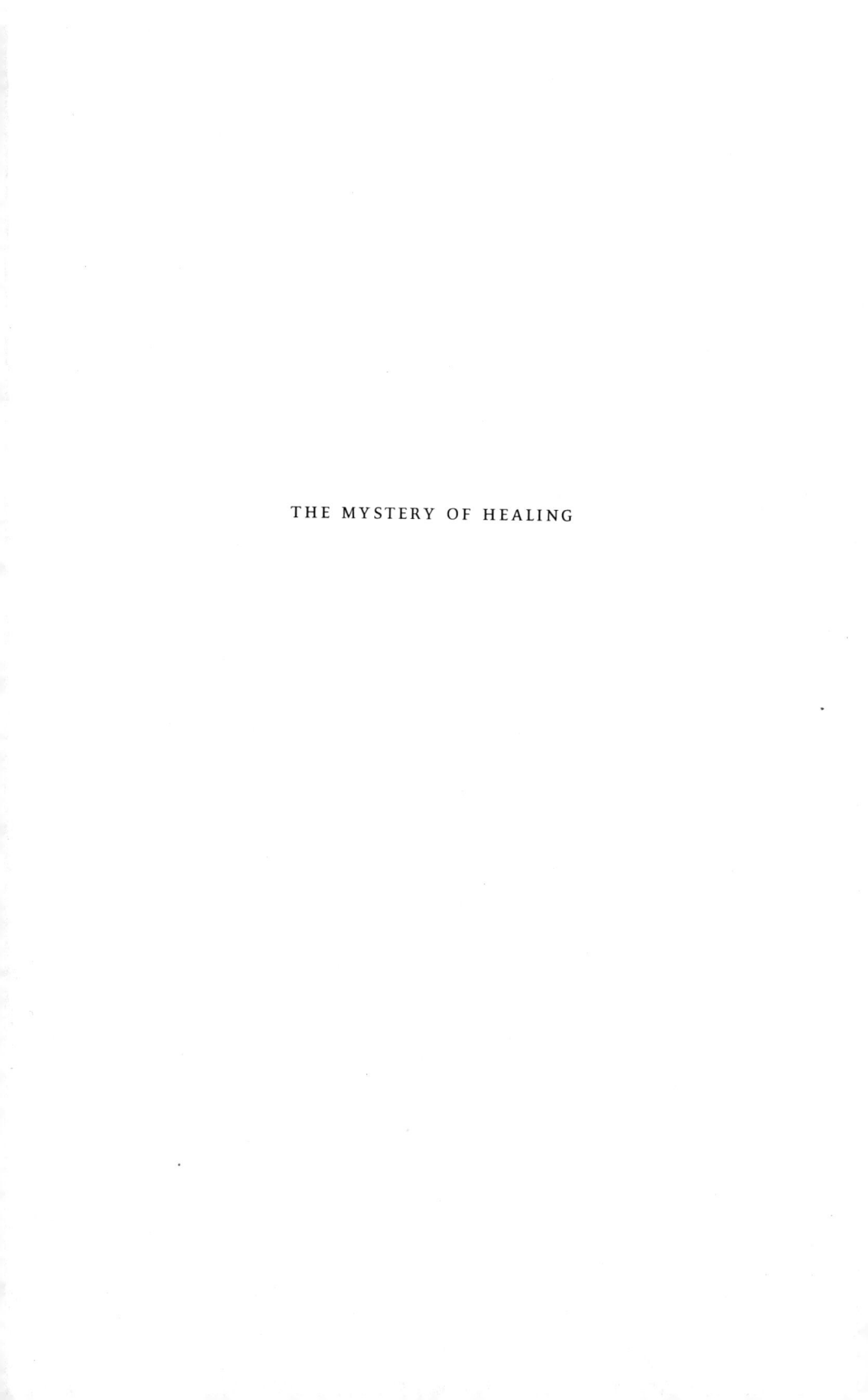

THE MYSTERY OF HEALING

The Mystery of Healing

Journeys Through Alternative Medicine

Stephen A. Appelbaum, Ph.D.

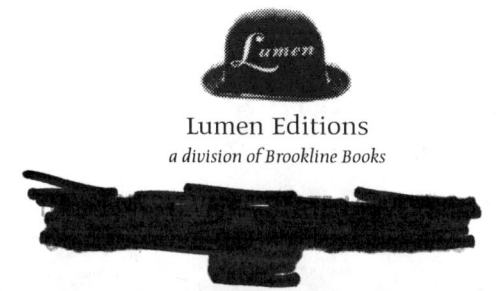

Lumen Editions
a division of Brookline Books

Copyright ©1999 by Stephen A. Appelbaum.

All rights reserved. No part of this work covered by the copyright hereon may be reproduced or used in any form or by any means—graphic, electronic, or mechanical, including photocopying, recording, taping, or information storage and retrieval systems—without the permission of the publisher.

ISBN 1-57129-062-1

Library of Congress Cataloging-In-Publication Data
Appelbaum, Stephen A.
    The mystery of healing : journeys through alternative medicine / Stephen A. Appelbaum.
        p.   cm.
    Includes bibliographical references.
    ISBN 1-57129-062-1 (pbk.)
    1. Alternative medicine--Miscellanea.   2. Healing--Miscellanea.   I. Title.
R733.A65   1998
615.5--dc21   98-38700
                                                              CIP

Cover design by Kate Rubin.
Cover illustration by Nathan Budoff.
Book design and typography by Erica L. Schultz.

Printed in USA
10 9 8 7 6 5 4 3 2 1

Published by
Lumen Editions
a division of
BROOKLINE BOOKS
P.O. Box 1047
Cambridge, Massachusetts 02238
Order toll-free: 1-800-666-BOOK

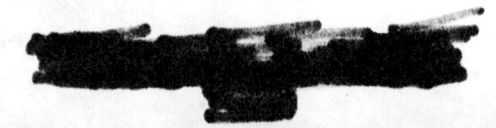

Contents

CHAPTER ONE
The Mystery of Healing 1

CHAPTER TWO
The Spirit Is Willing: Meetings with a Medium 7

CHAPTER THREE
Georgia On My Mind: Surgery in a Trance 18

CHAPTER FOUR
The Magical Mystery Tour: Philippine Psychic Surgery 30

CHAPTER FIVE
The Laying On of Health: Some Who Heal by Touch 63

CHAPTER SIX
But Faith In What? God's Healing Delegates 85

CHAPTER SEVEN
Dealing with a Dread Diagnosis 109

CHAPTER EIGHT
Affairs of the Heart: A Cardiovascular Adventure 153

CHAPTER NINE
That Old Black Magic: Voodoo Healing in Haiti 159

CHAPTER TEN
C. Norman Shealy and Friends: A Holistic Healing Center 173

CHAPTER ELEVEN
Exploring the Personalities of Psychic Healers:
A Psychological Test Study 189

CHAPTER TWELVE
Kinesiology: Bodily Truth and Consequences 199

CHAPTER THIRTEEN
Olga, Ambrose, and Robert: A Convention of the Unconventional 204

CHAPTER FOURTEEN
Tripping the Light Fantastic: The Possibilities of LSD 216

CHAPTER FIFTEEN
Beating the Bushes: Folk Medicine in Belize and Beyond 251

CHAPTER SIXTEEN
Endings and Beginnings: Conclusions 257

References 274
Index 277
About the Author 285

To Brooks and Eric

who will find here their editing, and occasionally their own words. With fatherly pride and gratitude.

Chapter One

The Mystery of Healing

I HAVE BEEN A HEALER, specifically a psychoanalyst, for over three decades. I know that people get healed — not all of them and not in every way, but healing is real and blessed. Still, on my desk as I write this is a brochure advertising a conference entitled "How Change Comes About in Psychoanalytic Psychotherapy." With all the years of experience with people's being healed, with all the panoply and superstructure of degrees, professional organizations, academic appointments, scientific studies, insurance support, and prestige accorded its practitioners, we are still having conferences to try to understand healing. And such a conference need not be restricted to psychological healing; it could just as well be held with respect to physical healing. It could be held in any one of the thousands of years of healing, and with respect to such healing interventions as incantations, eating animal entrails, bloodletting, laser beam surgery, and talking while flat on one's back on a couch. Such is the mystery of healing.

Healing is mysterious not only because it comes about through so many modalities, but because its effects are so unpredictable: people get better who, according to medical experience, should not, and people succumb who should get better. Diseases follow varying courses as if they have a life of their own.

A YOUNG WOMAN consulted me with complaints of intestinal pain from alleged endometriosis (inflammation of the lining of the uterus) which continued despite supposedly successful surgery, leaving her with a recommendation that she take painkilling drugs for as long as necessary.

While she had been in the hospital, a psychiatrist had appeared in her room without her prior knowledge and permission, asked to be there by her physician, at the instigation of her mother. The psychiatrist, according to her, had only discussed her mother's complaints about her, in an apparent attempt to convince the patient that she needed psychiatric treatment. She and I had one interview, and then arranged to meet again for a battery of psychological tests. At that second meeting, four days later, I occupied myself with the test materials and with thinking about her in psychological rather than physical terms — and so she had to volunteer the information that she *no longer had* physical pain.

How to understand this apparent healing? One way would be to consider what I had said, the content of the initial interview. That content included nothing apparently complicated or "deep." In addition to learning superficially about her physical symptoms, her occupation, her social life, I took up her use of the word "problems" with respect to herself. I told her that I tried never to use the word, nor its associated words such as "pathology," "sickness," and for that matter, "health." I figure people always do the best they can, and have reasons for whatever they choose to do. If we had all the information, we could see that their decisions made, in their own terms, a kind of sense. "Problems" exist only because they or others don't like what they choose, for social, religious, or legal reasons, and because the observer does not understand the purposes for the behavior. I suggested that a more helpful way might be to decide what one wanted for oneself, and then judge one's behavior according to whether it was likely to help achieve one's aims. It was her business after all to decide how she wanted to live, what in effect was "healthy" for her; neither I nor anyone else could be sure what made for another's happiness in the long run, or what life would be like if she did something different from creating her particular symptoms. As to her physical pain, I said that physical illness was a language; her pain was a way of saying something. If she could find the right words and feelings, she would not need the pain to speak for her.

Another way to try to understand her apparent healing is what *the fact of the interview* meant to her regardless of its content. When the patient's mother called me to make an appointment for the patient, I asked that the patient call me about the appointment. So in contrast to the unexpected appearance of the psychiatrist in the hospital (engineered by her mother and surgeon), she made her own arrangements to meet with me in my comfortable office instead of a hospital room. She might have gotten the idea from our meeting that help was available. She might have liked me. As a young child she had lost her father, and may have sensed in me a replacement.

I HAVE HARDLY EXHAUSTED the list of possible explanations of this seemingly miraculous healing. Even if I had, we would still be left with the mystery of how any meanings had stopped her nerves from sending to her brain signals which she reported as pain — or why she no longer reported and presumably experienced pain, whether or not pain-conducting nerves had anything to do with it. When one frees oneself from the well-worn pathways of the mind that accept the ways of healing unquestioningly, healing stands revealed as humbling, awesome, and mysterious. And so I set out on an odyssey to enjoy the awe, and perhaps dispel some of the mystery.

I selected stops along the way with the understanding that healing was bigger and broader than conventional Western medicine. Healings have not only been brought about by "designated" doctors, now and certainly in the past. Healers have included Jesus, kings such as Edward the Confessor and Charles II who were said to possess a healing "royal touch," and less sung practitioners including countless grandmothers. I determined to study the unconventional, the extreme, as a means of understanding the less extreme. One learns much about how the body normally works through studying its pathology. For example, studying the delusions characteristic of what is considered to be severe mental illness and the apparent bizarreness of dreams sheds light on the less conscious aspect of the normal mind. By that token, learning how the laying on of hands, for example, works may contribute to the understanding of how penicillin and surgery work.

I selected diverse healings to explore. If people can be healed through diverse (as well as seemingly improbable) procedures, then these procedures likely have elements in common, elements that might turn out to be the essence of healing.

I expected to have a lot of fun on this odyssey. Whether the trip for the reader is a pleasure trip or a business trip depends on the passenger's interests and sensibilities. As a pleasure trip, the tour is a geographical, psychological, and vicariously experiential voyage to places, people, and activities not ordinarily available to most of us. How many of us are familiar with healing by way of surgical passes done by a surgeon in a trance guided by long-dead physicians? Healing by breaking the neck of a chicken and dropping its blood and other excreta on the patient's head? Healing by having matter apparently taken from the body through apparent incisions made by the bare hands of the surgeon?

I travel with a romantic indulgence which decrees that *anything* might be true until proven false. I pack also a classical-scientific horror at the unsubstantiated which decrees that anything that might be true *isn't* until it has been shown to be so. (As Oscar Wilde said, the purpose of an open mind is occasionally to snap shut.) If this romantic–classical juxtaposition generates tension and improbability, then welcome to the ambiguous, perplexing, and endlessly fascinating world of healing.

ONE CAN CONSIDER all of life as a series of attempts to heal: people are engaged in healing whenever they try to find ways to move from disagreeable conditions to more agreeable ones. We try to heal ignorance through education, loneliness through sociability, hatred through love. Attempts to heal designated physical or psychological illnesses are but special instances of healing. Because such illnesses tend to be grave and frightening, they reveal much about all of life's healing efforts, and indeed much about life itself. What may seem on the surface like a routine trip to a healer for a routine symptom or examination is experienced, at least in the dim reaches of ourselves, as an issue of mortality and consequently of life's purpose.

Zealots tend to believe in single causes for complex events — it is all the fault of the labor unions, the economy, sunspots. Healing efforts and philosophies can make the same error, substituting simple-mindedness for complexity. Thus, one gets sick from overwork and is healed by drinking chicken soup. Healing includes a *technology*, those healing measures taken designedly in order to bring about cure, such as the administering of a medicine. And healing includes a *context*, which refers to other factors in the healing situation of which one may or may not be aware. Notable among such factors is the suggestion-placebo effects of, for example, receiving a healing agent derived from gleaming machines and administered by an impressively trained person whom society has designated as one who can "make it better."

Here is the case for open-mindedness with respect to unorthodox healing: nothing is known absolutely; we are all children of our time. Even science, so far the best way of making sense of the everyday world, claims only to approximate reality and stands ready to change its views as necessitated by new information.

Anyway, we cannot afford to be closed-minded about healing unorthodoxy when healing orthodoxy has failed us in many ways. Our health care system has produced at best mixed results, at increasingly unbearable costs. Successes in the treatment of infections and accidents are counterbalanced by failure in the treatment and prevention of cancer, diabetes, arthritis, and other chronic degenerative diseases. Deleterious side effects from medicine and hospitalization, iatrogenic disease, and medical errors are scandalously prevalent. It makes sense to consider alternatives.

One way to keep one's bearings amid the panoply of diverse healing procedures is to categorize them in terms of their emphasis on *body, mind,* and *spirit.* In modern Western medicine the body is the center of attention, as befits a culture saturated with Descartes's separation of mind from body which likens the body to a machine. According to that philosophy, ills of the body should be treated by actions on the body, such as surgery, radiation, or drugs.

Mind refers to consciousness. We use mind to heal by thinking inspiring and encouraging thoughts. We also use consciousness to heal body and mind with meditation, as yogis did for thousands of years. Freud turned our attention to the unconscious as a source of healing by making the unconscious conscious.

Spirit in healing is more tricky and elusive. In unorthodox healing circles, spirit is a fashionable concept and encourages feelings of elevation and trust. Spirit helps with the increasing condensation of religion and psychotherapy, as can be seen for example in pastoral counseling (probably more psychotherapy is done by pastors than by official psychotherapists). Spirit also refers to experiences we label rapture, glow, revelation, or epiphany, whether these accompany a healing or are experienced in church, when in love, or when communing with nature. Such moments are experienced as being apart from one's workaday self — as transcendent. Many people consider such experiences to be evidence of the Divine. Others consider them solely psychological. Many unorthodox healers see themselves as merely mediums, channels for the healing that comes from God. Whether psychological or supernatural, spirit plays a major role in many unorthodox healings.

IN HIS PRESIDENTIAL ADDRESS to the American Psychical Society in 1896, William James likened the study of the paranormal to a search for a white crow. If one could just find a single white crow, one would have to think differently about crows. If only one fully substantiated instance of the paranormal could be found, he said, then our ideas about reality, about how we know things, about the nature of the universe are open to question.

Orthodox healing practices can be considered black crows, for as anyone can see crows are black, and all are presumed to be that way (except for a few albinos). Instances of unorthodox healing, and the unorthodox version of reality in which such healing may be embedded, could be considered white crows, for they are believed to be impossibilities. To countenance a healing practice like the laying on of hands, for example, is to see a white crow.

Physical, psychological, and spiritual contributions to healing, singly or in combination, make for a complex problem — and moreover one that requires a suspension of disbelief, as we now consider what for most modern Western persons are alien ideas and strange events. But to spur you on there is the beckoning seduction that if you look quickly, if the light is right, and if you are willing to believe your eyes, you just might see wheeling across the sky a white crow.

Chapter Two

The Spirit Is Willing: Meetings with a Medium

DONALD GALLOWAY IS AN English spiritualist medium, or "sensitive." He serves as a conduit, relaying messages to mortals from the realms of the dead, what he calls the "other side." In the Bible and in the ancient world, the voices from that realm were considered to be non-human — the speakers were angels, demigods, demons, or subdeities. In recent centuries the spirits are said to be those of persons who were once mortals on earth and whose "passing over" occurred recently or within the last few centuries.

I was eager to get acquainted with Mr. Galloway, since the role of the medium shares basic assumptions with that of the psychic healer. Any paranormal activity that can be demonstrated as valid lends credibility to other paranormal activities. Moreover, most psychic healers claim that their healing power also comes from "the other side." They believe that they serve as conduits; the healer directs God's healing energy to the patient, while the spiritualist transmits energy from metaphysical sources. In fact, according to the jacket of his book *Inevitable Journey*,[1] Mr. Galloway did run a healing sanctuary in England before becoming an administrator at the College of Psychic Studies in London. When I knew him, he lectured and offered "sittings" in Britain, the United States, and Canada.

Mr. Galloway is a no-nonsense, straight-talking person who gets on with his work; he is friendly but remains strictly within the limits of his task of relaying information. The sittings take place in whatever hotel or motel room he is staying in. For me the juxtaposition of a Ramada Inn with the "other world" was jarring, but I am sure that Mr. Galloway would respond to that observation with, "Never mind, let's get on with it."

"Getting on with it" involves his taking a watch or a ring, holding it in his hands for a moment or two, and then speaking more or less nonstop for some 45 minutes. He says that holding the watch or ring gets him in tune with his client. Realizing that memory may be unreliable, he encourages the use of a tape recorder. I was encouraged by his willingness to put his work in a form in which it could be scrutinized by others, and from a temporal distance. I was less encouraged by his belief that some psychiatric phenomena, such as the hearing of voices or the developing of seemingly unsubstantiated ideas, were not pathological, but instead messages from the spirit world.

I had three sittings with Mr. Galloway, two and three years apart. I tape-recorded and transcribed each one. Before going over the tapes of the three sessions, I first assessed my memory of them. True to the often-remarked tricks of the mind, I found I remembered the seeming successes more than the apparent failures or inconclusive comments. Moreover, in memory I tended to exaggerate the successes by substituting somewhat more accurate words for Mr. Galloway's slightly less accurate ones.

In some ways, Mr. Galloway worked like a dream interpreter. That is, he would get images sent by the spirits and then translate them. That kind of translation is risky business. A psychoanalytic interpreter of symbols reduces the risk by getting the *patient's* views and associations rather than by depending upon universal meanings or solely on his own interpretations. Mr. Galloway just improvised. For example, when he saw colored lights, he thought that meant renewed energy, a profusion of new and vibrant ideas and feelings awaiting me. When he saw a white ladder, he thought it meant that the steps of the ladder were ideas, and so my development of new ideas was like climbing the ladder. In this connection, he saw the spirits dropping little keys in front of me, each one standing for an insight, for new information that would lead me on. Sometimes he saw me in images in his imagination; for example, he saw me in an office with huge windows, which he thought meant that I was breaking out of the confines of traditional knowledge and expanding my vision.

As is so often true with any kind of psychic reading, a good many of the comments Mr. Galloway made were likely to be true of anybody. The astrology readings in daily newspapers tend to be of that sort. Mr. Galloway told me that I was struggling to distribute my time between my private life and my work responsibilities. True enough, but likely to be true of many people. He said that I have intuitive powers, capacities to know people beyond what can be learned about them through their superficial self-presentations. That, too, is probably true of most people — indeed, those who believe in psychic phenomena claim that intuitiveness is potentially true of *all* people — and certainly ought to be true of most psychoanalysts. At any rate, it is the sort of thing people like to hear and believe about themselves. People also like to believe that they are sensitive, and Mr. Galloway told me that I was extremely sensitive, more than other people knew and even more than I knew. I was also alleged to be tired, need a vacation, and tend toward having an upset stomach. Mr. Galloway said that I should avoid acids, such as can be found in citrus fruits. The same thing was told to me by several of the nutritionists practicing in the context of holistic medicine, as described in my book *Out In Inner Space*, and I assume that they told the same thing to thousands of others. Needless to say, I have lots of company in having occasional disturbances of the gastrointestinal system. As to being tired and in need of a vacation, that is a problem the ubiquity of which helps to support the travel industry. Not only was I especially sensitive, according to Mr. Galloway, but I was rather special; I could have been an "ordinary doctor," he said, but I was more than that, and I should not doubt myself so much. In fact, I do sometimes believe that I am extraordinary, as many others sometimes believe about themselves. I also sometimes feel that I am ordinary at best, and I daresay I have lots of company in that respect also.

So far as I know, Mr. Galloway knew about me only that I was, as he said, "a psychologist, a psychoanalyst, or something of the sort." Some of his remarks could have been deduced simply from that fact, as well as perhaps from the way I look. That I as a psychologist and psychoanalyst was visiting a spiritual medium could, in and of itself, have suggested to Mr. Galloway that I was open to new ideas, broadening my horizons and extricating myself from conventional ways of thinking. In connection with my breaking out of such confinement, he saw me speaking in front of colleagues, about which he said disarmingly, "One doesn't have to be psychic to know that." One also doesn't have to be psychic to know that I might be interested in schizophrenia, which Mr. Galloway said I was. I was then probably no more nor less involved with schizophrenia than most people doing my kind of work. The same could be said for the interest in dreams that he said I had. That I was interested in reincarnation, as he suggested, was strongly implied by the fact that I was with a man talking to spirits.

A good deal of the apparent validity of psychic readings comes about merely through one's being able to find events in one's life that appear to correspond to those referred to by the psychic. The more general the psychic's statements, the more likely that this will happen. Some of Mr. Galloway's statements were quite general. But some were fairly specific; for example, Mr. Galloway said that I had taken on some piece of work begun by others, and that it had proved to be more than I had anticipated. In fact, I had ended up writing a book based originally on the work of others when they were unable to complete it. Mr. Galloway's repeated references to my developing new ideas and breaking out of the rigidities of my training is a little more difficult to assess. In a sense he was right, as can be seen from this book and my other studies of new therapies and new medicine. Yet that turn of mind in me could have been deduced from the mere fact that I was with him. His comment that I worked on my own rather than as part of a group is true of any author. He said that he saw me speaking at a lectern and being surprised at what I was saying, which he interpreted as my almost inadvertently coming up with new and useful discoveries. He could easily have guessed that I occasionally give talks, and I, like most people, would like to agree that I make new and useful discoveries. Perhaps he was referring to the discovery that I could be comfortable speaking in public. Perhaps he correctly sensed what I have often experienced: that I sometimes do not know what I am going to say, or even what I think, until I say it; at those times speaking is less the conveying of a thought than it is the creation of one. Or perhaps these "perhapses" are a good illustration of how one can find evidence seemingly corroborative of a psychic, even in those instances where the psychic may have not correctly divined anything (except perhaps that the subject will find corroborative evidence!).

But some of Mr. Galloway's inferences about me illustrate an issue that demands consideration in any evaluation of his or any other psychic's accuracy: the issue of what we mean by "accuracy." Mr. Galloway was quite sure that music was of great importance to me, and in this he was correct. He suggested that I was a pianist, and indeed I did take piano lessons off and on for about six years as a child, and occasionally now play a bit for my own amusement. The great importance to me of music, however, lies in playing the saxophone. His surmise about music being important obviously could have been a lucky guess, and would probably be right for a substantial number of people. The same could be said of playing the piano, which a number of people at least try to do as children. He was wrong in identifying me as a pianist rather than a saxophonist, but what is meant by "wrong" in this context? Do we insist for a judgment of rightness that he be specific as to instrument? Or, after due allowance for coincidence and lucky guess, could he not be considered more right than wrong in identifying music as a major interest? It may be that we need to apply a connotative standard rather than a denotative one; perhaps the phenomena of paranormal activity exist, but not in a way that allows a high degree of precision in any given instance.

A similar issue came up in connection with Mr. Galloway's mental image of me writing. According to him, I was writing more than I anticipated; I had started out modestly, but then the work got bigger and longer. In fact, my book on the new therapies began as a series of informal reports to Roy Menninger, the President of the Menninger Foundation, who sent me on several of my early trips to explore one new therapy or another. Only as the reports mounted, and the overall implications of them as a series became more clear and compelling to me, did I think of making them into a book. Once again, allowing for a lucky or an educated guess, Mr. Galloway seemed to have been essentially right. However, his timing was off. The book had come out shortly before the sitting, so the scene that he had visualized could have only taken place several years previously. To what extent do we evaluate his image as being correct, even though the time was wrong, or do we demand from psychics a very high degree of precision before allowing their comments to be persuasive?

Mr. Galloway saw me in a large gathering, behind double doors, with about a hundred people, getting an award that "had to do with the writing of a book ... something to do with the printed word ... I hear lots of pens scratching." I did receive a Distinguished Writer award some four years later. I do not know how much my demeanor could suggest a person who would one day receive an award for writing, but Mr. Galloway did know my profession and and know of my work as a sometime writer. The odds against a person in my profession, even among those who write regularly, of receiving a distinguished writer's award would seem to me to be considerable, though perhaps not astronomical. Another of Mr. Galloway's predictions was that I would do lots of traveling. True enough. But I was, in fact, in a different city from my own when I was with him, which he knew.

Mr. Galloway claimed to be in touch with a lady of moderate height, solidly built but not fat, who had something to do with my family. In her "earthly life" she was very much a family woman, much less interested in the outside world than with her own flock. She had very straight hair, plain hair, the whole tone of her is solid. "A photograph of her is still in existence," he told me, which is a somewhat curious thing to say since his description fit in every respect my paternal grandmother who lived and died when photographs were relatively uncommon. Nonetheless, I do have, as I subsequently found out, a single photograph of her.

Mr. Galloway saw her as putting in front of me "homemade cooking," and then went on to say, "in itself, that doesn't mean much; they give the sense of what they are trying to convey with that ... They are saying this is the way to substance, homemade stuff, everything good and pure, nothing messed up and tampered with." As it happens, this sitting took place the day before I was scheduled to make my first visit to the macrobiotic central office in Boston, where I would learn of the macrobiotic belief in the necessity of eating natural foods. In 24 hours I would have my first dinner comprised of such foods, no chemicals, no preservatives, "nothing messed up and tampered with," as Mr. Galloway said — an idea that was echoed by my macrobiotic guides. My spirit grandmother, according to Mr. Galloway, also cautioned me to be free of "acidic-citrus foods;" my macrobiotic sources likewise instructed me not to have citrus fruits or juices because these foods were too acidic.

I found this material about my grandmother to be moderately compelling evidence for mediumship. But for the next several years I exaggerated Mr. Galloway's accuracy by remembering that he had reported my grandmother saying specifically that I should "get back to natural foods," and meaning it literally more than metaphorically. Only when I listened to the tape of the sitting again did I realize that this was an embroidery of mine; "she" was not quite that specific. In assessing paranormal phenomena, one needs not only to beware of fakery, intended or not, on the part of the psychic, but on the part of oneself as well.

Mr Galloway had me not only doing lots of traveling (correct), but traveling "over water, I see you standing in front of a microphone." I was at that time scheduled to give a talk in Germany in two months.

Mr. Galloway saw, in his mind, energy emerging from my fingers as I put my hands to the head of another person. "I can feel it vibrating," he said. "The 'other side' is concerned that you start using your hands this way." I did, in fact, try my hand at psychic healing, as detailed in Chapter 5, and both of my first such instances had to do with the head. One was an ordinary headache, and the other a migraine that had been resistant to medical treatment. In both instances, for whatever reason, the patients claimed to have felt immediate relief.

Perhaps the most curious and impressive of all of Mr. Galloway's inferences did not take place during the sittings at all. Rather, on the night of one sitting he called me at my then-home in Topeka after having gone to the trouble of getting my number from the people who had organized his trip to nearby Kansas City. Such a phone call was totally out of character for him, and nothing like it occurred after the other two of my sittings with him. Mr. Galloway said that he just could not put out of his mind that I must be concerned about money and investments. The facts are that at the time of the sitting I was consulting an investment broker in Kansas City and was caught up in making an important financial decision, which I did on the phone just after leaving Mr. Galloway. He had made no mention of money or investments during the sitting, though he said on the phone that he had thought about it briefly. Nonetheless, the issue would not leave him, and so he felt that he must, for his benefit and possibly for mine, tell me about it.

It would be nice to report that Mr. Galloway's psychic or mediumistic abilities proved to be lucrative. He gave me no hot tips, nor was he entirely clear or convinced about what I should do. Rather, he said that it might be well for me to do nothing at the moment, advice which I had that afternoon acted on anyway. The decision, whether his or mine, proved to be inconclusive. But how in the world he knew how preoccupied with investments I was is difficult to say. Mr. Galloway doubtless would point out in his understated British way that the information was not "in the world" to begin with, and so I need not be astonished that it did not follow the rules.

Mr. Galloway was outright wrong in seeing me involved importantly as a child in a boys' group, "not the Boy Scouts." I could see no relevance to his seeing a big "s" having to do with a German or Austrian name connected with a living doctor, unless it was to my first name and my German last name. He claimed that in the next two weeks new ideas would be put to me, but I should resist them and stay with my own. Excepting those of the general run of idea hucksters, no such ideational temptations came my way in the next two weeks. Nor did anyone named Dora or Doris emerge in my life as he predicted. Yet some time later a Doris did emerge significantly. Is there a statute of limitation governing how long one must wait before judging whether a prediction of this sort is correct or not?

MY THIRD SITTING WAS remarkable, though not because of the accuracy or inaccuracy of Mr. Galloway's inferences about my life. As I approached that meeting I remember noting that I was in a bad mood. In addition, I was in one of those troughs of disbelief, one of those times when I would ask myself exasperatedly what I was doing here, and what the point was of pursuing such phenomena to the detriment of my other work. My glum and nihilistic mood was exacerbated by Mr. Galloway's early inferences. One of them was clearly wrong — he had my father's side of the family suffering from heart conditions and other circulatory disturbances, which they did not. He said that he was getting messages from a lady from the other side who had had bronchial or respiratory problems long before her death — also wrong. I became seriously morose when Mr. Galloway asked, once again, if I was having difficulty balancing my professional and private life.

I remember running out of patience with hearing wrong and repetitive material, and I felt ridiculous at even half-believing in what I was doing. In counterpoint to this mood, Mr. Galloway had a spirit woman "trying to create a sense of light and energy" to counteract my "flatness, plodding." Mr. Galloway asked rhetorically, "Why do I get a sense of flatness, dullness? Have you been under the weather or something? ... overworking yourself lately? I don't know why I'm trying to generate colored lights to you ... 'Don't be tempted to go over old tracks.' I don't know why I'm tempted to say that." Since I *was* troubled by his going over old tracks, he could have been saying that to himself as well as to me.

Mr. Galloway then said that he was "blocked completely, blanked out," that this sort of thing happened sometimes, and that one could not force information when it did. According to the spirits, he and I would have much greater success in September, though I would presumably have to find him in England to demonstrate that. The spirit-helper was "standing back," said Mr. Galloway, which is the spirit's way of saying that he could go no further with the reading. However, images of colored lights and messages to "lift, freshen and cleanse my mind" were sent as encouragement. Mr. Galloway said that he had gotten a sense of "flatness" that "floored" him. He had run into a "solid wall" in his mind.

I raised the question to Mr. Galloway as to whether he thought my mood or his mood had created the blockage. While being too politely British to accuse me, he did mention that he had had a particularly good session just previous to mine and had felt invigorated enough by it to start with me without his usual "recharging" time in-between.

It certainly looked as if Mr. Galloway had correctly sensed my sad and angry mood. He could, of course, simply have chattered on nonetheless, and collected his full fee of forty dollars. Instead, he refused to charge me for what he considered a failed meeting, but finally accepted half the fee. That he did not simply go on is a tribute to his sincerity and suggests that he does indeed have a sense of when he is in tune with the other person (or spirits relevant to that person) and when he is not. All in all, this event suggests that at the least Mr. Galloway is not simply a cynical faker, and it throws into sharp relief the question of how Mr. Galloway gets his information.

If anything is true in the way of his having access to information other than through the usual senses, then one or more of the following are true: (1) He is sincere, but gets his correct information by hunch, sensory cues, chance, or luck. (2) He gets his information from the other side, from spirit helpers. (3) Information that is known to me he gets by way of telepathy, and information not known to me he gets by way of clairvoyance or precognition. In other words, it may be that Mr. Galloway is neither a spiritualist nor a medium, but is indeed a sensitive. The whole superstructure of beliefs in the other side, spirit life, otherworldly guides, may be an elaborate misleading hypothesis to explain secular, worldly skills. Those secular worldly skills, however — telepathy, precognition and clairvoyance — while perhaps not as fanciful as spiritualism, are plenty fanciful enough themselves. I stumbled off into the late afternoon looking for colored lights.

SPIRITUALISTS SUCH AS MR. Galloway, at least in the United States and England, have a casual relationship to organized religion and religious doctrine. Not so with the Faith of God Foundation, a straightforward, if not frenzied, expression of fundamentalist Christianity. Among its outreach ministries are The Healing Ministry of the Conquering King, which conducts healing through the laying on of hands and so-called distant healing, in which members pray for patients whom they know only through being on a list of people to be prayed for. Another of the Foundation's outreach ministries is the Ministry of the Angels of Christ. Among other activities, members of this ministry transmit information from one's Guardian Angel. Adherents claim that mere spirits, such as those invoked by Mr. Galloway, are under the direction of guardian angels; so in getting an "angel listening" I was taking my case to a Higher Court.

Magdalen St. Claire, Guardian of the Ministry, requires a picture or handwriting which she meditates on until she receives the angel's message, To get anything from handwriting such as mine is, in the opinion of some, miraculous in itself, to say nothing of getting spiritual messages from it. I rather think that Magdalen, as she is customarily called, knew from an intermediary about my background and work; in any case, the main points that the angel made to me, through her, would fit a good many people, and particularly those with letters after their name. She described me as being impatiently rational rather than contemplatively thinking according to the wisdom of the Son of God. The result was that I was vulnerable to worry, pressure of time, and a sense of clouded vision. I was said to long for the peace of non-involvement while entrapped by the forces of rationality. If I was to give up this rationality, I would, after a brief period of disorientation, overcome weariness, be released from a nagging sense of not quite getting hold of things, and in effect be on my way. My best means via Magdalen for "achieving these gifts is to enter into prayer more regularly, and with an actual belief that I was being heard."

I was assured that this Guardian Angel is always available to me, and when I am in particular need I can call on "him." (Nothing sexist about this; his message included the intelligence that he happened to be "male in nature.") I was given a word with which I would be able to reach my Guardian Angel. The word is "Tzenianan," which was helpfully, and perhaps meaningfully, spelled out for me phonetically as follows: "TZEE-nee-a-nun." It so happens that at that juncture in my life an ex-nun was playing a significant role, and "thee-need-a-nun" could be considered to make sense in that context. My angel's final comment was that I was considering embarking on a project that drew my interest despite there being no logic attached to it, which, however, I should follow up on since it was a pull from my soul.

This discussion took place near the beginning of collecting information for this book. (I choose to believe, however, that there is at least some logic attached to it.)

Just as Western healers can be separated into those who work with the body and those who work with the mind, so too can spirits. Both Galloway's spirits and Magdalen's angels work by way of the mind; they offered information, insight, and inspiration. Other ethereal entities concern themselves with the practice of medicine in the sense of purporting to cure *physical* ills. In the next section, I will recount my experiences with what amounts to the practice of medicine by spirit physicians.

Chapter Three

Georgia On My Mind: Surgery in a Trance

As I write this, I am flat on my back in a lavender-decorated bedroom in Toccoa, Georgia, where I am recovering from my morning's "surgery." The postoperative rules are that for 24 hours after surgery one is to subsist only on fluids, and move as little as possible. I am not precisely sure what was operated on. Some of my complaints were deemed by the "surgeon" to be inoperable. As far as I can tell, he tried to correct chronic low back pain through work on the spine. Right now I have a good deal of low back pain.

How did I get here? The proximal explanation is by twin-engine Apache, the surgeon's private plane, flown by him. As I was leaving Kansas City for Atlanta's Peachtree-DeKalb airport for private planes, my well-wisher said, "If he seems strange, promise you will not fly with him." "Sure," I agreed, lying, since what did she think I would be able to do at such a juncture? It never became an issue, anyway, as the pilot-surgeon, my host, was solid-looking, warm, and welcoming. His plane had two engines and looked reassuringly shiny. And his friend who was to accompany us on this hundred-mile trip was also a pilot. The total ambiance was so comforting that I hardly gave a thought to the implications of the pilot's forgetting to pull the chocks out from under the wheels, the homemade spring helping the handle of the door next to me to close, and the errant mileage indicator. Before surgical operations people get anxious about lots of things unnecessarily, I thought to myself, and proceeded to enjoy the trip.

A more distal reason for my post-operative condition on was that the name, Reverend William C. Brown, had been included on a list of major healers supplied to me. As luck, providence, synchronicity, or coincidence would have it, I was invited to lecture at a psychiatric center in Columbus, Georgia, some 175 miles from Toccoa, which finally decided me on visiting Rev. Brown.

There are healers and there are healers, but "Bill" Brown is, he says (hyperbolically and incorrectly), the only practitioner of etheric surgery in the United States. (George Chapman is a well-known practitioner in England.) I learned something about etheric surgery from several books and articles about Reverend Brown, and from the description that he customarily sends to his prospective patients. I am not sure I follow the metaphysics of it, but the main point is that there is supposedly an etheric body occupying some six or so inches of space around the physical body. Surgery done on the etheric body is duplicated in the physical body. The "etheric physician" does not use physical operating instruments nor even touch the body. Or, as Reverend Brown writes, "the instrumentation that they must use is fourth dimensional which is not recorded by the physical senses to the degree that one can see the instrumentation that they use with the physical eyes. However, those who have had and do have extended vision, i.e., clairvoyance, have seen the entire process from its inception to its end."

During the telephone negotiations for my visit, Reverend Brown spontaneously offered information which he says he gets more or less involuntarily by reading it off what he describes as a kind of internal movie screen. For example, he interrupted our conversation to ask whether I had any French artifacts in my office, perhaps a vase. (No, but mediumistic readings of my past life have placed me in France.) Mr. Brown "saw" a scroll and key suggesting that I was a member of Phi Beta Kappa (no scroll, but I am a member of another scholastic honor society whose key, unseen for years, lies buried in a drawer). I was also told to get blood checks on any schizophrenic patients that I might have, which would reveal their lack of copper. If I should have any cracking around my mouth (I do not), I should use zinc. Reverend Brown asked why my left eye was bothering me (it was not). One of the introductory letters, written by Reverend Brown's wife, Maria, used guidance for college-bound people as an example of what could be learned from reading the Akashic Records. (The Akashic Records are fabled books allegedly recording each soul's excursions, which can be "read" by those gifted to do so, among them Reverend Brown. A reading of his own records reveals that he lived in Atlantis, Egypt, England, and that he tried and failed to practice etheric surgery in at least five previous lifetimes.) Was it just coincidence that my own children were just then deciding what colleges to apply to?

In a subsequent phone conversation, which included my son on an extension phone, Reverend Brown alleged that my son had capacities to become a healer, and suggested that I feel the heat from his hands. I did think that I felt such heat, as much as one can tell by a quick observation under those circumstances. He thought that my son had done some sculpting (correct), in particular of a horse (not true), and had done a bust of me (no, but several drawings). He thought my son had a headache on the left side (no), perhaps the result of "cranial bone slippage." He thought that he had "penetrating eyes that looked right through you," that he had unusual powers of concentration on things of interest to him, and might frighten people with his penetrating eyes and mind so that they would retreat from him (largely correct). Reverend Brown was sure that my son was uninterested in following in my vocational footsteps (true), and was involved in, or should be involved in, architecture.

In this telephone conversation, Reverend Brown alleged that I had lived a past life in Egypt. Such clairvoyances are more difficult to evaluate than they might at first seem. A day or two after Reverend Brown's remarks, my son reported that he thought the reference to architecture might reflect his intense absorption at that time in the architecture of the pyramids, which in turn might reflect the comment about Egypt. One can usually cast about and find seeming confirmation of a psychic's powers: the man chiefly involved in my training to become a psychoanalyst, with whom I would be expected to identify, was Egyptian.

In that same telephone conversation, my son quipped about my having a garlic over my head, referring to the supposed properties of garlic to ward off the dangers of evil spirits. He added that he had just had a salad with garlic dressing — all of which may or may not have had something to do with Reverend Brown's saying on our first night together, out of the clear blue, that he figured that I liked garlic.

UPON INQUIRY, REVEREND BROWN sends prospective patients a packet of instructions, along with introductory information about etheric surgery and about himself that includes the following:

PREPARATIONS FOR HEALING:
ETHERIC SURGERY

If you are going to visit a healer, make this a moment to remember. You are going to see a man who is a psychic. If he were on top of a mountain, you would have a sense of occasion. If he were wearing a white nightgown, burning incense and chanting holy words, you would have a feeling of awe.

A healer looks like an ordinary sort of person. He isn't. Through him you are going to link with the life force, with a power greater than the hydrogen bomb. You are going to touch the end of a wire that carries a trillion volts. The healer is the insulator that prevents this power flowing too strongly, or too soon. You are going to receive the power that flows from God.

Before you go, wash and cleanse your body. Put on fresh clothing, and clear your mind of all negative thoughts, then empty it. Go in the healer's room with humility. Say to yourself, "I am here; I am ready; I wish to be healed." This is a moment that can change your life, mend your body, re-orient your mind. Prepare yourself.

If you write to a healer, first wash your hands, sit at a table and relax. Breathe slowly and regularly and try to induce a sense of tranquility. This letter may be the most important you have written. Then write shortly and to the point. You have an illness. The symptoms are such and such. You have had it for so long. You are ready and willing to be healed. Seal and post the letter.

Enclose a stamped addressed envelope. The healer gets so many letters it helps enormously not to have to write envelopes and to decipher addresses. After you have posted the letter, find a time to sit for a quiet moment each day. You are being sent healing. Put yourself in a condition to receive it. The state of mind that a patient needs is one of serene acceptance.

A healer is daily seeking attunement with the life force. He seeks it not for himself, but for you, so that you may plug yourself in to the power that can flow through him. *It is up to you to reach up to his spiritual level, not to pull the healer down to yours.*

Reverend Brown, my pilot-surgeon and host for the next four days, is a fairly short gentleman with a youngish man's body and the face of a man well into his sixties. He sounds like Lionel Barrymore, and looks like Eric Sevareid. His age, according to his wife, is 56; according to a magazine article about him, he is 65; and according to him he is ageless, "like you, like everybody," by which I assume he was referring to the eternal spirit. His response is a sample of the way he often deals with questions, in parables, jokes, allusions, metaphors, changes of subject that later, however, may turn out not to be changes of subject after all. The youngest of three brothers, he was born in Pittsburgh, Pennsylvania, and lived most of his life in Florida. As a World War II member of the Merchant Marines, he lost most of his hearing and became paralyzed, but he was cured of both of these afflictions through the arcane means that he now employs with others. He received a minister of philosophy degree from the Spiritualist Episcopal Church in Flint, Michigan. After a brief time in the real estate business, he entered a five-year self-training program at a spiritualist retreat in Georgia.

Devoting his life to spiritual, psychic, or extraordinary healing was a logical, if not preordained, development for Reverend Brown. He first realized his special powers when at the age of three he encountered the spirit of John Jeffrey Spaulding, a Presbyterian minister, who had died around 1800. Dr. Spaulding took the three-year-old under his generative wing. Some months later Brown met a Sioux Indian, Thundercloud, who showed him, for example, the electromagnetic fields around plants, which plants were toxic, and how the antidotes for toxic plants are found in their immediate vicinity. To Reverend Brown this was a metaphoric teaching about good and evil, about the capacity to repair what is broken, and about sickness and health. Reverend Brown learned to keep his clairvoyant, clairaudient, and psychometry powers to himself until the employment of these became his way of life. For a long time his schedule was to do Akashic readings in the morning, psychotherapeutic counseling in the afternoon, and etheric surgery in the evening. In recent years he has restricted himself almost entirely to three etheric surgeries in the morning. He has performed some 7,000 such surgeries over a period of 26 years.

Reverend Brown objects to any intimation that *he* is the surgeon. Rather, shortly after the healing sessions begin, he as a self leaves the sessions. His body remains to perform the surgical acts, speaking the words and thoughts of the 28 medical specialists from the "other side." The body was trained by Thundercloud, and the discarnate team is composed of three Americans, two Irishmen, and 23 Englishmen. The neurosurgeon of the group is Harvey

Cushing, the famed contemporary Boston physician. Reverend Brown reports that, in ordinary life, Dr. Cushing's nephew complained to Reverend Brown about the claims that his uncle was working as a spirit, but when confronted with information that Reverend Brown likely could not have gotten in any way other than from Harvey Cushing, the nephew was mollified. The discarnate physicians evidently have ways of keeping up with medical knowledge; they dispense modern information and techniques, as well as homeopathic remedies, and other information not yet known to contemporary medicine. I adjusted, during my visit, to what became the informal, conversational references to what Dr. So-and-So said about such-and-such, and whether he ought to be consulted about one or another problem. This is what Reverend Brown's wife meant when she said over the phone that I would be meeting "the doctors."

Tape-recorded consultations with one or another doctor have yielded information such as the following: Never use aluminum pans, aluminum foil, or Teflon-type pans, as all these deposit harmful substances on food; old-fashioned cast-iron cookware is best. Vitamins should be taken before eating and with water only. Never use dairy products, according to Dr. Murphy; when asked if only a little would be harmful, he has replied, "You would like to introduce just a little strychnine into your system?" According to Dr. Murphy, dairy products set up a paste in the intestines that attracts and holds wastes, and these wastes over time become polyps, benign or malignant. Dr. Murphy refers to the body as a giant lung that needs free movement between inside and outside, and should therefore not be blocked by talc and aluminum as found, for example, in underarm deodorants. Dr. Spaulding echoes recent holistic medicine views on the causes and prevention of cancer, indicting refined foods, chemicals, preservatives, and additives, along with air pollution. He recommends a high-fiber diet and colonics in order to keep the gastrointestinal system clean. Dr. Fredericks, the cardiovascular specialist, has designed a retractor made with a reverse caliper for use in retracting ribs for heart surgery, which includes a gauge in order not to exceed the level at which ribs break. He has offered a diagrammatic picture of this invention, drawn, of course, by the hand of Reverend Brown.

IT WAS WELL PAST midnight before I fell asleep in what was to be my recovery room. The morning alarm was unwelcome, as was the groggy recognition that today was operating day. There was little time for lugubriousness, however, since all three patients and their supporting friends or spouses gathered at 7:15. We filled out a form that included space for complaints, release of responsibility, and some restrictions on publications (though they knew I was there collecting information for a book).

The operating or healing room looked to be a converted dining room, with incense burning and quasi-religious and esoteric pictures and artifacts scattered amidst desks, typewriters, and other office paraphernalia. In the center of the room was the portable operating table. Reverend and Mrs. Brown were dressed in white uniforms. We patients were covered only by hospital gowns. We were instructed and reminded by Mrs. Brown to keep our legs and arms uncrossed so as not to impede the flow of energy. The session began with stereophonically recorded organ music, followed by the group's reciting the Lord's Prayer, and an invocation by Reverend Brown. He then explained a bit about catalepsy and told us not to worry when we saw him slump forward in a cataleptic state, for that was when he would be leaving his body and turning it over to the doctors to be used for diagnosis and healing. Shortly after, when he did indeed suddenly slump forward in a rapid, convulsive, movement, I was grateful for the warning. A few moments later he sat back and announced that he was Dr. Spaulding. Dr. Spaulding seemed to be something of an *éminence grise*, introducing the proceedings and taking the responsibility for the safety and good treatment of Reverend Brown's loaned body. After being introduced to the patients by Mrs. Brown and greeting all of us, Dr. Spaulding turned the session over to Dr. Murphy, the diagnostician. "Top of the morning," said Dr. Murphy, who intersperses his diagnoses with stand-up-comic routines. But at times he, like the other doctors, can sound irascible and indignant — not unlike Reverend Brown himself on occasion.

I observed five operations in two days, plus a sixth which I observed from the vantage point of being on the operating table. The patients were clearly concerned with their illnesses, which is understandable enough. However, I thought several times that they crossed the line between understandable concern and hypochondriacal preoccupation. The Browns report that many of their patients come to them as a last resort, and this was true of at least one of the group that I observed. The rest seemed to come simply as a preferred alternative to conventional surgery; they had picked this doctor rather than another one. Some were returning after a number of years, and others were returning with spouses who now required treatment. Several were longtime believers in spiritualism, seemingly convinced not only that the surgery was therapeutically beneficial, but that they were in effect under the care of the spirit doctors.

Some of the treatments were directed toward complaints that the patients brought. Others were directed toward illnesses or deformities that Dr. Murphy diagnosed whether the patient had been aware of them or not. These difficulties included scoliosis, uneven length of legs, aneurysm in the abdominal aorta, angina pectoris, hernia, imperfect closure of valves of the heart, and other heart ailments. Mental illness, diabetes, and structural deformities of the hands and legs are not treated.

The examinations all began with Dr. Murphy's scrutiny of the sitting patient's back and of the rotation of the patient's head to the left and to the right. Reverend Brown's eyes were closed throughout, regardless of the diagnostic treatment procedures being enacted with his body. So, Dr. Murphy, in the form of Reverend Brown, made his diagnosis with eyes closed. Sometimes he ran his hands down the patient's spine. Sometimes he recommended a chiropractic adjustment, to be made later by the patient's chosen chiropractor. Sometimes Reverend Brown's arms made an adjustment on the spot.

The procedure for anesthesia was for the patient to count backwards from ten to one, with Reverend Brown's hands looking as if he was administering a hypodermic needle. One of the patients claimed that he felt a slight pain from this injection. Operations were performed by Reverend Brown's arms several inches from the patient's body as — with quick movements that resembled actual operating technique — he cut, passed and received instruments, and reached for thread and sewed the incisions. I irreverently thought of children at play imitating doctors. But Reverend Brown's operations were conducted with all the seriousness that befits health-giving procedures. Several times Reverend Brown's hands produced pain by pushing at the patient's organs, sometimes demonstrating a difficulty of which the patient had previously been unaware. One patient, he said, had no need for surgery: "I'm not going to do surgery just for the sake of doing surgery." He gave such bits of advice as recommending pancreatic enzymes and specific dosages of Vitamin A for a specific number of days, and recommending that a physician be used to drain bodily fluid. Several patients were advised to rid their body of worms by getting a colonic irrigation with the herb wormwood.

I was advised to get chiropractic adjustment of my fourth cervical vertebra to help even up my shoulders, one of which was supposedly lower than the other. The scoliosis that I was, for the first time, apprised of having was at one time described by Reverend Brown as a birth defect and at another time as compensatory to another anomaly. Whatever its etiology, the result was the low back pain for which I was to be operated on.

Mrs. Brown and some of the doctors were eager that I be given the opportunity to check on their work. So I was encouraged to listen with a stethoscope, touch spines, and probe intestines. No matter that I knew nothing of these procedures, and I rather disliked doing them — especially without an agreed-upon relationship with the patients. They probably had as hard a time saying "no" as I did. Half the time I was not sure what I was touching, feeling, hearing, or doing. When asked, I straddled a line between being agreeable and negativistically saying that I felt nothing. Nonetheless, I think I can reliably report that upon the introduction of the phantom hypodermic needle and the counting backwards, the patients' pulses became slower and slower. With one patient I heard through the stethoscope a whooshing rushing sound in the background of the heartbeat, while after the surgery the heartbeat was unaccompanied by such sounds. In another instance — as far as I can tell — the sounds remained. Mrs. Brown checked along with me and, though more adroit than I, seemed also to have difficulty at times making the judgments. At one point when she reflected some indecision she was told, tartly, by one of the doctors to make up her mind: "We can't tolerate imagination here."

The last patient to be operated on, namely myself, seemed to be in danger of getting short shrift. The attending doctor made several comments about having to hurry up, having to get finished. Reverend Brown later explained that his body gets tired and he can lend it out only for a limited amount of time. Nonetheless, all the procedures that I had seen done with others were done on me, all painless. At the end of the operation, a gentle-voiced Dr. David took over and closed the proceedings, whereupon Reverend Brown came back to his body and opened his eyes.

I left the other patients preparing to go back to their motel rooms for recovery. Mrs. Brown tenderly ushered me to my bedroom, there to instruct me in how to get in and out of the bed with minimal involvement of my spine. I was to lie flat on the hard bed, no pillow, for the next 24 hours. I was to consume nothing but liquids and eschew television and stimulating conversation. (This last was completely disregarded, as individually Reverend and Mrs. Brown visited me, with no diminution of their usual inclination to fill me with information.) I asked whether I could read, and was told vaguely that I could — the implication being, however, that I probably would not much want to.

The stack of reading material that I had planned to get through on a day that was to be devoted to nothing else did in fact remain largely untouched. I did just make it through a fat pre-holiday issue of the *New Yorker*. My reading was interspersed with naps, as my major post-operative symptom was fatigue, along with headache and by now rather severe low back pain. The headache could have come from reading with my head flat in poor light. The back pain could have come, according to Mrs. Brown, from the cure, with pain leaving my body; or it could have come from stretching out flat for so long. I also felt a general malaise, including mild nausea. Was Mrs. Brown joking that the nausea might be from the "ether"?

While I had had little sleep the previous night and two plane rides before that, the amount of fatigue and frequency of napping were in excess of what I would have expected. In short, I did seem to have a variety of symptoms, all or part of which could be understood as stemming from my operation. I later read that fatigue, sometimes including nausea, are characteristic of the day after etheric surgery. Moreover, according to the articles, those least inclined to believe in etheric surgery are most inclined to have post-operative symptoms. It is as if the powers that be are out to convince such skeptics. Mrs. Brown hinted that some strange things might very likely happen during the first post-operative night, particularly waking up and being unable to get back to sleep; this was later confirmed by my reading. She helpfully organized my pile of books and magazines and put it close enough so that I could read when I might otherwise expect to be sleeping. That night I did awaken a couple of times, but fell immediately back to sleep, with reading materials put off for another day or night.

Reverend Brown refused to let me run a tape recorder because, among other things, he said that it would not work; he offered dire stories of cameras becoming stuck and other electronic devices failing. During my first post-operative day, two sets of new batteries failed to energize my tape recorder. I heard a high-pitched radio sound, such as from a physician's beeper, when Reverend Brown came to sit by my bed. He claimed not to hear it. Some three or four times Mrs. Brown emerged in response to what she said was the sound of my bedside bell, which I had not rung.

The beeping sound turned out to be the alarm on Reverend Brown's watch. The tape recorder required only a trip to a Radio Shack where its batteries were finally inserted correctly. The summoning bell was never explained. Suggestibility being what it is, it is difficult to know for sure what my post-operative symptoms were symptoms of. I am willing to consider that the fatigue and malaise were symptoms of the procedure, especially as such symptoms were reported by other patients in person, on tape, and in publications. Less amenable to explanations such as suggestion were Reverend Brown's apparent clairvoyant powers. I overheard a *sotto voce* conversation at the Radio Shack between the manager, who was also a pilot, congratulating Reverend Brown on psychically locating a heretofore lost plane. Since we had come to Radio Shack at my initiative, Reverend Brown would have had to call ahead at the last minute to arrange such a conversation, which is really too Byzantine to consider seriously.

Reverend Brown's work offers at least five major possibilities. One is that he heals people. A second is that he does not heal people, and may even make them worse. A third is that he heals people through operating on their etheric body. A fourth is that his diagnoses and treatments are guided by spirit doctors. A fifth is that such spirit doctors inhabit his body while the essence of himself is "out of body." Reverend Brown may heal people to the extent that any psychic healer heals people, and be completely misguided about the usefulness of his operating procedures, spirit advisors, and the lending of his body. He may lend his body, receive spiritual help, perform operating procedures on the etheric body, and not heal at all. Or any other combination could also be true. The most parsimonious possibility is that he heals to the extent that any healer may heal, the other hypotheses being irrelevant or acting merely as powerful suggestive aids to the healing.

That *something* happens is implied at least by the reports, including mine, of seeming post-operative symptoms. To the extent that my nervous and ill-at-ease observations were valid, pulses did slow and the sounds of imperfect valve closure of the heart were silenced. One of the patients claimed to have increased freedom in breathing and relief from pain. This same patient, who seemed superficially at least to be a reliable observer, claimed to have felt some pain from the ministrations in the air above his physical body. That patients return after what they deem a satisfactory experience years previously, and bring their spouses for treatments, also implies that

Reverend Brown has healing power. I was shown samples of the literally thousands of testimonials received from the former patients of Reverend Brown, some of which have included meticulous reports of the changes and benefits following Reverend Brown's surgeries.

Reverend and Mrs. Brown were serious about the need for post-operative care, or "all our work will be undone." For example, they refused to allow me to patronize the best restaurant in Toccoa because it would have involved climbing several stairs — a prohibited activity for several days and preferably three weeks after the operation. Although a post-operative patient is allowed to be an automobile passenger, he is advised against being a driver. When the time came for me to leave Toccoa, by car, Reverend and Mrs. Brown arranged a driver for me, and tried hard though unsuccessfully to persuade me to use him. I continued to violate their prescriptions for good post-operative care, and so any benefit that I did derive may well be less than would have occurred had I followed instructions. The instructions are probably difficult for most people to follow — not driving a car, not climbing stairs, sleeping only on the right side after heart surgery, not bending after work on the spine, etc. — and so the effectiveness of the surgery may be regularly interfered with.

Incidentally, what does a healer do when he needs healing? While I was there, Reverend Brown accidentally stubbed his toe. He tried soaking it, then went off to a hospital for X-rays. There was some desultory discussion about consulting Dr. Murphy. Instead, I treated the toe myself with the laying on of hands. Reverend Brown said it felt better after that, and I thought it looked better. But then I hadn't checked it carefully before the healing. My eyes could have been playing tricks, or maybe Reverend Brown was suggestible or just being polite. It may be easier to heal a healer than to satisfy an experimenter.

Chapter Four
The Magical Mystery Tour: Philippine Psychic Surgery

I.

PSYCHIC SURGERY, PHILIPPINE STYLE, refers to the following startling procedure: A medically untrained surgeon appears to open the patient's body with his bare hands, plucks usually organic matter from the pool of blood covering the incision, closes the alleged incision (again with the bare hands), and leaves no scar. The procedure is done in non-sterile conditions, without anesthesia, and takes a couple of minutes. The patient walks off without side effects from the operation and, it is said, is cured of whatever the operation was for. The surgeons may or may not have known the medical diagnosis; they either make their own diagnosis, or just let their hands guide the procedure.

When I first heard of these operations, I could hardly believe my ears, and when I first saw one I could hardly believe my eyes. That such a thing could be done was staggering in its own right, but more so in its implications: it called for a massive rewriting of the rules of physics and physiology. A year or so later, one editorial reaction to my first draft of the following chapter included the observation that I seemed rather offhand about such wondrous events. One explanation of the change in me from total astonishment to relative equanimity is that when an event is too immense to be comprehended adequately, denial sets in. Resisting being bowled over, dizzied, I had shut down awareness. Yet unable to sustain that device — since after all I was embarked on an enterprise designed to become aware — I let familiarity breed, if not contempt, a subtle accepting philosophical recognition that the unreal could become real. It had become all in a day's work. Millions of other observers likely employed similar devices when the psychic surgery operations were shown on American commercial television, including *60 Minutes*. As with so much television-inspired consciousness, the effects probably lasted for something like 60 minutes, then slipped into that vast sea of unintegrated, undigested information surrounded by protective devices of the mind where it remains, I suppose, still flickering.

Such information is a bit harder to dismiss when one sees it on home movies, shown by the person operated upon, who claims relief from symptoms as the result of the operation. That is what happened to me. By chance I met along the consciousness-raising circuit a Kansas City healer, psychic, and inspirational teacher. There she was, cinematically and in person, in my own living room, a hole apparently being made in her previously aching back, something being taken from her body, the hole being closed and the blood mopped up. She emerged happy, even radiant, from her operation. She claimed that her back pain had greatly improved, as had the symptoms of many of the other people whose operations she observed. So now I had these testimonials from a person I knew personally. Moreover, I had seen a picture, which of course is worth a thousand words, isn't it? Well, no, it isn't, as any magician will attest. The eyes can be led to play tricks by pictures, just as can be done with words.

The drums were beating. Just imagine, not only would the practice of such surgery be a revolution in healing, but the existence of such surgery would call for a suspension of the usual rules of reality, thereby opening vistas of new information, the making of a new reality. Should I or shouldn't I suspend disbelief on this one? Writings of others on the subject did not help much with that question. They ranged from derisive dismissal to uncritical belief. William Nolen, a surgeon (who therefore, one would think, would be in a position to know), had gone to the Philippines and observed the operations and come back to declare them a fraud, perpetrated through sleight of hand.[1] But serious studies had been made by reputable scientists from the United States and Europe which at least allowed for the possibility that the operations were legitimate. For example, there is the work of Stelter,[2] a German professor of chemistry and physics, who, along with a number of other engineers, physicists, and physicians, studied Philippine psychic surgery during five trips over a four-year period. According to him, some of the openings of the body are merely illusions, and some are genuine, but in any case some healing takes place.

The putative openings may merely serve dramatic purposes. One of the signatories, Sigrun Seutemann,[3] accompanies European patients to the Philippines for psychic surgery and has observed more than twelve hundred of the surgeries. She estimates that 2 percent of the patients were healed instantly and that another 10 percent could be judged medically healed at the end of a ten-day to two-week stay. Thirty percent had at least partial success within the first month. Another 30 percent had some success, with medical tests substantiating improvement in three to six months. No follow-up was possible for 18 percent, and 10 percent seemed not to have benefited.

As usual, I emerged from reading the literature on psychic phenomena impatiently wondering why someone didn't design a good experiment and settle the matter.

AS LUCK, OR SERENDIPITY, would have it, during the time that I was considering whether and how to pursue the topic of psychic surgery, I learned that a Philippine healer was to be in the United States to serve as the subject in what might be the "crucial experiment." Not only would the machinery of science be brought to bear, but it would be done in the United States, and I would be saved the time and rigors of a trip to the Philippines. What could be better, I thought, than to have the arcane mysteries of the Orient examined by Western science and medicine on its own turf?

That turf was to be Oakland University, in Rochester, Michigan. My initial phone conversations with the experimenter, anthropologist Phillip Singer, fanned the research flames. Singer has traveled widely in foreign terrains, geographical and experiential. He ignited my curiosity and hopes for miracles with offhand remarks about his experiences in India — for instance, a pumpkin being changed to a statuette in his hands by Sai Baba, who also produces food by rubbing his hands together. He piqued my scientific curiosity with his description of the projected experiment: Television and movie cameras would be trained on the operation. The subjects' illnesses were to be certified by their doctors, who would also be observing the operations and would follow up the results of the healer's treatments. Best of all, a magician-observer was to be there, as a representative of the "truth squad" of magicians who follow healers and psychics (notably Uri Geller) and demonstrate that they can do with magic everything that the psychic claims to do with special powers. Here was a chance for a magician to observe and intervene under laboratory conditions. He would, Dr. Singer told me, be empowered to halt the proceedings at any time, look at the materials, suggest changes in the procedures, and be in a position to detect any fakery. I was invited to be an "official witness," to observe and be interviewed afterward along with Drs. Norman Shealy, a physician and author on the frontiers of medicine (see Chapter 10), and William Nolen, the previously mentioned debunker of Philippine psychic surgery. The official witness triumvirate failed to materialize — the healer changed the date of his arrival, and Shealy could not make the new date; then, at the last minute Nolen was unable to interest a periodical in supporting his trip, so he decided not to come. I turned out not to be much of an official witness either, but that is getting ahead of the story. The magician did come, and as it turned out played a key role.

This side of the Baskervilles, Detroit and its environs may be the grayest spot in the Western Hemisphere. It certainly seemed so after the hour or so of driving in fog and rain to Rochester, the home of Oakland University, some 20 miles from Detroit. I briefly met at the motel a gentleman who, it turned out, was to appear that night in a movie taken in the Philippines; the film recorded a huge tumor being removed from his neck by Juan Blanché, the healer to be studied the next day. His companion was his son-in-law, who it turned out was to be operated on during the next day's healing experiment. The driver of the car, who was to guide me to Dr. Singer's home for a pre-experiment meeting, also became a Blanché subject the next day.

Out beyond the street lamps, past fields and woods, we drove through the rainy outskirts into what seemed to be another world. It was not only the weather and surroundings that gave rise to my eerie feeling. I felt myself on a threshold, with mingled hope and fear of exploration and discovery. Slogging on foot through the mud on the way to Dr. Singer's renovated farmhouse, I saw outlined by headlights on the fog screen the dark shapes of others in front of me, a band of pilgrims trying to find their way to familiar landmarks. The country silence and wet gray were suddenly punctuated by an open door to a room full of eating, drinking, talking people. I was swept in by the rich stentorian tones of the welcoming Phillip Singer and by the equally stentorian size of his Saint Bernard. In no time at all, I was seeing faces from which moles and warts had been removed by the healer, was shown a picture of a huge neck tumor, by its owner, in preparation for seeing it removed on the movie screen, and was given a book of photographs and texts by the author of a healing trip in the Philippines. I learned the sad tale of American reluctance to fund psychic research: Dr. Singer turned down the original grant to support the experiment because, he said, the grant-giving agency was interested in controlling the results of the experiments for its own publicity-seeking purposes. Thus, he was passing the hat in our group. Whether on credit or through deficit spending, Juan Blanché was there, with his assistants Mr. Rodrigo and Miss Hernandez. Tall and lofty for a Filipino, Mr. Blanché smiled benignly for my photographs and at his many questioners.

The movie shown was in many respects typical of the genre of home movies taken of Philippine healings such as I had seen in my living room — wavering film, goodbye scenes at the San Francisco Airport, quick shots of early moments in Manila, then down to the business of healing. But Mr. Blanché's healing, as demonstrated in the movies and during the experiment, was different from those I had observed in other movies. In those other healings the operations left no scar, though the body was said to have been opened, as evidenced by a pool of blood and by organic matter allegedly taken from inside the body. How the healer got in and out without surgical instruments and without leaving a scar were piquant questions raised by the procedure. With Mr. Blanché an actual incision unquestionably was made, which left the expectable scar. He made that incision, however, some two feet from the body with a slicing action of his hand, and did the same thing by moving other people's hands similarly. The movie showed him removing the neck tumor, with alcohol as a disinfectant, a lit candle for cauterizing, and a forceps for yanking out the tumor.

The next morning did not dawn bright and clear; after all, it was still Michigan. But at least it wasn't raining. The emerging daylight gave promise that mysteries, too, would also be cleared by the crucial experiment. The operating theater was a television studio, complete with wires, cameras, and lights, the last of which were to play an unexpected part in the proceedings. When I first arrived, the operating table had on it cotton balls, towels, and a spoon, which looked like the spoon I had seen in the previous night's movie that had been used to spoon out some fluids from the body, in particular in the treatment of diabetes. Shortly after, a physician brought armloads of bandages, cotton, towels, all as part of the certification that the healer could not use any of his own possibly doctored equipment. On either side of the operating table, and to the front, were bleachers. These were used by patients, their physicians, and the magician. Although there was room there for me, an alleged official witness, I was instead seated in the audience section flat on the floor, at some distance from the proceedings but with television monitors to allow a closer view. I later learned that another "official witness" was similarly situated. I never did find out the reasons for these seating arrangements. The previous night's movie with its explicit views of blood and guts had prepared me for viewing gore at close range. The geographical arrangements precluded that possibility, even for the magician and others in the bleachers. The surgical field was partially shielded from most views. A number of physicians, however, did leave the bleachers, or stand up for a closer look, and presumably were able to see as much as they wanted. The magician took it upon himself to wander around and view the proceedings from various angles.

Dr. Phillip Singer was admirably suited for the role he chose to play in chairing the production of the experiment. Wrapped around his high-volume, commanding baritone voice is a tall, imposing, silver-maned frame. Words like "impresario" and "ringmaster" came to my mind, although he started out in a suitably low-key scientific manner describing the experiment. He told of the physicians in attendance who would certify that their patients to be treated by Mr. Blanché and his assistants, Mr. Rodrigo and Ms. Hernandez, did indeed have the physical ills of which they complained. The physicians would be on hand also to assist in case of medical emergency should that be necessary, a reassuring possibility after the bloody procedures I had witnessed in the previous night's film. Any organic matter taken from the patients would immediately be turned over to the nearby hospital medical laboratory in order to ascertain whether such material actually came from humans, specifically from these patients, rather than from animals, as had often been suggested in critiques of the work of Philippine surgeons. Dr. Singer then introduced the healers, the physicians, and finally the magician. He announced that if the magician should see any sleight of hand, or wanted to raise any procedural issues or get a better look at anything, he should say so to Dr. Singer, and if it appeared that there was any evidence of fraud, Dr. Singer said that he would immediately stop the experiment. The magician had been suggested by the Committee for Scientific Investigation of Claims of the Paranormal, a supposedly objective group of scientists who have, however, been accused by Dr. Singer and others of being out to debunk psychic phenomena. At any rate, we could assume that the magician was not to be an especially friendly witness. Although the situation seemed part court of law and part theater, Dr. Singer reminded us that we were engaged in a dispassionate, objective, scientific inquiry. We were to go beyond simplistically affirmative and negative positions and develop a "collective judgment."

Ms. Hernandez began the healing proceedings by adding still another dimension. We were engaged, she said, not only in scientific activities but in spirituality, and she led the group in prayer. The prayers, she said, are necessary to give Mr. Blanché his healing power, for the healing is ultimately done by spirits, "saints," and "angels." She also slipped in the intelligence that Mr. Blanché had recently operated successfully on the daughter of the then-President of the Philippines, Ferdinand Marcos.

The first subject was a physician with multiple myeloma, a debilitating cancer of the bone marrow. He had had this disease for two years, one result of which was a series of broken bones. Mr. Blanché chose to treat this man by moving his hands around the subject's body. As if to counteract the assumed disappointment of the group at not immediately seeing surgery, Ms. Hernandez explained that Mr. Blanché's treatments may include the laying on of hands, he may open the body, or he may "just pluck something out without opening the body." As if to counteract any boredom in watching Mr. Blanché merely move his hands over, around and upon the patient's body, Dr. Singer announced that all the surgical equipment had been brought by the physicians in attendance — "no props here."

The atmosphere was formal, respectful, even hallowed, as would befit a look into a new dimension of existence, new realms of healing, indeed the possibility that this presumably doomed cancer patient might be rescued.

The first actual operation was done on the son-in-law of the ex-tumor patient, whom I had met the night before. He had several benign lipomas remaining after many others had been removed by conventional methods. In the film of the previous night I had seen Mr. Blanché apparently make an incision in the air a foot or so from the patient's body; now he used one of the physician's fingers to make the incision the same way. He later was to use the magician's finger to make a similar incision.

I could not see the operation clearly, even with the aid of the television monitor, but those who passed behind Mr. Blanché could, and they did indeed certify that a surgical operation was taking place. All seemed to be going well despite several complaints from Mr. Blanché about the heat from the television lamps. Dr. Singer asked whether the physicians in attendance or the magician could explain what they had seen. "They cannot explain it," he repeated for the audience. Presumably what they said they could not explain was the making of the incision from a distance, the relative lack of blood, and the remarkable absence of apparent pain. The patient had responded to Dr. Singer's inquiry during the operation that he felt calm, and experienced only "a little tugging," despite the fact that the only anesthesia was alcohol spread around the wound. The medical technologist made a cursory examination of the tissue and affirmed that it appeared to be from a human being. One of the physicians, a veterinarian, was asked by Dr. Singer whether there was any possibility that the tissue was of animal origin, and was told, "not at all." In response to Dr. Singer's questions, the subject responded that he felt "perfect," that he had hardly any pain. Dr. Singer reminded the group that samples of the blood were being taken and compared with a sample of the patient's blood to make sure that blood had not simply been slipped in, as alleged by those skeptical of psychic surgery. I failed to see what this particular fuss was all about, since it was clear both from the movie last night and from today's witnesses that Mr. Blanché did in fact make actual incisions. Yet it became increasingly clear that Dr. Singer was inclined to seize upon any event to drive the point home that we were in the presence of legitimate phenomena. He seemed at times barely able to restrain his enthusiasm, repeating and emphasizing, like a daytime television host, what he apparently wanted the audience to notice. He paid proper scientific obeisance by saying that we were reserving judgment, then added, "We will see at what point we no longer need to reserve judgment." Presumably the judgment he had in mind just then was that psychic surgery was legitimate.

The next patient had recurring ganglionic cysts on both forearms. He had had previous operations on these recurring cysts, and he told how uncomfortable those operations were, all of which stood in sharp contrast to his reports after this operation. About an hour later I chatted with him in the hallway, and there was no doubt in his mind that the cysts had been removed; he was free of pain, comfortably going about his business. Perhaps he was benefiting, also, from Ms. Hernandez giving him energy, what she called "prana."

How was this possible? Hardly any pain, with gaping bleeding holes and the removal of internal tissue, recovery room time cut from three days to zero? I felt exhilarated, on the verge of being able to believe, not only in the effectiveness of psychic surgery, but in the limitless possibilities that would then open up once the barrier of disbelief and conventional explanations had been crossed. It seemed to me mere cavilling that the magician suggested that there were too many people around, making it difficult for him to get an adequate view of things, and that he wanted at least 30 seconds between the last time the patient's body was touched and the making of the distant incision. In other words, he suspected the incision was made by some agency other than the moving finger that was monopolizing our attention — for example, a blade hidden in the healer's hand.

The next subject was a professor of parapsychology at Oakland University who also had a ganglionic cyst, as certified by his surgeon, who was there. The magician, more ostentatiously now, examined the hands of Juan Blanché and his assistants. Ms. Hernandez said that the projected operation would result in a lot of blood, so she wanted everyone to pray very hard. She and the others moved their Bibles around, holding them over the head of Juan Blanché, and the magician asked to see their hands after they touched the Bibles. Ms. Hernandez was troubled by the lack of healing power, and increased her efforts to have the audience pray along with her. She suggested that we repeat the sound "om," which she said means God. There was much waving of Bibles as Mr. Blanché tried to work the cyst out of the subject's arm. Dr. Singer commented at the confluence of cultures — Indian, Philippine, Christian, science, medical, and magical: "This is, indeed, the spaceship Earth." More complaints from Ms. Hernandez and Mr. Blanché on the drain of healing power by the overhead lights, more entreaties for power-rejuvenating prayer. Ms. Hernandez read from John 17:1-26, and she asked various of the physicians to hold Bibles here and there. Evidently there was a considerable problem getting the cyst out, and time started to hang anxiously heavy. More requests for prayer, and finally the comment "No more power," which resulted in a Bible again being held over Mr. Blanché's head. There was a consultation between Dr. Singer and the magician; the latter then moved his position around the table, asked to see a kidney tray, and examined it. There was now a drum roll of complaints from the healers about flagging power, more requests for prayers, and Dr. Singer commented several times how ironic it was that the person who most believed in parapsychology was having the most difficult operation. The subject remonstrated that he was a believer in parapsychology, not necessarily a believer in psychic surgery, but that hardly seemed to faze Dr. Singer's enthusiasm for what he took to be high irony. The subject then said that he felt pain like a razor blade slicing him, and the magician swooped down upon a ball of cotton to see whether a razor blade was hidden in it. The subject said that he had a clear feeling of having had another incision, and shortly after, the cyst was successfully removed. Mr. Rodrigo put a flame to the site of the wound, which brought an anguished "ouch!" from the subject. In the grand surgical tradition Mr. Blanché walked away from the operation, leaving his assistants to finish up. Dr. Singer announced that because of the lessening of healing power, Mr. Blanché would require an interruption from the present (12 o'clock noon) until 1:30.

Dr. Singer then announced an immediate meeting of the physicians and the magician. When I asked Dr. Singer in my presumed capacity as official witness for permission to attend this meeting, I was told emphatically that I could not. I substituted for that meeting hallway discussions with the physicians and subjects, and took the magician to lunch. He filled the lunch hour with denunciations of the whole procedure as well as psychic phenomena in general. "Utter chicanery," he said, going on to explain that the incision allegedly made from a distance was faked through misdirected intention, which he demonstrated by producing coins from my lapel. According to him, while we were watching the upraised hand, an incision was made just like anybody would make an incision, by drawing a sharp object across the skin. If he were doing it, he said, he would use a blackened piece of piano wire honed to surgical sharpness, which he would then drop on the floor after making the incision. He said that he should have brought along his 50-pound industrial magnet, stuck in the bottom of a cane, with which he could have swept the floor to discover whether in fact a sharp object had been dropped there.

"When did you skin your knee?" he asked, thereby attempting to demonstrate that most everybody had skinned his or her knee sometime or other, so that could be a pretty safe prediction, and he could appear to be a seer. He went on to tell about the chicanery that he said underlay the work of his friend, the stage personality Dunninger, on radio and television, and about the generalities offered by psychics and mediums which in a large number of instances could hardly help be true, or seem to be true to beguiled people. When I brought some instances to his attention which could not be explained in these ways, he pooh-poohed them, evidently completely convinced that any variety of paranormal phenomena was fakery. When I raised the issue of the seeming lack of pain of the subjects, he remarked on shipboard operations, old-fashioned surgeries done on countless farms through the years by laymen, and claimed that anyway most pain was "psychosomatic." According to him, the great problem in removing the cyst of the college professor was entirely explicable. The razor pain was, according to the magician, from a second incision made because the first had been too small to allow for the removal of the cyst. A properly applied finger by the assistant could control the amount of bleeding, just as a judiciously placed golf ball under the arm could lower the apparent pulse rate. He told how his own finger had been operated on by his stepfather, bound tight with a tourniquet to control the blood, with alcohol taking care of the danger of infection — procedures similar to those of Mr. Blanché. The magician said that he had closed his magic shop to come to this experiment, expecting only to stay the morning, but now that he was becoming the central figure he felt obliged to attend the afternoon session — if there is to be an afternoon session, I said to myself, thinking that the healer might very well claim a continued insufficiency of power and head back to the Philippines.

I felt terrible. An hour or so ago I had thought myself to be on the threshold of a new world, and now I was playing around in magic shops. How could I be so dumb, I thought, and yet ...

I had company. Upon returning to the television studio I learned that Mr. Blanché required an additional hour, but would be ready to resume at 2:30, and so I set about eavesdropping and conversing. The physicians milling around the hallway represented the spectrum of my own contradictory opinions and feelings. One maintained that pain, being a subjective phenomena, could not be adequately assessed by the observer, and gave several instances of patients who failed to complain of pain during procedures when others would have been in pain. Still another said that he could see no explanation for why the subject who had the lipoma removed, for example, would not be "screaming bloody murder," with that forceps tearing at his tissue in an open wound. When I raised the question of infection, the veterinarian laughed indulgently as he related how he does operations on dogs who then go immediately to the kennels and roll around in dirt and feces without becoming infected. Assuming comparability in this regard between dogs and humans, the conclusion seemed to be that the great care taken in conventional operating rooms against sepsis is largely unnecessary.

Just before the second session was to begin, Dr. Singer came by grumbling, "Magicians, I know all about them!"

At the beginning of the second session, Dr. Singer reported sketchily on the meeting of the physicians and the magician, and began to ask questions of the magician. However, he interrupted the magician and kept diverting the discussion, never really giving him the floor, and so the magician's opinion, so vociferously and comprehensively stated to me at lunch, was not made to the assembled group. Rather, Dr. Singer took up some tangential and assumed objections, asking the magician, for example, to examine the Bibles and showing him the trash can in which resided various materials from the morning work. At one point, he said, "We will satisfy whatever doubts may remain."

I made an inner prediction that no further surgery would be done that afternoon. Blanché asked for the return of the morning cancer subject and repeated his laying on of hands treatment. He asked him to read from the New Testament, to which the patient replied he would not since he was Jewish. He did, however, read from Acts 28.

Another subject came with the complaint and diagnosis of gallbladder difficulty. Mr. Blanché ignored that obvious invitation to do an operation and instead plucked a number of papillomas from her neck, causing her some obvious pain, and dotting her neck with alcohol-soaked puffs of cotton. In his best Bert Parks manner, Dr. Singer asked one of the physicians whether he had ever seen anything like that before, the plucking off of papillomas from the neck, to which the doctor replied sensibly enough, "I've never seen it done."

The woman professor at the university who had guided and driven me here and there turned out to be blind in her left eye, had a fibroid growth over the retina, and had been unable to read without special glasses on her right eye for many years. I had seen pictures and movies of Philippine surgeons operating on the eye, plucking the eye out, working on it and putting it back, and for a horrible dread moment I thought that Mr. Blanché was going to do this to this subject's eye. Instead he seemed merely to stroke it. She said that she "felt pressure, high energy, and no pain." Mr. Blanché was joined by his assistant in working on her with a laying on of hands while asking her to pray. Ms. Hernandez predicted that "little by little she will see." Shortly after, she reported that she could indeed see light areas in her heretofore blind eye, and she then read from the Bible without the glasses on which she had been dependent for reading. It seemed an odd time for Dr. Singer to put aside his usual enthusiasm in favor of objectivity: "I am neither advocating nor denying."

Dr. Singer asked for more volunteers, people who needed incisions, and singled me out in particular. No, I said, I have no complaint that would allow an incision. I was too diffident, or something, to suggest that I would like my low back pain worked on (so long as no incision was involved).

With no further volunteers for healing, Dr. Singer drew the proceedings to a close. As the meeting was breaking up, and I was confirming with the subject of the eye treatment her history and experiences, I heard a mild altercation between Dr. Singer and the magician. Dr. Singer was holding the trash can which included the materials from the operation and exhorting the magician to take the can with him and examine its contents. The magician was saying that he did not have any laboratory, his taking the can would prove nothing, and he didn't want it.

I asked Dr. Singer how I could have a look at the results of the laboratory investigations, the follow-up of the patients, and all the data from the experiment, and he said he would be writing it all up. In other words, it was not for me to see firsthand. I gently remonstrated with him that during the experiment he had hardly sounded objective. "Oh, that," he said. "That was just for the occasion," or words to that effect.

Trudging off in the mists of Michigan, I thought to myself I would have to go to the Philippines after all.

Upon my return to accustomed surroundings after one or another of my trips to study healings, I not infrequently become more objective and dispassionately critical. The insidiousness of group contagion, the unaccustomed surroundings that tend to suspend customary thinking and ways of living, diminish as the facts (at least as they stand in memory and notes) are required to speak for themselves. Something of the reverse occurred upon my return from Oakland University. I wondered whether I had been too hard on Dr. Singer and the experiment, whether what I had remembered seeing was really as scientifically objectionable as I had thought. I was reassured that I had not been unfair some time later when Dr. Singer sent me the report of the other supposed "official witness," Richard Kammann, co-author of *The Psychology of the Psychic*. Mr. Kammann's observations coincided neatly with my own. They were so persuasive to James Randi, the well-known magician member of the Committee for Scientific Investigation of Claims of the Paranormal, as to prompt him to write a letter to Dr. Singer, also sent to me by Dr. Singer, which can only be described as scathing. ("The 'thoroughly scientific' and 'objective' test you promised was obviously a farce.") Also included was another secondhand report of a second demonstration by Mr. Blanché at Oakland University some five days after the one that I observed, and a follow-up on some of the patients. The net impression of Mr. Blanché's work was inconclusive. Dr. Singer also sent me copies of his replies to the Committee for Scientific Investigation of Claims of the Paranormal in which he substantially reiterated his belief that he had designed and conducted an honest and reasonably efficient experiment to examine Mr. Blanché's work.

In a way, the whole discussion, imbroglio, and demonstration itself were beside the point, assuming the point was the validity of psychic surgery. Mr. Blanché made no attempt to demonstrate that he could open and close the body with his bare hands. Basically, he had only offered a demonstration of folk healing, with such psychic frills as the incision made from a distance.

I put in a call to my travel agent.

II.

MY ENTERPRISE RECEIVED A sobering blow when a travel agency, which I had been led to believe specialized in trips to the Philippines for healing, informed me that the Federal Trade Commission now forbade the selling of tours or tickets to the Philippines for that purpose. Indeed, an injunction against such tours had been issued by Judge Daniel H. Hanscom, who had declared that psychic surgery was "pure and unmitigated fakery." Case closed? No — it never seems to be with respect to psychic phenomena. In a masterly dissection of the ruling, Krippner and Villoldo[6] first note supporting evidence for the ruling such as *Time*'s review of Dr. Nolen's *A Doctor in Search of a Miracle*, and the *National Enquirer*'s own repertorial study of psychic surgery. Then they examine, raise doubts, and dismiss the logic and scientific conclusions of the critics of psychic surgery, even their basic facts. They go on to offer their own and others' firsthand observations. They conclude that all the evidence of fraudulent psychic surgery does not dispel the possibility that there is genuine psychic surgery.

Their second main conclusion boggled my mind, which by then I thought had reached its boggle limit. Krippner and Villoldo suggest that it makes no difference whether the material apparently extracted from the body is human or animal, whether the fluid is blood or vegetable dye, or whether the body is opened or not. What is critical is whether the appearance of material apparently taken from the body during the operation is explicable to orthodox science or requires explanations or beliefs not included in orthodox science. What they have in mind in the latter regard is "materialization," or "apportment," the producing or moving from one place to another of material brought to observable reality by means unknown to conventional reality.* In other words, the hypothesis of psychic surgery could be explainable through recourse to yet other psychic hypotheses. More and more, the crucial experiment was becoming a detective story.

Four years after the ruling that restrained travel firms from promoting psychic surgery tours to the Philippines, an article appeared in the industry house organ, *The Travel Agent*. The author of that article reported that the Christian Travel Center, of Manila, arranges for about one hundred foreigners (mostly Americans) to visit the Philippines and to be booked for healing sessions and education in healing and related topics. Presumably the Christian Travel Center is able to conduct its activities only because it is based in Manila, far from the U.S. Federal Trade Commission. I was advised by letter from the Christian Travel Center that from October through February the healers would be very busy, and that access to them, for my purposes, would "be quite impossible." But the Center was willing to do business with me at any other time. I had learned, by then, that the Christian Travel Center was owned by the wife of the most famous, if not infamous, of the psychic surgeons, Tony Agpoa.

Dr. Nolen complained often, in his book, about the heat of Manila. Indeed, his negative conclusions about psychic surgery could have issued as

---

* In Iceland, a country said to be hospitable to psychic phenomena, a local college professor-psychologist showed me a ring that he had seen materialized by Indian holy man Sai Baba.[4] With due respect for the treacherousness of informal observations, he struck me as a sober, knowledgeable, objective reporter.

much from his spleen as from his judgment. For me, the heat was nothing compared to the traffic and noise. The problem was magnified by the hours I spent in taxis in the midst of automotive havoc pursuing healers throughout the farflung reaches of that teeming Asian city. Unlikely as it seemed at the time, I was in only one automobile accident, in which I suffered only minor injuries.

Irony and misery governed my first experience with psychic healing. An acquaintance in the United States had asked that I deliver some materials to a a relative of his, whom I shall call Mr. Vargas, who was seriously ill with cancer. My acquaintance asked, also, whether I might try to be of some help to Mr. Vargas since he knew that I had been working with cancer patients. Mr. Vargas was terribly ill, and insufficiently clear of mind for me even to try to be of use through psychological means. His family arranged for me to talk on the phone with the patient's physician, whom I shall call Dr. Ibarra. Like the man who claimed he had not borrowed his neighbor's lawnmower and anyway it didn't work, members of Manila's medical establishment knew very little about psychic surgery, and anyway it was a fraud. Dr. Ibarra, however, seemed at least tolerant of the possibilities and mentioned healers with whom he was acquainted. Although later he told me that the surgery was just fakery, I was told by others that he had sent members of his family to Alex Orbito, a psychic surgeon many of whose operations I was later to watch.

The next day, I fought my way through jet lag and traffic to a middle-class residential street bathed in sunlight. On that street was the home, operating room, and chapel of Virgilio Gutierrez. Reverend Gutierrez' older sister, a lawyer, met me at the door of the family bungalow and directed me down the driveway at the end of which was the chapel. A Doberman Pinscher was barking in front, cocks were crowing in back, children were running about and shouting from under the pews. Yet the simple whitewashed room struck me as sincere and dignified, as did the people attending the service. The operating room was a cubicle with a glass window, presumably for viewing, though now covered by a drawn cloth. In response to sounds from the back of the hall, I swiveled my head around to see Mr. Vargas being half-supported, half-carried by his wife and child down the aisle toward the operating room. The Vargases had not told me of their intention to have Mr. Vargas healed by Reverend Gutierrez, nor did I tell them that I would be visiting Reverend Gutierrez. A serendipitous opportunity, I thought, to learn from Dr. Ibarra, who would be following the patient's condition, what, if any, change took place from the healing. But this self-serving and dispassionately scientific thought was quickly overcome by the vision of Mr. Vargas' wide, frightened eyes as he was led down the aisle. Mrs. Vargas spied me and motioned to me to come into the operating room, but I caught myself up in a spate of diffidence. How could I, bedraped with cameras and stuffed with scientific interest, get in the way of what might be this man's last chance for life? About fifteen minutes later, Mr. Vargas emerged from the operating cubicle, rather more walking than being dragged or led. Reverend Gutierrez later told me that Mr. Vargas' aura was basically good, and that he would live. I learned from Dr. Ibarra the next day that just about when Mr. Gutierrez was telling me that good news, Mr. Vargas had died.

I WAS TO RETURN several times to Gutierrez. I took still photographs and movies of several of his treatments, including surgery, and I interviewed a number of his patients. Among the latter was a seemingly astute, sophisticated American who claimed to have obtained great relief from his first heart operation, done by Gutierrez, and had returned for a second. A European, now living in the United States, was also a steady customer of Gutierrez, but try as I might I could not ascertain exactly what his ailments were. Such unclarity illustrates one reason why it is difficult to learn about the usefulness not only of psychic surgery but of all treatment interventions. In order to measure change one has to be sure what the difficulty was in the first place.

Gutierrez and I broke bread together in the kitchen alongside the chapel. He invited me to an all-night meditation retreat of healers, to take place in Pangasinan, a country town some fifty miles from Manila which is a center of psychic healing and surgery — an invitation that I regretfully could not accept.

Despite all of Gutierrez' friendliness and informality I could get no further than the bland assertion that what I was seeing was actually taking place, and a polite but insistent refusal to be pinned down; e.g., what difficulties were easiest or hardest to treat, what rate of success was there for any of them, how were the diagnoses made? I got the same reaction in talking to his sister, a lawyer, who in a most unlegalistic way offered the same blandly obscure answers to pointed questions.

Mr. Gutierrez seemed to be somewhat of a generalist, or general practitioner, rather than solely a surgical specialist. He treated some people with gentle massage, others by fluttering his hands over their ailments, others by the cupping and burning procedure that Blanché as well as countless grandmothers have used. With one partially blind man he poked and prodded around the eyes — arousing again the fear in me that he would remove (or even appear to remove) the man's eye, as I had been told sometimes occurred. He reported to me that the man now could see after being blind. One would think, under those circumstances, that the man would have called out, "Eureka! I can see," or the equivalent in Tagalog, but he merely got up and left in an unremarkable way. I would have to bet that his was not a miracle cure. Whatever the validity of the healing, I began to wonder whether Mr. Gutierrez was not given to exaggerated claims, emanating from at least a dash of grandiosity. It would be difficult for any grandiosity not to be summoned by hundreds of people entreating one for help.

Without warning Gutierrez began to knead a patient's abdomen. As his hands seemed to dig in deeper and deeper, a spurt of what looked like blood erupted. It looked as if he had opened a hole in the abdomen, and he appeared to pull some matter from that hole. The blood seemed to vanish almost as quickly as it had come, the last remaining traces being wiped up with cotton by an assistant to reveal an unmarked abdomen. The patient showed no particular reaction. In this and every other psychic surgery that I observed, with a variety of surgeons, instead of crisp commands for scalpel, forceps, clamps, the surgeon merely nodded for assistants to swab the operative field with coconut oil and mop the area with cotton. The other, and in the view of many, most important piece of equipment was a Bible, often held open over the patient. Not one of the thirty or so surgeries that I observed took place without cotton, coconut oil, Bible, and assistants. All of these have been suspect as contributing to chicanery.

BY CONTRAST WITH THE homey atmosphere of Gutierrez' work, Alex Orbito heads an enterprise that is much more like surgery in the grand tradition. I got to him under the auspices of friends of friends of friends in a chauffeured Mercedes. Filipinos share with many other countries once colonized by Spain not only Spanish names but a similar economic structure, which features lots of poor and a few very rich. Well-connected and well-appointed as my hosts were, they had never seen the psychic surgeons, though many of the upper class are said to know and use them. Nevertheless, many Filipinos are unfamiliar with the psychic surgeons. Indeed, I was to appear on the Manila equivalent of Jay Leno's televised *Tonight Show* because of my presumed expertise in the study of psychic healing that was so little known to so many Philippine viewers.

The most fashionable and famous healers live in Manila; the unfashionable ones live in the countryside. Orbito was, clearly, a fashionable healer. Between 100 and 200 people were sitting in the chapel at the side of his comfortable house. At least a third of them were foreigners. His brother led a brief prayer service, which one might expect from Orbito's business card: "Grace of the Holy Spirit Society — Phil. Spiritual Help Foundation. Reverend Alex Orbito Spiritual Leader." On what would have been a dais there was a room with a large picture window. Through that room could be seen the operating theater. The word "theater" seemed most appropriate, as a European cinema crew was making a documentary of the proceedings. I, with only my hand-held Super-8 movie camera, nonetheless gamely filmed alongside the professionals. The room itself consisted merely of a table, a stool for the surgeon, and a chair. The procedure was for patients to be led in, one to lie on the table, another to sit in the chair, while Orbito would operate, turning from one to the other. Patients sometimes said what ailed them, or pointed to the offending part. Other times they did not. It seemed to matter little to Orbito, as he later told me his hands tell him where to operate. Before beginning the operating series he read a few lines from a Bible, seemed to go into a slight trance for a moment, then gestured for the first patient to lie down. Most, but not all, patients received operations.

His technique was the same as that of Gutierrez. Surrounded by assistants, Bibles, cotton, and coconut oil, he would apparently rub a hole in the patient, extract matter and throw it into a bucket, and close up the patient. What he took out was anybody's guess except for one startling instance: he pulled from a woman's abdomen a couple of feet of hair. I was told that he and other healers might also extract palmetto leaves, lizards, and vegetables. Such articles, according to my informants, were taken from people who had been bewitched. The lady who yielded the hank of hair was somewhat overweight, which made it difficult to know whether Orbito's fingers were in her body, or just lost in rolls of fat. The psychic surgeons are often accused of doing their surgery on overweight people, the better to create the illusion of opening the body. He did, however, appear to open the body of thin people, and over bone primarily covered only by skin. Orbito was perfectly willing for me to take slides and movies at just about any distance I chose, which, especially with zoom lenses, made possible close-up pictures.

In part, I busied myself with photographic and journalistic chores in order to divert my attention from what I was observing. These were not pretty sights. Some of the people's infirmities, such as external tumors, were obvious. So was the worry on many of their faces. Whether or not the red fluid was blood, it looked it. One after the other, minutes apart, in dizzying succession, blood was spurting from what looked like fresh wounds, bodies were being exposed, hopes were being headily gratified or bitterly disappointed.

In all of my studies of the new therapies my procedure was to participate in all of the activities; thus, I had entered into Gestalt therapy groups, and I had spent a week at Esalen during which I was massaged and went nude swimming under the stars. My body has been offered up to the manipulations of Rolfers, to the practitioners of the Alexander technique and bioenergetics, and to nutritionists. I was less afraid of all of them than I was of being operated on by a psychic surgeon. A Philippine friend, who had tennis shoulder, was less timid. He emerged from his operation with only a thin red line and sheepish grin to show for it. It was now a matter of pride as well as scientific and journalistic conscience that I, too, be operated on.

But operated on for what? For reasons having to do with pure terror, I immediately chose my extremities rather than my head, chest or abdomen. Although the light has to be right to see it, I do have a somewhat enlarged leg vein that unless I get more exercise could one day qualify as varicosity. The problem suited the surgeon just fine. I rolled up my pant leg while others manned my camera equipment. During this first operation I lay back and tried to get all of the uninterrupted sensations that I could. In that position I did not see any blood or material removed from my leg, though both appear on film. I felt merely the pressure of Orbito's hands, perhaps a slight burning. A couple of minutes later I rolled my sock over the slight reddening that was the only visible souvenir of the experience.

On another visit to Orbito, now flushed with survivor's euphoria, I had the same operation done on the other leg. This time I swiveled my upper body around to get a close look at the proceedings but was told by Orbito to lie back. That was the only time that he objected to any of my viewings. Whether he did so in the interest of my health or to prevent my getting that particular, perhaps revealing, view of his work is at the heart of the matter: *What the hell was going on?*

It was a question I was to ask many times. I asked it of one of Orbito's assistants, a young woman who turned out to be a physician. She had been working with Orbito for several years, understood clearly and sympathetically why I was asking the question, and answered it: What I thought I was seeing, I was seeing. She was aware of instances of trickery, but absolutely clear that the phenomenon could be done genuinely and *was* done genuinely in the operations that I had been observing.

As befits an Asian Michael DeBakey, Orbito had the style of someone holding court. When he was not operating, people pressed themselves in upon him, seemingly hanging on his answers. He was, however, generous with his time in several talks with me, took parts of the Rorschach test, and told the following story out of — well, the *Arabian Nights:* He had been summoned to do an operation on one of the members of the royal family of Saudi Arabia. Once there, however, he was told that if the operation failed, he would pay with his life, and on that basis he could choose whether or not to proceed. The operation was a success, which was good news, presumably to the patient and certainly for the surgeon.

Orbito sees hundreds of patients per day. After finishing at his home, he goes to hotels where he treats foreigners who want extended sessions in the comfort of their own quarters. If Mr. Orbito were to see that many patients in the United States, he would require large tax shelters indeed. The financial aspects of psychic surgery are, like everything else connected with it, mysterious. Orbito and most of the others ask no fee; they merely make a contribution box available for those so inclined. The many poor people that Orbito treats offer the equivalent of pennies. Foreigners may leave modest amounts of dollars. Surely, this is no way to get rich, and so it is difficult to accuse the surgeons of financial exploitation. Yet I heard of grand sums being collected for the hotel work, and there are those who say that psychic surgery can be a lucrative business indeed. Its main value, according to Orbito, is, however, neither financial, nor as treatment either, in a way. Rather, he sees healing as a means of focusing interest on and increasing spirituality. A spiritual rebirth is necessary, he believes, in order to avert World War III. More healing power to him.

IT HAS BEEN SAID that if two people are marooned on a desert island, they will shortly set up competitive churches. So it is with spiritual healers in the Philippines. The main issue that divides the "Union Espiritista Christiana de Filipinas, Inc." and the "Christiana Espiritista de Filipinas" is that healer members of the latter are inclined to be paid for their work. For the most part, members of the former believe that healing is a theological exercise, should not be paid for, and indeed if one is paid, one is likely to lose the healing power.

As it happened, the Union Espiritista Christiana de Filipinas, Inc. was having its annual convention during my visit. And while at other conventions that I have attended some strange speeches have been made, none in my experience was made by a discarnate entity using the voice of a medium. (In these surroundings "the media" were not magazines and television, but one hundred mediums, each attached to a spiritualist center that was a component of the Espiritista Union.) The medium at this meeting was a tall, imposing middle-aged woman. Whatever language the spirit spoke in, the medium spoke in Tagalog. Later, in English, she told me she had no idea what she was going to say before the talk. Rather, she had just gone into her usual workaday trance, and let the spirit do the talking. As she explained it, the spirit's message was only a little clearer to me in English than it was in Tagalog, but in that respect was not substantially different from many other theological messages I have heard.

I had a little more communication success with another member of the Union, a professor of philosophy. He believed that the laws of nature, physics, and "clean morality" led to health. He suggested that there was only one absolute rule — to love your fellow man; any expression of that would be moral. After asking forgiveness for a little "sophistry and blasphemy" he said that God stole Adam's rib, so God is a robber. In the *Summa Theologica*, Aquinas wrote that man is essentially good, so whatever man does is good. Where, then, does evil come from? To define something as evil involves a judgment, and no one is in a position to judge, he claimed.

Whatever the merits of his theology and philosophy, this man was clearly an intellectual, so I was eager to get his considered opinion of psychic surgery. Everything is vibrations, he said, and a high rate of vibration can penetrate a low rate. The psychic surgeon's hand is capable of a high rate of vibration, thus the penetration. And where does the material, apparently removed from the body, come from? It was a thought form, he said, slowed in vibration to a point where it was physical to the naked eye. In short, it was materialized. I could have snorted that all this was unsupported theorizing, unconfirmed speculations, airy rationalizations for what one needed to believe in the first place. I lowered my dudgeon by reminding myself that if this professor had attended some professional meetings in which I have participated, he might well have justifiably said the same.

Whatever the ultimate origin of psychic surgery, its penultimate source seems to have been the town and surrounding area of Pangasinan. A number of healers have emanated from and many still do practice in this dusty, rural town. My travelling companions were Florida, a professor at the University of Manila who had been trained in the United States, and her long-time friend whom I shall call Estrellita, who was fluent in Tagalog; both of them were knowledgeable believers in psychic surgery. I thought at first that Florida's daughter, Marita, was along just for the ride. It turned out that Marita had considerable pain from a hip injury, had hardly been able to stand for the last several days, and hoped for relief from one or another of the healers. We found, at Pangasinan's Spiritualist Center, Rosita. This handsome middle-aged woman, touted as an up-and-coming though not yet famous healer, spoke only in Tagalog. Her conversation with Estrellita developed into an impromptu prayer service. She then was ready for her first patient, who turned out to be me.

Maybe I was too thin for purposes of demonstrating psychic surgery, but for whatever reason she claimed that I did not need an operation. I did, apparently, need a sharp twist of my head to the left, and then to the right, each time producing what to me seemed a deafening crack. She arrived at her diagnostic conclusions with what healers euphemistically call an X-ray. The X-ray procedure was to put a sheet over my back and then read the inner workings of my body as they appeared to the healer on this sheet. Or maybe instead she got her information from her guiding spirit who, Rosita said, had told her about our coming and our purposes.

For Florida's treatment, a Bible was held over her head, the healer's hands were waved over Florida's hands, and she was given instructions as to continued care by the spirit who serves as Rosita's medical informant.

Only Marita, with her specific vexing symptom, was operated on. As I was busying my movie equipment preparatory to the operation, Rosita sharply waved me away. It was not that she objected to my filming as close as I wished, but I was standing between the operating field and a banner on the wall. The banner, commemorating the Union of Healers, can be found on the wall of all members of the healing group. Healing power is said to emanate from it, and that power is diminished if one blocks the path from it to the patient. Rosita's surgical technique turned out to be like all the other psychic surgeons. As recorded on my film, she produced something that looked like fat from the buttock and then the presumably offending matter. While the fat looked like fat, the other matter was like nothing else that I had ever seen: brownish, vaguely organic, bug-like. I asked whether I could take it, and was told that I should not, as it was poisonous and evil and would be harmful. Maybe it *was* harmful, for after its removal Marita maintained that her pain had decreased. Later in the day, we climbed up and down steep concrete steps, which she managed nimbly and comfortably.

The next surgeon, Juan Flores, has been written about in many books reporting on psychic surgery. He lives in what elsewhere might be called a suburban development, though the term has the wrong associations for his collection of shacks and dirt paths. Wandering up and down the paths were villagers, chickens, pigs, and a water buffalo. Off to the side a mother was breast-feeding her baby. Flores could be seen working out in the fields under his broad-brimmed straw hat. He farms in the morning, and does his healings in early afternoon. As I observed, he goes from the farm to the operating room without pausing to wash his hands. His healing takes place in a crude stone chapel which is regularly packed with people. Part of Flores's popularity stems from his giving of "spiritual injections." Each of the lined-up visitors is the recipient of a stabbing movement, at the end of which they feel the sting of a prick. When my turn came, I too felt this moderately painful sensation. A cunningly placed pin could have been responsible. If so, it was too cunningly placed for me to observe despite my best efforts.

Several published accounts attest to the seeming legitimacy of the healer's capacity to produce a pinprick without a pin. Dr. Fernandez, a reliable observer whose research is described toward the end of this chapter, also experienced pain when Flores wielded the "pin"; so too reports Tom Valentine, a journalist, in his *Psychic Surgery*.[7] Lyall Watson writes of a similar experience, with the addition that he found a tiny puncture wound and a drop of blood though the shirt area above the wound was undamaged.[7]

Flores's operations somehow seemed more serious than those of some of the other healers. Perhaps it was because he refused to allow films to be taken, and he operated at some distance from the audience. One of his surgical patients was a young German woman who had been operated on by Flores several years previously, with considerable benefit to her, for a slow-growing cancer of the hip. She was here for another operation, to take place under the eyes of her husband, placed right near her, who was a surgeon. Here observing the operation at close range was a man who ought to be able to know what was happening medically. I could hardly wait to meet him after the operation. Of course, he might want to believe in anything that was beneficial to his wife; then again, because his wife was the patient, he might have observed with special care what was happening to her and thus be a sharp critic of the procedure. At any rate, when I did meet him, I pushed my face closer to him than I usually do in conversations, looked him straight in the eye, and asked whether the psychic surgeon's hands had, in fact, entered his wife's body. He looked back at me, just as forthrightly, and replied, "I don't know." He knew enough, however, to credit her progress of several years to psychic surgery and had backed up that belief with this repeated arduous and expensive journey. In other words, whether or not the hands of the psychic surgeon entered his wife's body was less important to him than the fact that she benefited.

Benefited from what — from the trip itself, from the belief that she was to benefit, from the operation, from a master healer's therapeutic touch? And so we leave the clearing in the jungle that is Pangasinan with a jungle of questions.

Perhaps Mr. Hoya, who tells fortunes from cards, will answer the questions. He was a member of the *Esperitista* group, in training to become a psychic surgeon himself, for a year and a half. Thus, he could be expected to give me the inside story. The inside story he told me was that psychic surgery was a fake. What appeared to be blood was simulated with betel nuts, bicarbonate of soda, and food-coloring dye, often placed under the long and dirty nails of the surgeon or in the omnipresent cotton. The equally omnipresent oil when mixed with the dye produced sanguinary liquid. He, too, was not allowed to take for examination any material ostensibly removed from bodies. He quit the group and the pursuit of the practice indignantly. Nonetheless, he continues his work as a psychic, continues to believe in miracles, and estimates that only eight of ten psychic surgeries, or other paranormal healings, are fakes.

That the greatest number of psychic surgeries use trickery seems to be generally agreed upon (see Krippner & Villoldo,[6] Watson,[8] Meeks,[9] Nolen[1]), yet it is difficult to find anyone who is willing to say that there never could be an instance where what one saw is not what was happening. Moreover, trickery to the Western mind is different from trickery to the Oriental. According to Hoya, while many Filipinos are naturally psychic, they have a colonial mentality, they need to impress foreigners. While they may do this for materialistic reasons and to bolster their self-esteem, their main goals are to cure and to persuade others of the power of spirituality. For them these ends justify the means, and because the ends are noble, so are the means.

Alien as such a point of view may be to the Western mind, at least such attitudes about what constitutes trickery and its moral implications take place within the same context of reality. There are those, however, who say that psychic phenomena are real or not real depending upon the nature of the reality of the viewer. For example, if one becomes interested in psychic phenomena, then all at once it seems psychic phenomena turn up everywhere. Is that simply because one is looking for it, others know that one is interested in it, or in fact has the interest created a reality in which psychic phenomena do in fact occur? If there is anything to the latter, it may help explain the apparent effectiveness of diverse health care systems the world over. In a health care system in which the throwing of bones is an accepted form of treatment, then the throwing of bones is effective not because of one or another variety of suggestion, as the Western mind might explain it, but because in the reality of bone throwing *as* medicine, bone throwing *is* medicine.

Was it the laws of chance, as viewed by a Westerner, or the reality of Philippine mysticism that resulted in Hoya's comments about me when reading the cards? Among the things that he said correctly were that I had two children, that I had a pain in my left foot, and that the first ride in a car that I would have upon my return to the United States in the next three weeks would be in a white or red car (I was picked up at the airport in a white car with a red interior), that within three years my son would travel in Europe (he did two and a half years later), that I would be involved in a property transaction with a person in whose names "R" and "L" were prominent (I was involved in such a transaction with a man named Rolley two years later), and that I have a sister (true).

IN THE SPIRIT OF Philippine mysticism, as well as scientific curiosity, Father Bulatao recommended to me that I study, in effect, exorcism, a major form of treatment in the Philippines. Despite being a psychologist trained in the West, who teaches at the Ateneo de Manila University, he was confident that people do get healed through psychic surgery and other interventions exotic to the Western mind. He was convinced of the reality of telepathy, clairvoyance, and precognition (though skeptical about psychokinesis), particularly when done by people in at least a light trance. He shared, also, the fairly common Filipino belief in the existence of *dwende*, or dwarfs. His incisive mind and sophisticated background made it difficult to dismiss out of hand any of his recommendations, and so it was that I found my way to Armong Frank.

I found Mr. Frank incongruously at home in a Manila residential subdivision. His shoulder-length pageboy hair parted in the middle, his six-foot shepherd's crook, his street-length robes of red and blue velvet, and the plastic lamb he held in one hand conspired to make him look like Jesus, albeit a bit more worldly.

The resemblance is no accident. Frank's healing work is a prime example of what might be called fundamentalist Catholicism, which is characteristic of much of the indigenous healing of the Philippines. At the front of his house there was a six-foot statue of the Virgin Mary. "Jesus Nazareno" is printed on the backs of the t-shirts of Frank's associates in his healing movement. Pictures and plaques on the walls all attest that the healing is an expression of Jesus's healing. That belief is joined with the belief in evil spirits which can be exorcised. The best way to do this is through a medium.

In order to observe a medium at work, Frank suggested that we travel to a storefront medical clinic run by his organization. Since Frank's clinic was part of the health care system of the Philippines, exorcism had better work. With few medical doctors and little money, the Filipinos have no choice but to take advantage of indigenous healings of many kinds. I saw people of all ages bring their physical complaints, receive healing procedures, pay their fee and leave. Anyone walking the sidewalk could observe the healing through the glass fronting on the street; few records were kept, and diagnostic procedures were not apparent. Yet in its essential activities this establishment was fundamentally like any medical outpatient facility.

Exorcism, by way of a medium, is done this way: Maria, the medium on duty that day, was strapped into a chair with heavy wooden arms, one of the straps being an airline seatbelt. Next to her sat the patient. Maria went into a trance in order to receive from the patient the evil spirits that were causing the patient's illness. When the evil spirits were shifted from the patient to Maria, Maria went into paroxysms of uncoordinated movement, thrashing and flailing around frighteningly. It was the job of Frank, or one or another of his associates, to summon or exorcise the spirits in turn from Maria. This was done by growling, shouting, making threatening movements in response to which, in-between her jerky movements, she cowered like a small, frightened animal. Then, she suddenly sat back in the chair, relaxed, out of her trance, and free of evil spirits. A moment later, she put on her glasses, greeted a mother and infant, briskly performed a brief healing using stroking and oil on the infant, and collected and recorded the fee in a ledger.

I am not sure how to take this, but — when my turn came to be exorcised and I took the patient's chair next to Maria, after a while she told me that I didn't have anything to be exorcised. Rather, I was inhabited by good fairies. Should I need help at any time, I should consult my main good fairy whose name, if I recall it correctly, was Mary.

IT WAS LIKE THAT SCENE in the Oscar-winning film *Treasure of the Sierra Madre* where Walter Houston is summoned to treat a child in a primitive Mexican village. Unsure of whether he is to be received with friendliness or hostility, he walks uneasily past the staring eyes of silent banks of people. All light-skinned 6'1" of me draped with camera equipment walked down the silent street in a dusty, remote Philippine village, past scores of smallish, dark, staring natives who, at any moment, could have surrounded me and made me a candidate for, rather than an observer of, healing. The crowd grew thicker as I approached a longish shed-like building, against whose partially open walls throngs were pressed watching the healing activities inside. This was the domain of Colcol, a renowned healer of the area.

Whether he was renowned for his healing abilities or his showmanship was difficult to ascertain. As soon as he became aware of my mission, crowds parted, doors opened, and I was ushered into the hall around whose walls sat patients and patients' relatives. The walls were decorated with pictures and notes of gratitude from patients who I was told were prominent in the government. The long arm of electronics had preceded me. Colcol did his healing *shtick* with microphone in hand. With it he would call new patients to him and also ones that he had previously healed who would offer testimonials. He waved the arm of an arthritic patient who, he said, had previously been unable to straighten out the arm at all. He had another patient stand up from his wheelchair. All of this went on to the counterpoint of his chatter delivered through glistening teeth wreathed in a huge self-satisfied smile. He showed his favorite stunt of reversing the healing process by immobilizing a previously immobilized limb. The healee, understandably, failed to see the humor as he once again was unable to extend his arm until Colcol gleefully, with a touch of his hand, healed him again.

I submitted an aching muscle to his ministrations. Since he failed to heal it, he could not unheal it either. With others Colcol's Hollywood hoopla may have contributed to his apparent healing success. It may have detracted from the possibilities of healing me, or maybe it was irrelevant. I thought that Walter Houston's make-believe was more believable, but Colcol's patients, relieved of their ills, had found their therapeutic treasure.

III.

I MET DR. CONSTANZA Fernandez at the Espiritista Convention, which she was attending in connection with her Ph.D. research, entitled *Tooth Pullers Among Filipino Folk Healers: An Exploratory Study of their Psychology and Practice*.[10] When she told me about what we may call "psychic tooth pulling" I thought, for a moment, that she was engaged in materialistic leg pulling. What she was studying were dental extractions done by mostly rural, medically untrained healers, using forceps, bare hands, or fingers wrapped in a handkerchief. Such extractions are made without anesthesia. They take only a few seconds, although difficult teeth might take a minute or more. Only minimal amounts of bleeding occur, and the pain is far less than what one would expect without anesthesia. Just after the operations, patients are usually made to wash their mouths with calamansi (a local fruit) juice or salt water. Despite the non-sterile conditions, patients do not become infected. Here we go again, I thought, as Dr. Fernandez and her husband drove me to the hinterlands outside Manila and to the hinterlands of another clinically bizarre means of healing.

We found Rodolfo Laganzod Caminong, known as Rudy, in his modest wooden hut. A man in his early thirties, with his mustache, beard, and long curly hair tied at the back, he resembled an American '60s hippie. He welcomed us with friendly informality. He was obviously proud of the literally thousands of teeth that he had collected in jars or spread on the floor in the shape of a star. He was informal and jovial during the tooth extractions. The "office" was nothing more than a chair set on the ground in the open. In the two extractions that I observed, he approached the patient from the back, leaned toward the side where the tooth was to be extracted, raised the patient's head, and grabbed the tooth firmly with a forceps, making a quick lateral motion before pulling the tooth out. (Rudy uses only his fingers when extracting children's teeth.)

One patient had a tooth pulled in a few seconds, with what appeared to be minimal or no pain and without bleeding. Before the operation I was invited to assure myself that the tooth was firmly anchored in the gum, which it certainly seemed to be. The second patient, who looked to be in her late teens, had six teeth removed in rapid succession. She seemed to be in considerable pain, or perhaps it was shock at having so many of her teeth removed. I could get no convincing explanation for the mass extractions, "they were all bad" being the closest approximation to a diagnosis. Despite the many gaping holes, she hardly bled at all. On the basis of what I saw, I was happy in this instance to break my longstanding practice of personally experiencing what I was writing about. Even if I had an ailing tooth for which a recommendation for extraction had been made, I rather doubt that I would have been intrepid enough to let Rudy have a go at it.

While I cannot offer a first-person account of psychic tooth pulling, I can offer a second-person one. During the time of her researches, Dr. Fernandez received a recommendation from her conventional dentist that she have extracted a supernumerary tooth which had erupted in a narrow space, causing irritation in the gums. The tooth's crown was not yet fully exposed, thus potentially making the extraction somewhat difficult. The dentist was unwilling to do the extraction at the time, because Dr. Fernandez had recently given birth. What a grand opportunity, she thought, to be a participant observer, except that when the time came it did not seem at all like a good idea. She asked Rudy if perhaps it might not be better to wait until the tooth emerged completely, but Rudy assured her that there would be no problem in his extracting it right then. Still hoping against hope, she asked him to proceed with another patient first. She then observed Rudy's extracting many teeth in rapid succession from the other patient. Three of them came out easily. Two came out with some difficulty. But with one, despite his applying great strength, the tooth would not come out. It finally broke and came out in pieces. Now pale and trembling, she began to leave until the healer told her authoritatively to sit down in the dilapidated operating chair. He seemed especially eager to perform the operation since a U.N. official was there to take movies of it. Pressured also by her scientific soul, she fought off her fear and after repeating that she only wanted one tooth out, opened her mouth. She felt a quick, sharp but not painful sensation, and in a few seconds the tooth was out. In a few minutes it had stopped bleeding and there was no pain or infection afterwards.

I got this account, and other accounts and data, directly from Dr. Fernandez and from her written report of her research. From my knowledge of her and her work, I would say that these second-person sources are as reliable as most firsthand ones. I believe that her extraction happened just as she reported it. The same can be said for her report of her friend's having a wisdom tooth extracted by Rudy. As a subject and observer of such Western operations myself, all followed by days of pain, I can only envy the account: a four-rooted wisdom tooth came out in about five seconds with slight pain during the extraction and none afterwards.

Dr. Fernandez observed several hundred extractions done by five tooth pullers. Most were done with forceps (Rudy had begun his career working with electrician's pliers), though one tooth puller almost always used his bare hands wrapped in a handkerchief. Of 41 subjects questioned by Dr. Fernandez, 26 of which involved multiple extractions done in a single session, 17 subjects (41 percent) reported no pain during the extractions, 10 subjects (24 percent) reported little or slight pain, and three subjects (7 percent) said they had pain but it was bearable. Only five patients (12 percent) reported strong pain. Of 20 follow-up cases, 16 reported no post-extraction pain, and four said they felt post-extraction pain in the area where the tooth was for some time. No patient developed an infection as a result of the extraction.

Unlike psychic surgery, which leaves no obvious residual evidence that anything has occurred other than sleight of hand, patients of tooth pullers have holes in their gums and the teeth that came from these holes. How is it done? All of the tooth pullers, as with most psychic healers, claim that the power that makes the operations possible comes from God and is merely channeled through themselves. One of the tooth pullers proposed that Dr. Fernandez prove to herself the existence of a special power by his transferring that power to her so that she, too, could perform a painless tooth extraction. The patient selected for this purpose was a 23-year-old man having six teeth extracted at one time. He gave his permission for the fourth one of these to be extracted by Dr. Fernandez. The tooth puller, Mang Celso, whispered some prayers over the forceps wrapped in a handkerchief. Then he blew strongly on Dr. Fernandez's fingers before enfolding them around the forceps. He prayed over the forceps again and pressed her thumbnail strongly with his right thumb. The tooth to be pulled was a mono-rooted pre-molar on the lower right side, the fifth tooth from the middle, blackish, badly decayed, with little crown left. However, she ascertained with her finger that what was left of the crown was firmly in place. Her first attempt to extract the tooth suffered from her nervousness as she failed to grasp it firmly. On the second try, the tooth came out unexpectedly while she was testing whether she had a firm grip. In other words, once she had grasped the tooth firmly with the forceps, it came out without her applying nearly the degree of force that she expected she would have to apply. The patient did not show any sign of pain. Mang Celso pulled the remaining two teeth uneventfully, if one can call such extractions uneventful. In a subsequent interview, the patient said he had felt a little pain when one of the molars was removed, but no pain with the other five extractions, including the one done by the researcher.

In 1905, Einhorn and Uhlfelder synthesized Novocaine. Through the ages before that, teeth were pulled without anesthesia. Australian and African Aborigines did it by placing a chisel-like tool against the offending tooth and pounding with a stone. The Romans used what they called a "mystic forceps" made of soft lead; it was unlawful to extract teeth that were not loose enough to be taken out with the soft lead instrument. The Greeks used a device to loosen teeth which were then pulled out by hand. In fifteenth- and sixteenth-century England, tooth pulling specialists plied their trade without a general knowledge of dentistry. In the *Chinese Medical Journal* published in China, in 1979, a dentist, Gong Xuehin, of the Liaoning Institute of Traditional Chinese Medicine, wrote of extracting more than 30,000 teeth by finger pressure at acupuncture points. He did all these extractions without the use of drugs, with patients claiming none or only slight pain and with little loss of blood. Some dentists conventionally trained in Western medicine now extract teeth using hypnosis as their anesthesia.

The fact that teeth can be extracted more or less painlessly and with minimal bleeding through hypnosis opens the door to the existence of esoteric capacities, abilities that transcend conventional knowledge of physiology. Secular theorists are thrown back upon explanations having to do with suggestion, placebo, and altered states of consciousness, which enable some laws of physiology to be repealed by the person's mind. To those who believe in parapsychology, tooth pulling without anesthesia is no more remarkable than healing hands affecting the growth and behavior of plants, enzymes, and human and animal physical symptoms. All these are an expression of a reality that exists beyond the five senses, a reality such as propounded by Buddhism where the mind is a sixth sense, capable of seeing without eyes, hearing without ears, or smelling without noses. To the tooth pullers themselves it is more simple: God is the Novocaine of the masses.

Chapter Five

The Laying On of Health: Some Who Heal by Touch

I BEGAN MY OWN CAREER as a psychic healer in a theater, just before swing clarinetist Benny Goodman was to perform. My daughter complained of a severe headache that might necessitate her leaving. I reached over and put my hand on her forehead for several minutes and imagined that I was sending healing energy to her. She soon reported that she no longer had a headache, and we went on to enjoy the concert.

That is a tribute to healing energy, to suggestion, or to the strength of a father-daughter relationship. Whatever the explanation, I thus joined a line stretching back to antiquity of putative healers who heal by touch.

It so happened that not long afterward I began to work psychologically with a woman who had ovarian cancer. After a remission, she had a recurrence of tumor growth which necessitated hospitalization. On several occasions she overcame intense pain during and following my laying on of hands. At one point she was close to death from renal insufficiency. Following my laying on of hands, her kidney functioning went from a near lethal 7.0 to a still grim, but much improved, 3.5. This up-and-down pattern continued until she finally did succumb to the cancer. An endocrinologist reviewing the laboratory studies said he could not understand how she had lived as long as she did. That she was not cured does not in and of itself obviate the possibility that the healing procedure was effective up to a point. Only lustful hopes are responsible for the assumption that healing must be all-or-nothing, healed or not healed. The operation can be a success — pain can diminish, time can be gained, readings can change favorably — even if the patient ultimately dies.

Like most medicines, psychic healing may be insufficiently powerful for a particular illness in a particular situation and still not totally invalidate itself. Or, as Stanley Krippner[1] suggests, "cure" can be defined as remission of all symptoms without untoward aftereffects, while "healing" can be defined as a movement toward wholeness whether of body, mind, or spirit.

Another patient was being treated in a hospital for pain from a migraine headache. After I held her head in my hands, she claimed immediate relief from the pain, relief which continued. How was it, she asked, that the whole hospital armamentarium failed to bring her the relief that my hands did? I wondered the same, though with less questioning of the hospital's failures than of my success.

My method was to take a few deep breaths and count backward from ten to one. With each number I imagined myself sinking deeper and deeper into — what? the depths of myself? altered consciousness? meditation? Or I might concentrate on a nonsense word, a mantra such as the one I was given when taking a course in Transcendental Meditation. Sometimes I would just relax and imagine that my hands were sending healing energy. My hands would become red and hot, though I was unsure how much of that came simply from prolonged physical contact.

To try to answer that and related questions, I had myself studied in a biofeedback laboratory. In order to establish a base rate, various psychological measures were taken while I rested for five minutes. Then I meditated for ten minutes; the measures were repeated at the beginning, middle, and end of the meditation, then compared with the base rate. These results are reported below along with a comment by the laboratory technician.

	Heart Rate	Left Hand Temp.	Right Hand Temp.	Blood Pressure
Beginning / base rate	64 BPM	95.1° F	96.1° F	132/80
End	69 BPM	95.4° F	96.4° F	
Mid-meditation	71 BPM	96.7° F	97.0° F	
End	66 BPM	97.0° F	97.0° F	120/78

"Other changes include a reduction in frontalis muscle tension to a level approaching deep relaxation, a lessening of autonomic (sympathetic) nervous system activity (as measured by galvanic skin response) and an increase in peripheral blood flow volume which co-related with rise in hand temperature."

Whether or not one is interested in being a healer, the strong implication here is that meditation is a safe, inexpensive way of lowering blood pressure.

If no physiological changes had occurred during the meditation, it would imply that either I was not really meditating, or that despite such changes during meditation being claimed by most others, my readings did not change with meditation. The achieved results, however, suggest that I did change my bodily functions with meditation, including a warming of my hands. A full-scale scientific investigation would require that these procedures be repeated frequently enough to know whether such changes were merely periodic variations which would have occurred even without meditation. And even if such changes could be established, we would still need to know whether the changes had any effect on the patient's symptoms — whether a meditation level of consciousness is the same as a healing level of consciousness.

I got self-reports of relief from several randomly chosen subjects suffering from a variety of ailments in addition to headaches: sequelae from medical operations, disabling back pain, lymphatic swellings, flu, and colds. A noted educator and clinician in cancer treatment went out of her way for a second laying-on of hands treatment from me of a mysterious swelling in her neck — which we did in a busy airport — because she said she had gotten so much help from my first one. A few people claimed not to have gotten any relief from my ministrations. I am unsure what to make of the reports of those who claimed that they did obtain relief. Having been on the patient's side of such encounters, I know how hard it is to tell the healer that he or she has failed, even though most psychic healers do not ask, seemingly unconcerned about "results," and anyway assuming that either results will occur some time after the laying on of hands takes place or they won't.

My experience doing the purported healings ranged from the feeling of an open, loving attunement with the person, to a wandering mind and an awkward sense of the peculiarity of what I was doing. It would be good to know whether such differing attitudes made any difference in the alleged healings. For what it's worth, I don't think they did, but researchers, please heed these hypotheses.

Just imagine — if one seemed to be able to heal others without their incurring side effects, with little effort and a small expenditure of time, would one not be expected to pursue such healing busily, enthusiastically, and never miss a chance to offer and experiment with such a remarkable and beneficent skill? Yes, but such was not true of me. I would forget about the possibility for many months at a time. When I did remember, or was reminded, it came as something of a surprise, so completely had I put it out of my mind.

One explanation might be that such activities were so different from my usual work and identity that I could not comfortably integrate them; my sense of myself simply would not allow it. And then there was the awkwardness of letting it be known that I was available for psychic healing. I further think that my reluctance to pursue this healing modality had to do with a fundamental anxiety about the implications of such an activity. I had noticed such anxiety whenever I was in the presence of what was, or seemed to be, paranormal phenomena, whether brought about by myself or anyone else. On the one hand I had the wish to observe and be persuaded by such discoveries that could open doors to the limitless possibilities of a new reality. On the other hand I felt the need figuratively to cross myself, as if threatened by a mystifying and vaguely dreadful supernatural. Perhaps that reaction on the part of others contributes to the animosity and derision often shown toward the paranormal.

If healing by touch works, how does it? To many psychic healers the question is irrelevant, even blasphemous. When paranormal phenomena are studied in laboratories and fail to work, apologists claim that the scientific world view is inimical to the work of the paranormal and spoils it. That may be a sorry excuse, or it may be true. More impressive is the fact that many healers refuse to charge for their services on the assumption that such crassness would interfere with their pristine capabilities. But with due regard to the sensibilities of healers, one also has to consider the sensibilities of the common-sense and scientific worlds and try to understand what is going on here. Explanations for healing by touch can roughly be categorized as follows:

(1) *Physical:* An actual and measurable energy is transmitted from healer to healee, a purely mechanical transaction independent of any other

factor. The capacity to heal by touch is rooted in the physiology of persons, perhaps all of us to a greater or lesser degree, which has atrophied through the years of evolution as other functions have superseded it, much as happened to the sense of smell. Less evolutionarily sophisticated lower animals, who heal each other through touch, have maintained this primitive capacity to a greater extent than have humans. Healers are either those who have selected themselves for that work, perhaps no more adept at it than would most others be, or they are persons who have maintained the biologically-given capability more than others have. By the same token, healees may vary in their receptivity to healing depending upon the degree to which their primitive capacity to absorb treatment has survived evolution.

(2) *Religious:* Most healers that I have encountered are religious. They are more or less straightforward about their belief that healing is evidence of God's grace; it is an answer to explicit or implicit prayers, a reward for good works. As surgeons were once barbers, and educators were once priests, so too were healers people of God. There is no need to posit such a construct as energy that only clutters the sublimeness of the relationship between God and persons.

(3) *A Combination of (1) and (2):* Healing comes about through a transfer of energy, but that energy comes from God. Many healers back away from a conception of their having great power by humbly claiming that they are merely vehicles or mediums for God's healing energy. (I have a lot of trouble resonating to their humility, since God, after all, has seen fit to choose *them* as His representative, or they have chosen themselves for this awesome task. But that may just be me.)

(4) *Parapsychological:* There are cause and effect mechanisms, not necessarily using energy, that preclude the familiar concepts of time and space; e.g., thoughts can be transmitted, objects can be moved by thoughts, the future can be predicted correctly — and people can be healed by thoughts or touch.

(5) *Psychological:* Leave God and energy, from whatever source, out of it. Benefits from healing through touch come about through little-understood but powerful "forces" generated by the psychological effect that occurs between persons. Such an effect may otherwise be known as placebo or suggestion; these terms merely elide the point.

People are social animals. They begin in the womb as a social unit, and indeed the fetus is "healed," or maintained in health, from the beginning by another. The mother whose stroking "makes it better" exercises a healing capacity rooted in human nature. While such a capacity probably plays a role in all healing, permeating the context of healing, its effects are usually masked by the technology of healing, whether that technology consists of administering penicillin or the alleged transfer of energy through one's hands. (I address these issues more fully in the last chapter.)

For now, let us note some of the researches supporting the facts of, and some possible explanations of psychic healing.

Two of the most famous researches in healing are famous in part because they are two of the very few creditable laboratory researches available in the field. The researchers are Bernard Grad, Ph.D., and M. Justa Smith, Ph.D., both using as healer in their experiments Colonel Oskar Estebany.

Oskar Estebany was a Colonel in the Hungarian Army who discovered his healing powers by healing cavalry horses, later healing people during the Hungarian Revolution when medical doctors were in short supply. I met this courtly gentleman in the course of my visits to Grad and Smith, and he served as a subject for the psychological test research on the personality of healers in Chapter 11.

Dr. Bernard Grad is a biological researcher and geriatrician at the Allen Memorial Institute at Montreal's McGill University. His research on healing by laying on of hands is creative and meticulous.[2,3] He inflicted wounds on the backs of three groups of mice and measured their rates of healing from these wounds. Colonel Estebany, the healer, held the cages of one group daily over a period of time; he did not hold the cages of the second group; and he did not hold the cages of the third group, but their cages were warmed mechanically to the same degree as those in the group whose cages he had held. (The last procedure was to control for the possibility that heat from the healer's hand alone would produce any observed changes.) The wounds of those mice whose cages were held by the healer healed significantly faster than the wounds of mice in the other two groups. Thus, the laying on of hands seemed to have contributed to the healing of wounds, and whatever brought about that result was something other than simply heat. In a second experiment one group of mice was treated by Colonel Estebany as in the first experiment, another was untreated, and a third was treated by several people who claimed not to have healing abilities. Again, the wounds of mice treated by the designated healer healed faster than those treated by people who did not identify themselves as healers, and still faster than the untreated mice. Grad then used barley seeds instead of mice as subjects. The healer simply held a beaker of water in his hands which was then used to water the seeds, while ordinary water, not held by him, was used on matching pots of seeds. Seeds watered by healer-treated water grew in greater number, weight, and yield than those watered by water not treated by the healer.

M. Justa Smith, Ph.D., a Franciscan nun, is a biochemist at Rosary Hill College in Buffalo, New York. She maintains that bodily health is related to the proper balance of enzymes, and so any capacity to heal the body should be matched by a like capacity to influence enzyme activity. Colonel Estebany held in his hands a vessel containing a solution which included enzymes. He increased the enzyme activity in the solution as compared to an identical solution which he had not treated. He had "healed" the enzymes! In another experiment the enzymes were damaged, i.e., made unhealthy by ultrasound irradiation at a damaging wavelength, and Colonel Estebany again "healed" the enzyme as measured by its becoming as active as undamaged enzymes treated by him.[4,5]

Presumably mice and barley seeds were not responding either to God or to Colonel Estebany as a person. God may have chosen to intervene in this experiment, perhaps to demonstrate the power of unorthodox healing, as some would claim. Apart from whatever the participants may believe about themselves, healing, and the universe, so long as they did not wittingly or unwittingly intervene unfairly, the experiment demonstrates effects whose explanation is consistent with a mechanical, secular transfer of energy.

Colonel Estebany believes that he can impart energy into a letter whose handling by others will allow them to absorb his health-giving energy, and recommends that one expose oneself to such a letter once a day for one-half hour. He recommended that I do that with his letter to me confirming our appointment. I read and answer my mail conscientiously, but I proved to be a bust at remembering to expose myself regularly to his letter.

Unlike most healers who use laying on of hands, Colonel Estebany adopts different hand positions for different ailments such as hemorrhoids, ulcers, and sinus. And also unlike many other such healers, he acknowledges that there are illnesses that he cannot cure, such as diabetes.

Dr. Grad's specific interest in healing stems from a more general interest in psychic phenomena as well as from a longtime admiration of Wilhelm Reich. Reich was a major proponent of the belief in a life force, an energy which he called Orgone and which he claimed to be able to collect in boxes. Grad, too, believes that when Estebany healed wounds and enhanced the growth of barley seeds he did so by directing an energy which is different from energy as conventionally understood, but which nonetheless is a biophysical reality.

Dr. Justa Smith told me that through her professional life as a biochemist she had been skeptical of that which cannot be measured, manipulated, and controlled in a laboratory. Now, after working with Colonel Estebany and circulating in the world of unconventional healing, she says that she has eliminated "impossible" from her vocabulary. She has not, however, eliminated a hard-headed attitude toward professional matters from the presentation of herself. I found her no-nonsense mien inspiring of confidence in her work whose design in and of itself impressed me with its rigor. For example, after reading her careful analysis of vitamins, using a chromatographic technique, I am inclined to believe her conclusion that there is a difference between natural and synthetic Vitamin C, and that natural is better despite Linus Pauling's opinion to the contrary.[6]

I was even inclined to believe her answer to my questions about Colonel Estebany's ability to break up clouds in the sky by concentrating on them: she was convinced that he could. Now that is not ordinarily a question that one thinks to ask. I asked it because Grad and I had apparently done just that by concentrating on a cloud that to its misfortune presented itself at the window of the hotel room where we were carrying on our discussion. When I rather sheepishly asked Dr. Smith's opinion about such powers, she recognized my timorousness as once her own. Now, as far as she was concerned, Colonel Estebany could without a doubt bust clouds with only a steady gaze.

I report this bit of cloud-busting intelligence after some deliberation. For some people it could fatally weaken their readiness to at least consider unconventional healing as a reality. Whatever feeling of validity may have been created by Grad and Smith's esteemed laboratory studies might then be eroded. These are the feelings with which I had to deal when I was with Grad and Smith, and subsequently. The situation is but an exaggerated and dramatic example of the tension generated when a lifelong conception of reality is confronted by claims of a different reality. The situation was made even more eerie by the juxtaposition of two impressive practitioners of the scientific method asserting something so fantastic. Wilhelm Reich had said that he could control the weather, and he published research with photographs to prove it. Surely he cannot be believed on that — or can he? Many people would also have bet against Grad and Smith's showing that under controlled conditions the laying on of hands could hasten the healing of wounds, the growing of barley, and the altering of enzymes.

Dr. Robert Becker, an orthopedic surgeon and pioneer in bioelectricity, has demonstrated in the laboratory that the human body radiates a weak electromagnetic charge.[7,8] He has published his findings in *The Body Electric: Electromagnetism and the Foundation of Life*. At a convention of aquarian healers in Washington, D.C., I saw him present his findings that suggested the possibilities of regeneration of limbs as a function of the body's electric nature. As a consequence of his belief in the ubiquitousness of energy, he is concerned that electrical equipment in the environment has a deleterious effect on human energy fluids and therefore on the body.

Dr. Robert N. Miller has a Ph.D. in chemical engineering, holds two patents, and is a published author in his research fields of metallurgy, high polymers, fluid flow, and heat transfers. I have not met him and know his work only through his writings. However, as noted in Chapter 13 and elsewhere in this book, I have studied Olga Worrall, whose reported abilities Dr. Miller measured as reported below.[8,9,10]

A cloud chamber is a glass cylinder with an aluminum bottom and a glass for viewing across the top. When it is put on a block of dry ice and methyl alcohol is put into it, a mist of alcohol is created. High-energy atomic particles generate vapor trails when passing through this zone of alcohol mist. By holding the unit in her hands, Mrs. Worrall produced a moving wave pattern in the chamber. She again produced a wave pattern when she was six hundred miles from the chamber and merely directed thoughts in order to produce the motion. The latter finding supports her contention that she can produce healing from a distance, so-called absent healing. (She tells patients to relax and receive the healing which she sent at 9:00 P.M. Eastern Standard Time.) One can conclude from Miller's studies that thoughts are things in the sense that they produce physical effects. Dr. Miller demonstrated that while Mrs. Worrall's brain waves under ordinary circumstances show a preponderance of beta waves, as expected, when she is engaged in her healing activities she produces a preponderance of alpha waves, which is the consciousness of most people just before sleep.

Mrs. Worrall's hands produced changes in cupric chloride solutions as compared to controls; she reduced the surface tension of water, and brought about changes in hydrogen bonding in water. She, like Colonel Estebany, was able to speed the growth rate of seeds, by holding in her hands a container of water which was then used to water the seeds, relative to comparable seeds which were watered with water not held by her. (Water exposed to a magnet did even better in enhancing seed growth, which suggests that healers send electromagnetic healing energy.)

A brief aside about scientific experiments: They often sound authoritative and make a good impression; they glow with mystique. To the uninformed about the details of research design, which includes most people, formal research may be overpowering in its persuasiveness. Truth to tell, it is a bit of a con game. Evaluating research is a specialty; even many researchers are unskilled at it. For evidence of this, one might simply have a look at the journals where experiments are debated. Even prestigious researchers argue back and forth about whether an experiment is sufficiently well-designed as to yield the conclusions claimed to be derived from it. Researchers testing the same question frequently get opposite conclusions. Belief in the results of a single experiment is usually ill-advised; even a few repetitions may not sufficiently safeguard against error. Science proceeds by successive approximations of the truth over time and with repeated formal and informal observations and experiments until a body of knowledge congeals. Even then, every once in a while surprises occur as discoveries are made that create shifts in understanding and raise doubts about that which has gone before.

The experiments reported here seem to me to be bold and respectable steps on the tangled, treacherous path to knowledge. But let us not be beaten into submission by their arcane numbers and esoterica. They are merely part of a process of attempting to document a view of reality.

It is plausible to conclude on the basis of the Grad, Smith, and Miller demonstrations that there is indeed an energy emitted from the hands of a healer — and from magnets — which is different from the energies known to conventional science. Such an energy seems to operate independently of psychological factors, and so is part of the technology of healing much as is an antibiotic or surgery.

The word, idea, concept, assumption of *energy* weaves in and out of scientific discussions and ordinary conversation among those interested in paranormal phenomena and psychic healing. Many people believe that life force or healing energy flows through unseen pathways called, in some traditions, *meridians*. Its gathering "points," the targets of acupuncture, are called in some Eastern religions *chakras*. These correspond somewhat to glands in the endocrine system. Besides having physiological effects, chakras determine a person's level of psychological development, character traits, and symptoms. It is the stuff of which the etheric body is composed, that body which, in paranormal circles, is said to interpenetrate the physical one. Its extension beyond the physical body can be seen by some psychics who call it an aura; and it is said by the general run of believers to be photographed with the Kirlian method, though hard-headed researchers of Kirlian photography may disagree. Some people conceptualize humans as nothing but energy, the so-called structures being merely congealed patterns of subatomic particles vibrating back and forth between energy and matter. Under a sufficiently high-powered microscope, what appears to the naked eye to be solid reveals itself as swirling movement.

Life force, or healing energy, has had a long and varied history. For Bergson it was *élan vital*, the Chinese call it *chi*, Indians call it *prana*, Russians call it *bioplasm*, for Reichenbach it was *od*, for Reich it was *orgone*, and Freud named it *libido* in his early formulation, in which he believed that an actual energy proceeding according to hydraulic principles caused symptoms. M. Justa Smith notes simply that energy distinguishes the living from the dead, and she credits it for bringing about all healing whatever the externally applied curative agent. Thus, designated healers may simply stimulate the patient's energy, or add to it if it is depleted. Since life force is the essence of the person, its existence lends credence to those who believe in the capacity of the essence of the person to get out of one's body (as in near-death or other out-of-body experiences), to go to heaven, or to be reincarnated.

To see energy around the edge of the body does not require a high-powered microscope or any complex machinery. It requires only a simple device invented by a Soviet electrician named Kirlian. This device passes a high-frequency electrical current through the subject, usually a hand, which is placed directly on Polaroid film — a kind of photography without a camera. The resulting picture shows the subject with flares extending beyond its boundary as seen by the naked eye. One might assume that the photograph is of energy indigenous to the body; at least as likely is that it is something introduced by the machine itself. The first Kirlian photograph that I saw was my own, taken when I was a demonstration subject at a Silva Mind Control meeting. Soon there were those of several other people, all different. The black oval pads of my fingertips were surrounded by an approximately quarter-inch bluish-green halo; those of other people were orange, yellow, purple, as well as bluish-green; some swirled off much further from the fingers than did mine. What, we wondered, did the differences mean? Some Kirlian adherents claim that all the different shapes and colors represent diseases, degrees of fatigue, and character traits; others disagree. Workers at the Polyclinic Medical Center in Harrisburg, Pennsylvania have found correlations between finger pad auras and emotional status and physical disorders including cystic fibrosis and cancer. Such correlations likely reflect something in nature, but not necessarily the effects of energy.

Other researchers claim that what is being photographed is not energy, but minute variations in skin conductance and electrolyte balance which reflect metabolic or physiological changes associated with illness. Still others claim the photographs are of electricity or moisture. Yet the same pattern persisted after drying of the hands. The objections further pale when confronted by the "phantom leaf": part of a leaf is cut away, yet the aura around its edge before the cutting remains. This is taken by some as proof that there is an energy body which duplicates the physical leaf, extending slightly beyond it and remaining, for a time at least, after the physical body is removed. There are, however, other plausible explanations for the phenomena. There are sharp differences of opinion about energy and Kirlian photography, as might be expected about a new and remarkable observation. For a comprehensive survey and even-handed analysis of various views, see Krippner's *Human Possibilities*.[1]

I, too, may have photographed psychic energy, not with the Kirlian device but with an ordinary camera on ordinary film. The subject was Uri Geller, the famed psychic, who is particularly known for his capacity apparently to bend keys and spoons by stroking them gently. When I visited Geller in his Manhattan apartment, I was hardly through the door before he set about bending keys and sending messages telepathically. I photographed these activities with a Rollei 35 mm pocket camera. Later, I photographed him simply posing at his desk. The posed picture turned out to be gratifyingly clear and sharp. The pictures taken while he was doing his psychic work have long, spidery streaks across them; same camera, same roll of film, same photographer, approximately the same time. Neither my photofinisher nor the Kodak company (which apologized for selling me what they called imperfect film) had an adequate explanation for the streaks, which were unlike the imperfections occasionally seen in many photographs.

Parenthetically, I made another trip to Geller's apartment in order to give him some psychological tests. When we were finished, he proposed — no, Geller tends to order with childlike exuberance more than propose — that he draw something and then telepathically send the image of what he drew to me, and I would confirm the reception of that message by drawing it myself. On the first trial what I drew failed to correspond to what he had drawn. He seemed surprised, even insulted, and insisted that we do it again. I suggested that he calm down and give me time to meditate briefly. Under these conditions, tranquil for me if not for Geller's impetuous soul, I drew a fork, which was what he had previously drawn. (What are the odds of a fork being drawn by chance? The odds are in fact pretty good, as are the odds that people will draw a sailboat.)

So according to those who believe in universal energy, we are all sending and receiving sets of an inherent store of energy. But just as television sets and ears have to be in good working order for there to be effective transmission, so too do the psychological condition of healer and healee. Dr. Justa Smith repeated her study within a year after the first one, and this time Colonel Estebany was unable to affect the enzyme. This result could be interpreted as the real one, with the first an artifact. Instead, Dr. Smith notes the following: At the time of the first study, the college where the study took place was at its relaxed summer pace. Colonel Estebany had comfortable quarters on campus and was attended to regularly by herself and many students with whom he became a personal favorite. The second study took place between Thanksgiving and Christmas, a hectic time; Colonel Estebany had to live off the now-packed campus, the Buffalo weather was foul, Dr. Smith was exceptionally busy and unable to attend to him, and in addition Colonel Estebany was suffering from some publicly unrevealed personal difficulty. Dr. Smith concludes that Colonel Estebany's frame of mind interfered with his healing powers.[13, 14]

Dr. Grad in the design of his research had taken into consideration the possibility of psychological factors playing a part in his research. Following the demonstration of Colonel Estebany's ability to speed the healing of wounds and the growth of barley seeds, Grad studied the effect on plant growth of people with presumed differences in mood. He selected a psychiatrically normal man, a neurotically depressed woman, and a psychotically depressed man, and had them hold in their hands the bottles of water used to water the seeds. As a control, some seeds were watered with water that was not held by anyone. His hypothesis was that a person in an untroubled mood would help seeds grow better than those in a depressed mood, and better than seeds not treated at all. That hypothesis was supported; the seeds treated by the psychiatrically normal man grew better than did all the other groups of seeds. Thus, an additional finding was that Colonel Estebany was not the only healer around; perhaps lots of people have similar healing powers. When the mood of the neurotically depressed woman improved she, too, showed an ability to influence the seeds. Thus, it seems that the mood of the healer makes a difference, and what is crucial is the mood at the time that the healing is being done rather than a more general cast to the personality; a positive mood promotes healing as measured by seed growth. Similar findings have been demonstrated among psychotherapists; therapists whose patients do well have been shown to be empathetic, therapeutically genuine, and to view patients positively; the patients of therapists rated as not having such qualities do less well. In other words, there is objective evidence for the healing properties of a good "bedside manner," for psychological factors influencing the effects of presumed deployment of energy, whether that energy is conceived of as being spiritual or secular.

The same seems to go for the patient. Grad demonstrated that mice made calm through stroking and letting them get used to their treatment boxes benefited from the laying on of hands treatment of their subsequent wounds. Mice that continued to be tense were shown to be resistant to the healing of their wounds. Here is at least some inferential support for the often-observed fact that hopeful patients tend to heal more successfully than hopeless ones.

Presumably mice and barley seeds are not suggestible, yet they were healed through the laying on of hands. Thus, support is lent to the hypothesis that healers do send energy. At the same time, that hypothesized energy may be enhanced or neutralized by psychological factors. Is there contradiction and chaos here? No, not any more than there is when one conceptualizes psychosomatic illness: sometimes the body falls ill with little or no encouragement from psychological factors, just as sometimes energy alone can bring about change. Sometimes psychological factors can promote illness with little or no contribution from physiological causes, just as psychological factors can bring about healing with little or no help from energy supplied by external sources. A reasonable way to conceptualize the interplay between psychological and energy factors would be that healing psychological factors release blocked energy which has contributed to illness, a process which can be aided by energy externally supplied through the laying on of hands.

I HAD MY FIRST personal experience with the laying on of hands when seated at lunch with Reverend Rosalind Bruyere, whose workshop on such healing I was attending in Boulder, Colorado. For some time I had been mildly troubled by soreness in a third finger knuckle which my physician said was due to arthritis. The associations of that term with infirmity and old age hurt worse than the finger did. Reverend Bruyere continued with her gay lunchtime chatter, with me and the others at the table, while she reached over and held my offending knuckle. I felt intermittent jolts like a mild electric shock. The healing result, assessed over the next months, was a waxing and waning of the soreness, an improvement but no cure.

Reverend Bruyere looks like someone one might meet at a backyard barbeque rather than on a church dais. Nor does she look particularly likely to head a healing center, to act as a consultant to medical doctors, or to be a university lecturer, a student of electrical engineering, and a private practitioner of psychic healing. She looks even less like a member of Hell's Angels, which she used to be. (She claims to hold some sort of record in motorcycle jumping.) That is all in her present life. In her past life, she told me, she ran a plantation alone during the Civil War while her husband fought in the Union Army, a husband, incidentally, whose spirit she maintained later inhabited her father.

Her Healing Light Center, near a shopping mall in Glendale, California, was in some respects like other suburban medical clinics. She has a staff of fourteen healers who see their patients, clients, or healees usually for a session each week. However, the resemblance to one's familiar suburban clinic stopped short for me with the information that every now and again medical consultants in the form of a country doctor, Dr. Johnson, now deceased, and Dr. Chang, an Oriental physician very long deceased, could be sensed, or as staff members would say, they "were around."

In addition to being a center for treating patients the Healing Light Center is a school of healing and metaphysics in general, and awards a degree and ordination to ministers. This Pastoral Healing program offers the degree of "Bachelor of Natural Theology in Sacred Healing." Apart from its subject matter, its program description is much like any other college catalogue (categories such as application for enrollment, completion requirements, tuition and fees, grading and probation). If for no other reason, being an ordained minister is useful in that it supplies a legal umbrella for what otherwise might be prosecutable as practicing medicine without a license. Or its practitioners could suffer the fate of clairvoyants in nearby Long Beach, who are forced to buy an annual six-hundred-dollar license and whose activities are restricted to a central business district near adult bookstores. Here are titles of some courses offered by the Healing Light Center: Quartz Crystals; Window of Light; The Ceremonial Shaman; Creative Imagery; Creating Medicine Shields. Required courses for the Pastoral Training Program include: Consciousness Seminar; Meditation Perspectives; Introduction and Intermediate Healing Technique; Intuitive Awareness and Development. Some other titles of courses offered: Intermediate Psychic Development and Natural Healing; Advanced Psychic Development and Natural Healing; Consciousness Raising; Health Perspectives Through Psychic Awareness; Acupressure; Zone Therapy and Reflexology; Introductory Astrology; Spiritual Astrology; Huna: The Religion of Ancient Hawaii; Autogenic Training; Yoga; Polarity Therapy; Massage.

When I visited Reverend Bruyere at her Center, she said she would get serious about the finger that she had previously treated informally in Boulder. She put me on a standard examining table and then stroked my finger for about ten minutes. She commented, as had others, that I was fighting the healing, that I was turning back the energies. However, I felt, or thought I felt, a cracking or moving of the knuckles, at which point she said, "Now I have got it." As it turned out, she had — or something had. Of course, the cure could have been the result of suggestion, even pique at being accused of turning back healing energies, or simply the salubrious course of a self-limiting ailment. At any rate, I no longer have signs of arthritis.

I then asked to "meet" one of her spirit guides. She thought that could be arranged, since she thought Dr. Chang seemed to have been around recently. She let it be known around the office that she was going to get in touch with Dr. Chang, and several of her colleagues gathered. She quickly went into a trance and began to speak, in English but with an Oriental accent and in an unaccustomedly guttural voice. That was said to be the voice of Dr. Chang speaking through Reverend Bruyere. I was introduced to Dr. Chang and given the opportunity to talk with him, but it was not much of a conversation. In part that was because upon the invitation to speak to this discarnate person I felt as linguistically awkward as I am when talking to an answering machine. But mostly it was because Dr. Chang demonstrated a mixture of Oriental inscrutability and typical healer evasiveness. I was cast as the uptight West and he the unflappable, opaque East, and with a bit of the knife out for me also. For example, he was inclined to answer my questions such as what he did, for whom, where he was, by calling attention to my lack of "accepting spirit" and suggesting that I needed to get in touch with my own guides. He said that it was difficult for me to ask, and him to answer, questions because so much was foreign to my experience. He did not think much of my thought processes either, which he described as being involved with "intricacies." As he said, he was not sure where I was "coming from." I wondered where that bit of California patois had come from; either he has picked it up in the environs, or maybe Reverend Bruyere lent not only her voice but her speech patterns to the translation of Dr. Chang's thoughts. Dr. Chang had a mildly encouraging sense of this book, which he thought could be "monumental" if it changed many people's consciousness. I had to decide, he said, whether to finish it quickly or slowly, and seemed to recommend that I take my time and immerse myself in the material.

Dr. Chang described himself as a philosopher, deferring to Dr. Johnson, apparently a crony in the spirit world, for narrowly medical questions. Anyway, he figured Reverend Bruyere, as a psychic, did not require much help with specific questions. He evidently thought himself to be more needed and helpful to the Center's students who did not have their own guides and could consult him through meditation. He predicted that he would speak to me again next year (which for all I know he did, in his own way and unbeknownst to me). He ended with the following: "I give my love to you. You give it back to me. I give it softly, sweetly, lovingly. Good afternoon."

Reverend Bruyere snapped out of her trance and resumed her usual manner as we sat down to do the psychological tests. That is, we began the tests, but a telephone call interrupted us with the request that she help with an emergency at the famed Burn Center at Sherman Oaks Hospital. Reverend Bruyere drove there in the manner of an ex-Hell's Angel motorist, and immediately went to work on a patient there. She alleges that she can turn flesh cold, with consequent healing benefit to burn victims, and can also regenerate burned flesh. The medical establishment at the hospital was sufficiently impressed by her work to open its doors to her ministrations, and to have begun a research project on her healing there.

In a fashion typical of such healers, Reverend Bruyere is difficult to pin down with specific questions such as what condition she is most and least able to heal, the length of time the healings take, and whether she follows up any of the healings to see whether successes have continued or whether apparent failures have later turned into successes. At the time neither she nor her staff of healers kept progress notes or records of their sessions, though I am told that now they do. But from what I could gather from hours of informal discussion with Reverend Bruyere ("interviewing" suggests far greater discipline in these meetings than I could achieve), she claimed to be able to cure just about any affliction. She mentioned specifically: arthritis, cancer, leukemia, removal of a bullet from a spine, eczema, multiple sclerosis, kidney stones, sexual frigidity, the physical sequelae of infantile paralysis, rotating a uterus thereby making conception possible, and epilepsy, which she says is especially easy to treat. She can also read past lives, make physical diagnoses on the basis of her X-ray vision, and see auras from which she can deduce a person's physical and mental condition as well as what they are thinking.

Such a multiplicity of skills and beliefs is unsurprising, for these skills and beliefs often appear together. That may be because they stem from the common reality of the participants, and the group contagion which can be expected to be especially powerful in an often derided sub-group. Or, as Reverend Bruyere believes, such skills come from a common source in the mind which most people have squelched with psychological barriers. For whatever reason, healers, sensitives, and psychics have simply not put up such barriers to the natural state of being psychic. One price such people often pay for these retained abilities is to become, in her words, "spacy." The light which she sees emanating from people, their auras, is, she says, the same for healers as it is for paranoid schizophrenics. Since she had mental illness in her family she was concerned that I would find, with the psychological tests, that she too was mentally ill, by way of heredity. I did not. She was open to, if not needful of, an idiosyncratic way of perceiving things, but not disorganized in any formal way.

Among others of Reverend Bruyere's beliefs: illness is an attempt to achieve understanding, particularly "spiritual understanding" which is why so many physical treatments do not work. Everything in the universe is composed of energy, and that is all there is just as the quantum physicists and others say. We choose our parents and the lives we lead in order to fulfill grand designs or karma. (She even went so far as to speculate that Hitler's karma was to demonstrate the evils of racism; the six million Jews who went submissively to their executions chose to be killed as part of *their* grand purpose. These opinions unfortunately are asserted by others, also, in the unorthodox healing circles. This was one of the times I reflected that I deserved hardship pay for doing these investigations.)

Cancer, according to Reverend Bruyere, reflects an attempt to get a new consciousness, which may involve the death of the old one. It is treatable by changing the patient's ion field from positive to negative, through imagery on the part of herself while she works with the patient and on the patient's part, and through eating healthfully. Healing moves electrons, which in turn changes enzymes. Energy has a direction of its own, so a healer can touch a patient anywhere and the energy will go where it is needed, even apart from where the healer and patient intend it to go. Physical ills reflect psychological problems: breast cancer is a sign of indecision about sexual role; arthritis puts a hardness between the patient and the rest of the world as an expression of inhibition of sexuality; digestive disturbances come from not being able to stomach something; knee trouble reflects a lack of humility, in that the person is brought to his or her knees; chronic back pain stems from being inflexible; head difficulties come from awkward, pressured attempts to get ahead of oneself in an excess of drive and ambitiousness; throat difficulties stem from inhibited yelling.

She bases much of her thinking about healing and personality on the chakra system borrowed from ancient Indian philosophy. The chakra system's centers of energy, to which correspond personality traits and physical symptoms, resemble in some respects Freud's psychosexual conception of development. Development first proceeds from the rawly primitive, or kundalini, chakra, through centers of emotional, spiritual, celestial energy, to the ultimate seventh chakra in which one would have achieved the consciousness of Christ. In Freud, development proceeds from developmentally early and primitive to later and more sophisticated levels. Fixation at one or another chakra or Freudian nodal point reflects one's overall level of development.

Some of Reverend Bruyere's ideas are standard esoterica, which she might have absorbed from her subculture; or she could have gathered them independently, their commonality with those of the subculture reflecting their universal truth. Some of her ideas are supported by theories and researches independent of her. For example, there are a good many articles in conventional medicine which link cancer with difficulties establishing sexual identity, and as we have seen, Justa Smith has demonstrated that healing changes enzymes. Others of her ideas can easily be disdained as merely an elaborate conscious or unconscious scam, offering her self-aggrandizement and financial profit. In short, one can come away from an exposure to Reverend Bruyere, her personality, her work, and her philosophy, as with those of many other healers: dismissing them, being persuaded by them, or suspending judgment. But there is more to the Reverend Bruyere story than that.

Enter Valerie Hunt, who has a doctorate in education from Columbia University and is a professor at UCLA in its Department of Kinesiology. For those who are unfamiliar with kinesiology, as was I at the time, it is the study of human movement. In pursuit of that interest Dr. Hunt organized research on Rolfing, or Structural Integration. As I detailed in *Out In Inner Space*, Rolfing consists of manipulation of the body in specified order over ten sessions. Its purpose is to align the body in a direct line with gravity. In the course of the painful but strangely exhilarating procedure, it brings about changes in appearance, posture, feeling about oneself, and personality, recovers early memories which seem to have been embedded in the physical areas manipulated, and in my own case changed my somewhat reedy voice to a sonorous baritone (which lasted intermittently for several months).

Dr. Hunt took sequential readings of Rolfing subjects before, during and after the procedure to find objective laboratory evidence supporting changes through Rolfing. She measured energy emanating from the body with EEG and EMG recordings, D.C. Field recordings, and electronic recordings of the areas where chakras are said to be. Along with conventionally accepted means of measuring, she used Kirlian photographs and the reading of auras by Reverend Bruyere. Dr. Hunt's research proceeded from the following conceptualization of energy and auras.

Consistent with a holistic point of view of the universe and the new science of quantum physics and biology, electrobiologists, psychoenergeticists, and those knowledgeable about nuclear medicine believe that energy (i.e., electrical energy) is the primary substance of the cosmos, and that its patterning and organization provide the basic laws of interaction. All living tissues possess electrical properties. Wherever there is an electrical field, there is an electromagnetic one as well; all living things emit electromagnetic energy. The interplay of electrical and electromagnetic energy between man and the universe is unclear, though speculations have been put forth by counterculture New Age theorists to account for such relationships, and particularly those relationships between deployment of energy and New Age activities such as Rolfing and psychic healing. The famous Kirlian photograph previously mentioned — of a leaf with part of it cut away, yet whose natural border could still be seen — suggests that an energy field exists apart from the physical one. The aura which psychics claim to see is comprised of energy from such fields, independent of but related to the energy field of the physical body. Observations of such energy fields by Kirlian photographs and aura-healers are supported by light recordings by photomultipliers and through the use of chemically coated screens and lenses. There seems general agreement that auras are made up of colors which shimmer, vibrate, and form shapes in space.

Dr. Hunt found in her research that after Rolfing subjects showed greater dominance of the right hemisphere, that colors shown in Kirlian photographs change in consistent ways, that higher and freer flow of energy occurs, and that motor performance improved. Finally, changes in the energy field correspond to changes observed in the auras as reported by Reverend Bruyere. Uneven low-frequency and -amplitude emissions during the early sessions gave way to larger, lighter-color, higher-amplitude and -frequency waves in the later sessions. (According to metaphysical literature, each chakra has its associated color: red for kundalini chakra, yellow for spleen chakra, blue for throat chakra.) Subjects had emotional experiences, images, and memories connected with the different body areas Rolfed, giving credence to the belief that memory is stored in body tissue. The usual large blue or white emanations from the Rolfer's hands and arms gave way to red when the subject experienced pain from the procedure. Thus we have the first objective electronic evidence of emissions by frequency, amplitude, and time which validates the subjective observation of the human aura that has been described by sensitives for centuries.

While Dr. Hunt's main interest was in the changes brought about by Rolfing, she at the same time demonstrated that people who claimed to see auras really do see something. We are therefore encouraged to take even more seriously Reverend Bruyere's reports, observations, and actions. If she can see anything in that area spreading out six or so inches from the body, what she sees may indeed signify psychological characteristics and physical ills, and if that is so, who is to dismiss any or all of the rest of what she stands for, including her alleged capacity to heal? Perhaps in that darkened pre-Benny Goodman theater, I really did send health-giving energy from my hands to my daughter.

Chapter Six
But Faith In What? God's Healing Delegates

ONE CONCEPTION OF GOD is as an external figure, both loving and forbidding, who will grant healing, among other good things, if you are loyal to Him and follow His dictates. Another conception is of an internal God, part of the self. You are God, and God lives in every cell of your body; God heals, but only in tandem with your own healing potential, only to the extent that you believe in yourself, and ally yourself with God as a worker for good, however good is defined. A third conception of God is as a sort of generator, a fount of healing energy that is dispensed by way of spirits who act as guides for the healers who are mediums for the transmission of energy.

Different regimes for psychic healing stem from these different views of God and healing. Healing from an external God, rooted in fundamentalism, is represented here by Oral Roberts and Father Ralph DiOrio. The indwelling God of self-responsibility is represented here by the Unity movement in the person of Coletta Long. Spiritual healing is represented by the famed Englishman, Harry Edwards.

ORAL ROBERTS UNIVERSITY IS probably not what the city fathers of Tulsa, Oklahoma had in mind when they named two of that city's prominent avenues "Yale" and "Harvard." Instead of being the home of ivy-covered citadels, Tulsa is known as the place where another educational vision has come to pass. That vision is the one of evangelist, author, television personality and healer, Oral Roberts. The 500-acre, 4,000-student campus which bears his name was founded in 1963, not only as an institution for secular education but as a healing ministry and vehicle for educating what Oral Roberts likes to call the "whole man — mind, spirit and body." It is, to quote from one of its brochures, "a Christian institution with the distinctive charismatic dimension of the baptism in the Holy Spirit and the gifts of the Spirit." Particular emphasis is paid to "the baptism in the Holy Spirit with the accompanying Spirit-given ability to speak in tongues in one's private devotions as a deeper level of personal communication with God and upon the nine gifts of the Spirit to enable faculty and students to have that much more of the life of Jesus Christ reproduced and manifested through them to meet the needs of people."

Oral Roberts University is composed of wildly futuristic buildings, a blaze of jagged edges, spears, and lots of reflecting metals, especially those colored gold. The letter that prompted my visit, signed by Oral Roberts, announced the dates of a "laymen's seminar" and went on to say, "and because I have such a deep feeling for you as my partner, I am inviting you to attend." I was to learn that *partner*, as used by Oral Roberts, means just what it says: you join up in body, mind, spirit — and pocketbook. Gold was to play a more significant role than that of architectural decoration. The letter promised that Roberts would be sharing with me the "Word of God about the miracle of salvation, the importance of the Holy Spirit in my life today, and the Blessing Pact Covenant we have with God;" it included a prayer for my healing and the meeting of any other needs I might have.

What with the apparently handwritten signature on personal stationery, typing that looked like it had been picked out on an old portable, and the meeting being described as a seminar, I rather expected that I was being invited to a small working group. Instead there were three thousand of us.

It never did seem especially crowded, however. The meetings were masterpieces of planning and organization. The facilities were top drawer, including a 12,500-seat auditorium and lots of college students who kept everything moving and under control. Moreover, the participants seemed an exceptionally peaceful and quiet lot (their languid rhythm perhaps geared in part to the many halt and lame among us). Lodging was provided at motor hotels around the city, to and from which we were transported by chartered buses; all meals were supplied at the convention center. I wondered innocently how the astronomical bill for all this was to be paid. But more of that later.

Oral Roberts University has an accredited medical school, perhaps the only one in the world that includes prayer among its specific healing activities. With the help of a nurse on the faculty of ORU who knew of my interests in unconventional healing, and who had put my name on the list of partners, I was able to squeeze in some interviews with members of the medical school faculty. Other than that, I was pretty much swept up by the programmed juggernaut: the conveyor-belt agenda comprised teaching, preaching, entertaining, inspiring, collecting money, and healing.

The tenor of the meetings was evoked by the first comment that I heard, when I entered the auditorium a few minutes late: "He's a great God, isn't he?" If I tuned out the references to God, I could have swung through much of the program as though it were a musical show. Richard Roberts, one of Oral's sons, is a handsome singer, entertainer, and recording personality. He croons in the old style of vocalists with Big Bands, the songs were sprightly-upbeat and romantic treacle, and the taped orchestral accompaniment had a first-class studio orchestra sound — lush strings and piercing, goosebump-inducing trumpets. Richard was perhaps most effective in Oral's nationally televised show, with guest star Mel Torme — one of several filmed TV programs interspersed between the live activities. Oral's wife, Evelyn, participated also. An attractive woman in her fifties, she claimed to be thrilled because she felt that "so many marvelous things were going to happen to us" during that seminar. At times it seemed to me like a family sitcom, with Oral Roberts playing Oral Roberts larger than life impersonating "just folks."

We each received a Bible, an Old and New Testament which was regularly referred to as if it was incontrovertible evidence. Roberts made no bones about knowing precisely what God felt or thought or wished at any given moment. Throughout the three days God became, in my mind and presumably in the minds of all assembled, more and more like a person, and one who was growing ever closer to us. That He sometimes seemed to contradict Himself, and could be translated one way or another by Roberts to suit the purpose at hand, didn't seem to matter much.

Roberts emphasized here and there, and devoted one whole lecture to "seed-faith." What he meant, as he explored the ramifications of "whatsoever one plants, one reaps," was that if you contributed money to the Oral Roberts ministry, you could expect good things in return, perhaps miracles: "Give and it shall be given to you." It was not a matter of loyalty, he said, but rather a matter of investment. "You don't owe anybody anything, you just 'give off the top' and your seed will multiply." He equated such acts with God's giving his only Son. As the ultimate pitch to a health-conscious audience, he promised, "Give so you can receive everlasting life."

I could have done without the way he identified a contrary point of view about giving, namely giving out of gratitude rather than for investment, as a covenant good for Jews. "But I'm no Jew, I'm a Christian," he hollered, to the accompaniment of laughter from his audience. As if sensing the malice inherent in this interaction, he hastened to add, "I don't hate the Jews, I'm just glad I am a Christian."

Roberts often came out in favor of doubt, at least of a kind. "Don't be afraid to investigate," he railed at his audience. He, himself, he said, was a doubter. He examined the evidence, which I gathered was the Bible, and in that way he was able to distinguish true faith from gullibility. "I'm not afraid for you to investigate us," he cried, reminding me uncomfortably of another leader's comment — "Your President is not a crook."

An opportunity to gain everlasting life and other desiderata was provided by a program devoted to collecting money for the City of Faith, which is the name of Roberts's then partially completed medical complex. After taking the audience through a page-by-page brochure during which Roberts appended price tags to each illustrated part of the complex, he asked for donors to come forward to the stage with pledge cards, "and bring your wife." He started with $150,000 for a hospital floor and continued down through hospital rooms, EKG machines, and floor coverings. A small, aged woman came onto the stage and said she was on Social Security but still wanted to contribute $77, at a time when Roberts was working on $50,000 contributions. Roberts all but flung her back to her seat, to the accompaniment of the audience's nervous laughter. But except for such occasional crudities it was a slick, masterful operation. I lost track of the stratospheric amounts being collected, but clearly the meals, lodging, and transportation sowed by Roberts had reaped a bundle.

Apparently, Roberts had designed the basic plan of the hospital on the basis of his unhappy experience of having had five operations in other hospitals. His repeated references to his unhappy experiences in hospitals made it difficult not to believe that one of his motives in constructing the City of Faith was to find a decent hospital in which he could be sick. I can't fault him for that, nor can I really fault him for the whole production. The television, the show biz, the pitch went over extremely well with his audience and resulted in converts, enthusiasm, and funds. Issues of aesthetics, style, and intellectual niceties could all be considered irrelevant to his putative task, which was to propagate his version of belief in the Lord, the better to influence people's lives to the good.

Insofar as healing is concerned, the question is whether the whole massive enterprise is useful, harmful, or irrelevant to the amelioration of physical and mental ills. It certainly is not harmful or irrelevant in the opinions of Vernon Scholes, M.D., microbiologist and immunologist in the medical school, and George Treadway, M.D., Obstetrics-Gynecology. I was able to meet these men during a break in their duties as ushers for the seminar. That they spent these hours, over several days at this task, was in and of itself a testimony to their faith and commitment. In their clean-cut, clean-shaven, middle-aged way, when talking about medicine they were like most other physicians, imbued with the technicalities of medical practice and research. When talking about religious faith and its application to healing, they were indistinguishable from others of the zealous Oral Roberts community. Both had come to their religious convictions in the last few years. As Dr. Scholes put it, he had always walked behind Jesus; now he walked *with* Jesus. Apparently, the negotiations about his coming to Oral Roberts University Medical School were decisive in his changed attitude. These negotiations included being told by Dr. William Standish Reed, author of *Surgery of the Soul*, that he should go to Oral Roberts University, though Dr. Reed had no prior knowledge of his negotiations with Roberts. Dr. Treadway said he had achieved his greater conviction as a result of his having had an unspecified malady, presumably overcome through faith healing.

According to one of Oral Roberts's perorations, healing is best accomplished by medicine on the one side, prayer on the other, and Jesus in between. This was apparently what these men believed, and on what the City of Faith Medical Complex was to be based. The medical school staff employs prayer as if it were an entry in the U.S. Pharmacopeia. Dr. Scholes gives his patients the option of praying with him, in addition to his treating them according to standard medical practice. Dr. Treadway prays before each operation that he performs. The City of Faith Hospital is designed so that there is a room in each eight-patient alcove for prayer by patients and families with a person designated by the Hospital, in effect a member of the "medical" staff. Rather than being an alternative, or even in conflict with God, conventional medicine is seen as a means that God uses for healing. Thus, God performs direct healing in answer to prayer as well as indirect healing, whether one prays or believes or not, through conventional medicine: all healing, ultimately, comes from God.

Well, not quite. Early in our conversation, and shortly after I told about my experiences with laying on of hands, Dr. Treadway asked how I stood with regard to satanic healing. All healing, Dr. Treadway said, was either from Satan or God. Somewhat nervously, I asked how one could tell the difference. Dr. Treadway said obliquely that one criterion was in the scriptures. Healing, he said, may occur even though it is satanic. The problem is in what the long-term and derivative effects may be, either on healer, patient, or society.

Healing, according to these men and the shared understanding of the Oral Roberts group, is always successful. Its success may be immediately apparent, like those dramatic instances of people's throwing away their crutches on the spot. It may take awhile, like most medical healing; to ask that an alternative healing be immediate, when few other healings are, would not be fair. Or the healing may not take place until the next world. According to the latter formulation, the healer can't lose and the sick person can't either, unless one is stubbornly attached to the idea of being well in this world and soon.

According to these men, miraculous healings are all in a day's work. Dr. Scholes mentioned that while he was on duty at one of the Oral Roberts meetings, a woman with multiple sclerosis had fallen down due to the lack of coordination caused by her illness. He administered to her as a physician, doing first aid, and also as a minister of God; not long after, she was running around the audience demonstrating how her movements were free of the effects of multiple sclerosis. Just yesterday both men had treated a woman who had convulsions during the seminar, and with prayer in addition to their emergency first aid her convulsions stopped. The glow of these contributions to the annals of miracle cures is dimmed by such questions as whether the people were in fact sick to begin with, whether other possibly curative elements had played a part, and whether the cure lasted. Without documented answers to such questions it is no wonder that traditional physicians, when confronted with miracle cures, are often brusque, indulgent, or assume that something they did had some delayed effect.

The culmination of the seminar, and also my chief interest in the Oral Roberts enterprise, was the healing service on Sunday morning. However, I was unable to attend. There was some complicated business about airplane schedules, and my having to be away from my office an additional day if I did attend. I got descriptions from several people who had attended previous healing services, and I remembered having seen Oral Roberts conduct such a service on television. I knew that a long line of people would file down from their seats and across the stage, where they would be touched by Oral Roberts and others of his associates, including the two physicians I had interviewed. I had pressed for the statistics for "miraculous" healing and learned that I might see one such occurrence at any given meeting. I knew that I would at least half-believe that such an occurrence had been set up, just as I had half-believed that the first man who came forward and gave a $150,000 floor for the hospital was a ringer. Finally, in my list of excuses, I promised myself that I would return to attend such a service, and do so at a time when I might be able to arrange a private interview with Oral Roberts. (I no longer had much hope that he would agree to having psychological tests; he had already answered a letter from me in the negative about that. Moreover, I was repeatedly told that he was, in effect, quite defensive these days, especially as a result of legal moves to stop his building the City of Faith.)

On top of all that, I just could not face another day of immersion in Oral Roberts' way of propounding faith. *My* mental health, at least, might be better served by a return to an environment of non-belief, if not disbelief. That is no justification for poor data-collecting, certainly says nothing about the efficacy of Oral Roberts' healing, and surely fails to acknowledge the world view of those who genuinely and selflessly believe in the tenets of their faith. It only says something about my staying power in such atmospheres as the one up the road from Yale and Harvard Avenues.

THE UNITY MOVEMENT HAS its headquarters in Unity Village, in a suburb of Kansas City, Missouri. According to that movement, God has His headquarters in each cell of each person; thus, healing comes from within. The healing spirit, then, is identical to self-healing: that is the Unity philosophy. Yet prayer abounds among its members, and it is not always clear whether "the Father within" is really within. To judge from the sample that I observed and some revealing phraseology, it is likely that most of the movement's hundreds of thousands of members, when in trouble, gladly combine a vision of an in-dwelling and an external God.

The impetus for Charles and Myrtle Fillmore to found the Unity movement stemmed from Myrtle Fillmore's overcoming her supposedly incurable illness by way of prayer, and from her success in healing others the same way. From the humblest of beginnings the movement has grown to include two hundred affiliates through the United States and in many foreign countries. Annually, it receives a million prayer requests for various kinds of healing, and its publications total a million and a half each year. Positive thinking is central to its theory and practice. Members are encouraged as a daily regime and at times of crisis, to repeat "affirmations," which are assertions of good; and "denials," which are assertions that there is no bad, under the rubric "Like attracts like." In other words, whatever one asserts as true will become true. Affirmations of good and denials of bad are not only exercises in positive thinking, but like mantras they offer a focus that insulates against the clamoring of the outer world; they help people to take their mind off their troubles. Many Unity ministers also use meditations as part of their services.

Unity's theology shades into psychology. When one discovers God and the Divine Law, one makes at the same time a self-discovery. Such self-discovery results in the capacity to improve the quality of life in general, and to overcome and prevent illness in particular. By thus making internal what in most spiritual traditions is external, in heaven, Unity creates conditions for psychological analysis. At times its teachings are barely distinguishable from college classes in psychology. And in-between services it presents adult education classes, lectures, demonstrations, and workshops with a strong secular psychological emphasis. In keeping with its theology, however, the psychology taught in these educational endeavors exploits the conscious aspect of mind with persistent emphasis on the brighter side.

After reading several of Unity's publications I figured I could cope with an unaccustomed exposure to Sunday morning worship, this one in Unity Church, the chapel of Unity Village. Coletta Long, the minister, floodlights wreathing her ash-blonde hair and with a voice evocative of sincerity and goodness, radiated health-giving power. The usual announcements and pleasantries of religious services everywhere were followed by a series of Unity affirmations: "Ask and it will be given." "My life is transformed by the loving presence of God." "God does nothing for us, but *through* us." "With failure, failure becomes easier; with each success, success becomes easier." The program for the service included a sermon, called in Unity a "lesson." That linguistic practice reflects the Unity belief in the need to learn Divine Law and so to make available in daily life the in-dwelling wisdom of God. Rather than sermons on the right way to live, the lessons are designed to encourage people to discover and use their capabilities to find for themselves the right way, including educating themselves about human behavior. Even knowing this about Unity, however, I was not fully prepared for how academic a slant Reverend Long sometimes gave to her lessons.

She reminded the audience that Jesus learned his healing techniques and understanding from the Egyptians, by way of the Essenes, which might come as a shock to those who believe that Jesus's powers came directly from God. She delineated the left-brain, right-brain hypothesis, the left side of the brain being the center of logic and calculations, among many other characteristics prized in an intellectualized and technological culture; the right side of the brain being the center of creativity, feeling, intuition. For her the right side of the brain corresponded to the inner self, the God-like capacities for warmth, love, harmony, and innate knowledge. Included in such knowledge was the way to heal and be healed, all available to those who can release their undue attachment to left brain functions. She cited experiments done on such healers as Olga Worrall in which it was demonstrated that at the time of healing, and only then, the brain waves of both healer and healee emitted frequencies of 10.6 cycles per minute. According to Reverend Long, that key number is also emitted by plants, and is related to the measurements of the great pyramids, which supposedly have healing properties.

Reverend Long then led the congregation in a meditation which incorporated some, in effect, hypnosis-like procedures. In the midst of her hypnotic monotone, she mentioned how difficult it was to raise one's eyelids; though I suppose I could have if I really tried, it certainly was difficult, and since she had me feeling as if I did not want to try, for all practical purposes it was impossible. She ended the meditation with the suggestion that members of the audience were to be wide awake and alert, and I did feel much refreshed; to the extent that my sleeplessness and fatigue could be considered an illness, I was healed. The service ended with a traditional holding of hands with whomever was on the left and right while singing "The Peace Song." The message of that rousing song was that peace begins with the individual. The song was perfect for Unity's emphasis on individual growth, and for Unity's assertion that the way to secure the general peace, as well as for an individual to flower, is through love.

By happenstance, I was treated to a concrete example of the way Unity's philosophy, at least as used by Reverend Long, can be applied in healing through psychological counseling. While waiting in the lobby of the chapel to interview Reverend Long, I overheard a request that she see a young man who was said to badly need counseling. Despite her appointments with me and others, she saw the young man immediately in the lobby, and then in her office. With these actions she implemented the idea, suggested in her church service, that help was always available. During the sessions, as she later told me, she asked him to imagine that he had come into a movie a few minutes before the usual happy ending, and then imagine how he would feel while he was watching the movie from the beginning, with all its seemingly insoluble problems, and tension amid ambiguities about the ending. Would he not, she asked, by knowing the ending reduce the anxiety, confident that all would be well, that attempts to create a solution sooner or later would be successful? He could do the same with life, simply know that all would one day be well and that his efforts would be rewarded. She then encouraged him to say some affirmations and to use them in the future as needed; for example, "God is the only power in my life." As I had observed, she is capable of saying the affirmations so evocatively that the words take on the quality of immutable truth. She had him repeat with her, "I release all persons, places, things, and conditions that are not for my highest good, and they release me." She helped him to understand that when he released the dreadful aspects of his life, a vacuum would be created for good thoughts and deeds to fill. She then had him join her in prayer, sitting opposite from him with hands touching. As they prayed, he visibly relaxed, then burst out crying with relief.

Traditional psychotherapists would disapprove of such a session, just as a part of me does, for its overlooking of the sources of the patient's complaints and its wholehearted reliance on God's help and the patient's conscious intention. Yet, however inadvertently, Reverend Long was employing many theoretical and practical principles of psychotherapy.

> (1) The patient was in effect screened for this treatment by virtue of his membership in the Unity group and his attendance at the church service. He was, by definition, ready to believe and be helped by what he knew was available.

(2) He experienced catharsis through the opportunity to tell her his troubles, to let go of his emotions.
(3) Touch was made concrete by their holding hands during praying, and symbolic by her seeing him immediately, attending to him, behaving as if touched by, and thereby touching him.
(4) The positive affirmations were his to take away, giving him something *he* could do, thereby increasing his self-esteem and sense of mastery while also implicitly reminding him that she, in the form of the affirmations, was still available to him.
(5) Her earnest and sincere therapeutic stance functioned as a suggestion that there really was medicine here, a means of his getting better.
(6) The medium of saying something purporting to be psychotherapeutic, regardless of the content, summoned to it the power of placebo.
(7) The content of what she told him carried with it at least the possibilities for his developing insight. Her comments and questions provided for him an opportunity to see himself and his difficulties as an object of psychological study, something that could be understood and viewed from the perspective of observer as well as participant. He was given the opportunity to see that the collapse of one aspect of his life after another might not be coincidental or adventitious — that perhaps *he* was doing something to bring about these circumstances.
(8) He was most probably disabused of the common idea that if he told about himself he would be judged harshly. Reverend Long's steady, non-judgmental responses taught him that this fantasy about himself and others was incorrect; thus he had what is technically called a corrective emotional experience.
(9) Whatever he learned was most likely learned more effectively in the somewhat altered consciousness brought about by the quiet of her office, the hypnotic qualities of prayer, her soothing voice.
(10) He, too, had just undergone the same meditation during the service that I had. He, too, may have been tranquilized by it and, therefore, more receptive.

In a subsequent discussion Reverend Long agreed to the apparent relevance of all of these elements. However, she elaborated on the element of positive thinking to include what she called the "subconscious." Subconscious is usually used as slang for the Freudian unconscious, but for Reverend Long it is a thing apart. It is lodged in the right brain and is especially equipped to absorb the positive affirmations so central to her therapeutic work. Reverend Long had learned of the need for such systematic, ongoing affirmations after attending more than a dozen self-help educational classes, and observing how short-lived the results of such classes were, necessitating the patient or student's return for more of the same. So, she drafted a series of tasks and exercises designed to enlist the person in constantly applying positive thoughts to an extent and degree that penetrated to the subconscious, there to exercise long-term behavioral change as well as buffering for short-term relief. She had people repeat positive affirmations verbally, out loud and to themselves, and write them many times during the day. She makes tape recordings of positive affirmations as part of a meditation, with soft unobtrusive background music, thus encouraging subconscious repetition and absorption of the affirmations.

She also suggests that people play the tapes under the pillow at night, thereby applying a once-popular fad of learning while sleeping. According to Reverend Long, the fad should never have been just a fad. While one probably does not learn while asleep, the hypnoidal period between wakefulness and sleep does provide an excellent condition for subconscious receptivity. Learning in this way has been resurrected in the Lozanov teaching method now gaining adherents around the world, though Lozanov focuses more on his specialized classroom instruction than upon "sleep learning." Reverend Long uses the Lozanov method along with her other educational, psychological, and spiritual interventions to bring about decisive, and often startling, changes. She offered case examples of having worked with patients who were severely disturbed, and who made remarkable changes apparently by pursuing the program that she outlined for them. And she had similar testimonials from groups of children with learning disabilities, who, in a matter of weeks or months, made objectively measured educational improvement that had eluded them through years of frustration on their parts and the parts of their parents and teachers. Such gains were durable, and radiated out to include diverse behaviors as well as those attended to specifically during the treatment or educational process. Thus, they meet the criteria for what is known in psychoanalysis as "structural change," the definitive change that justifies the time and expense of psychoanalysis rather than one of the less demanding psychotherapies.

In the hands of Reverend Long, at least, mere positive thinking turned out to be anything but mere. In fact, positive thinking was not a matter of simply adjuring people to think positively, but a systematic training, exercise, and adoption by the mind, if not the right-brain, of new points of view and psychological skills. Even so, positive thinking in her view did not come to grips with the deeper sources of distress. Rather, she acknowledged that the deeper sources of distress can never be fully overcome, but they can be tamed, their effects can be made less injurious. By training the subconscious they can be detoxified, and their negative signs reversed to positive.

Such a point of view leads to the possibility of a combination of approaches. In principle, patient and therapist could gain insight into the unconscious sources of distress, and then learn and practice dealing with distress through training of the subconscious with positive affirmations. Such a combined approach would make use of the psychoanalytic power of discovery while ameliorating what may be its weakness, namely training in how to apply those discoveries in everyday life. By the same token, such an approach, while taking advantage of Reverend Long's cornucopia of skills in living, would add to her capacities for survey and discovery of the sources of distress, the better to make more particular and individual her affirmations as well as others of her psychotherapeutic interventions. In researching this program one would, of course, have to control for the self-selection of patients to one or another approach, for individual differences in skill in applying one or another approach, for the possibility of a negative interaction between approaches that might yield a result less effective than either one alone — in other words the litany of sources of error in any, and especially psychotherapeutic, research.

Finally, something within me railed against the activity, the busy doing and the naive-seeming simplicity of a positive thinking approach to psychotherapy — that is one reason why I had become a psychoanalyst. I daresay something in Reverend Long railed against depth exploration; presumably that was one reason she had chosen to involve herself in positive thinking, in working with altered states of consciousness and enlistment of the spirit. Our respective experiences dramatize how easy it is for healing to be fragmented rather than holistic, how difficult it is to cross boundaries, how easy it is to grind away at what is familiar and fits with one's training and personality. The practitioner's peace of mind can be served at the expense of scientific and clinical progress.

To the extent that Reverend Long's session with her post-Sunday morning service patient was effective, were the operative elements spiritual or psychological? Much of what passes for the spiritual in the body-mind-spiritual definition of holistic medicine can be considered as within the purview of mind or psychology, however unsystematically or inadvertently applied. Often Unity believers and others use "spirit" as a euphemism for psychology. Certainly her work could easily be seen as having been solely psychological. Embracing the hypothesis of an extra-psychological force — spirit, God — runs the danger of minimizing the psychological powers inherent in clinical interactions as practiced, sometimes only intuitively, by gifted pastoral therapists. Only from the philosophical or religious point of view can holistic medicine define itself as attending to body, mind, *and* spirit. From the scientific point of view, only body and mind, unwieldy as they are to study, are wieldy enough to be considered within the purview of scientific healing. One must take on faith the participation of spirit. Faith has to be taken on faith. In the meantime, however, and presumably totally uninterested in such questions, a young man in distress went to church, had a psychotherapeutic encounter, reports that he feels and behaves better as a result, and presumably has at least begun a path of exploration with a view toward changing his life. Compared to the ideal of what might one day be established as the perfect means of bringing about lasting improvement in his life, he may have been given short shrift. Compared to what would have been available to him in a society in which there was no therapeutic tradition of help through body, mind, and spirit, he was lucky.

With regard to the physical lens through which healing can be viewed, Oral Roberts comes out squarely in favor of an amalgamation of physical healing with his faith healing, as can be seen in his creation of a standard medical hospital within which the practice of spiritual healing has been integrated. As he says, healing is best accomplished by medicine on the one side, prayer on the other, and Jesus in-between.

The Unity movement has no such intimate, concrete connection with physical healing. Indeed, most of its teaching is inimical to it. In that way it is similar to Christian Science. Unity emphasizes creative self-responsibility rather than turning oneself over to the routine medical establishment. Unity members object to medicine's sometimes gloomy prognoses and scientific realism. Indeed, that anything could be *wrong* with one is anathema to Unity. For example, things are not lost, they are merely misplaced. Even thoughts about aging are avoided — some of its members refuse to discuss it, or even tell their birthdays, as if acknowledging aging would help to bring it on. Unity accommodates its self-help and antimedical biases by pursuing physical healing mainly through unconventional approaches. Its members tend to rely on chiropractors, colonics, food supplements, and nutritional lore. To what extent many of these are physical treatments rather than exercises in suggestion and placebo is at the heart of the research matter.

With regard to the psychological lens, on paper both Roberts and Long eschew psychological factors in favor of explanations of healing in spiritual terms. For both, healing comes from God. Whether or not Roberts is aware, or makes conscious use of it, his healing is likely the beneficiary of massive power of suggestion. People flock to him from geographical distances *en masse* and are treated to group rituals resulting in group contagion much as occurs at Lourdes. He seems such a good man, with such a good family, devoted to such good work; for many people it seems axiomatic that only good can come of his enterprises. In a much lower key, some of the same probably contributes to Unity healings. In addition Unity makes straightforward use of psychology, particularly as purveyed by Reverend Long, in its lessons, meditation, and individual counseling, though it may not always acknowledge psychological factors in their own right. Since, for Unity, God is in the person, a crucial question exists as to the respective roles of secular skills and spiritual force.

With regard to the spiritual lens both Roberts and Long would claim that their healing was brought about through spirituality. Both adjure their congregations to have faith in spiritual healing. Since they feel no need for evidence, except what is in the Bible, both are in a literal sense faith healers. Faith is so much acknowledged and so explicitly relied upon that it can be considered a technology of healing, even as its allied but unacknowledged aspects of suggestion and placebo go on quietly providing, by way of psychology, a healing context.

IN THE BODY-MIND-SPIRIT triumvirate, *spirit* is used loosely to refer to God, the supernatural, religiousness in general. To Harry Edwards, arguably the world's best known and most revered spiritual healer, *spirit* refers literally to spirits of once-living persons now "alive on the other side" who give counsel and direct healing force from God to the patient via the healer-medium.[2]

At a time when I was studying the psychological aspects of cancer I read of Mr. Edwards' reported success not only in working with cancer patients but in organizing a research to systematically demonstrate it. I wrote to him for information about his study and received a pleasant letter in return. He evidently was approaching the healing of cancer much like Carl and Stephanie Simonton (see Chapter 7) do in this country, as a disease with a considerable psychological component whose cure requires that a positive orientation to life replace a pessimistic, nihilistic one. He wrote in his letter that he was in the midst of collecting data. Before that task was finished, and before I could correspond with him further or meet with him, he died — or as he would say, he passed over and became a spirit himself. In a letter written to be read posthumously, he did in fact promise that he would continue his healing work from the other side.

While he may be doing that, thus far he has not made it back by way of direct communication. His successor, Ramus, or Ray Branch, has three acid questions (as he calls them) that he puts to anyone who reports having communicated with Edwards. Correct answers to such questions would pretty much guarantee that the communication was from the Great Chief, as Edwards is familiarly referred to. No one has as yet been able satisfactorily to answer the questions. Harry Houdini, the great magician, also promised to let the world know if there was life after death, and he has not definitively been heard from either. The prospects of such direct and recognizable communications seem not good at all.

Be that as it may, on the earthly plane Harry Edwards demonstrated healing prowess for over thirty years at countless public meetings from small Boy Scout meetings to audiences of six thousand at the Royal Albert and Royal Festival Halls. In such public demonstrations he usually picked people to heal who had obvious ailments such as deafness, blindness, and crippledness whose healing would be immediately apparent to the audience. He healed at individual sessions at his healing center in England. And he is said to have healed thousands through absent healing; that is, he sent healing in response to letters requesting it. Whether he healed successfully or not is, as usual, indeterminate: lots of testimonials, anecdotes, and demonstrations, but no controlled research. There seems little doubt, however, that many believe that he was a genuine healer, at least to judge from his mail — some nine thousand letters a week, or about a half million a year, in thirty years some fourteen million, many including financial contributions. He never accepted fees as such for any of his healings. He created enough of a stir to be hauled up for a joint investigation by the Archbishop of Canterbury and the British Medical Association. Asked to submit six cases to the commission for investigation, he submitted seventy-two. These were never investigated, however, or at least no report of such investigations was ever released. The official negative concluding opinion was apparently based more on prejudice than on study.

In testimony before the commission Edwards said that a healer is a person with no necessary personal ability to heal who is used as an instrument for healing by non-human agencies. "Intelligent direction" provides the healing force. Such intelligent direction may be a god who is reached by prayer. The other possibility, according to Edwards, is a spiritual life going on after death and retaining its mortal personality. Edwards cited a previous commission set up by the Archbishop of Canterbury which found in favor of life after death, a survival that is able to remove disharmony from the mind. Since, said Edwards, the mind is implicated in one-half of all illnesses that spiritual power can have considerable healing effects.

Despite the commission's negative report, unorthodox British healers in 1977 achieved a great victory. The General Medical Council, something like the American Medical Association, promised no longer to penalize its members for cooperating with spiritual healers. One result was to enable members of the National Federation of Spiritual Healers, of which Harry Edwards had been president, to do their healings in medical hospitals upon referral from physicians. That a goodly number of referrals are in fact made lends at least inferential support for the claim that spiritual healers do heal, whatever the source of the "intelligent direction."

Like Reverend Bruyere (see Chapter 5), Harry Edwards was a medium. He was aided by guides that spoke through him when he was in a trance. Among Edwards's guides were Louis Pasteur and Lord Lister. These two illustrious men did not speak aloud to others through him. That is unfortunate, for it might provide some badly needed evidence to those familiar with the ideas of the earthly Pasteur and Lister. Others of Edwards's guides were American Indians. How they got to England is an obvious, but to spiritualists an impertinent, question.

Edwards's more concrete theory of healing is that we live in a cosmic sea of healing energy. That energy is received by the psychic gland, a ductless gland or "condition," whose terminal is at the back of the nose. From there it goes down the spine, dividing off into the rest of the body as do the nervous and circulatory systems, and up to the brain where it links with the pineal gland and endocrine glandular system. It is thus similar to acupuncture meridians and the kundalini system of Eastern beliefs. Either Edwards is merely a copycat, or all the developers of these beliefs have discovered, or are responding to, universal truths that have thus far evaded orthodox medicine and Western thought.

On past the town of Wimbledon of tennis fame goes the train from London to the Harry Edwards Spiritual Healing Sanctuary at Burrows Lea, Guildford, Surrey. To a tennis fan and Anglophile, such environs have it all over the football-mad Oklahoma address of Oral Roberts, as well as most addresses of the world. To an aesthete, likewise, the building and grounds of the Sanctuary have it over most homes and offices. Built in the 1800s, Burrows Lea is three stories of tall windows and gabled facade, and includes garden and chauffeur cottages, a music conservatory, studio, game and billiard rooms, all of which are approached in the front by a long drive past sweeping lawns, and which in back cast shadows over fields on the way to Hurtwood Forest. The sight, if nothing else, is likely to be healing.

The Sanctuary is now administratively run by Ray and Joan Branch, longtime associates of Harry Edwards, who also do the healing. Before joining Mr. Edwards, Mr. Branch was an advertising executive. Ray and Joan both became healers, as did a previous heretofore non-healing couple, George and Olive Burton, in association with Edwards. This suggests several possibilities: anybody can become a healer, or anybody can behave like a healer, or by coincidence or for arcane reasons married couples who adventitiously cross Edwards's path have natural capacities to become healers.

On the day I was there, Ray Branch did his healing in a long white medical coat, as Edwards did when not in his more usual shirtsleeves. As an apparent result of Branch's healing, one patient had a noise in his ear lessened. Another had audible cracks in her joints vanish; another with shoulder pain that he described as stabbing claimed that his pain greatly diminished. Another with an inability to raise his arm raised his arm.

Branch's procedures, modelled on those of Edwards, included breathing exercises which the patients were enjoined to continue on the assumption that they encourage the receipt of healing energy, an old yoga belief. The procedures also included chiropractic manipulation such as rotation of arms and stretching of legs. They included also positive thinking and outright suggestion as, for example, "We will help you as we have helped others." Finally, they included what Branch described to me as love and compassion modeled on that between mother and child. As he said, "If we could muster up that feeling each healing time, we could do even better." And so psychoanalytic therapy is included in his modalities as well. As to the influence of spirits on healing, Edwards's sister perhaps said it best: "Oh, I think it was Harry's personality that did it."

A supposedly totally deaf patient claimed to hear sounds during the healing, though not words, and then only when Ray talked to him; he remained deaf to the voices of his wife and Joan. One can hardly avoid wondering if his deafness was not psychogenic in the first place, a means of turning off his wife or perhaps all women. This illustrates why one cannot with any sense of objectivity shout *Eureka!* at the apparent hearings that I observed. One does not know if the healees were organically injured in the first place, whether the improvements were valid in the second place, and whether whatever happened was a function of spiritualism, the deployment of healing energy, suggestion-placebo, or happenstance. Following my turn at undergoing the laying on of the hands of Ray Branch I felt pretty good, but the pain of unanswered questions about healing, and faith in what, continued.

IN HIS AUTOBIOGRAPHY, Father Ralph DiOrio lists Oral Roberts, along with himself and others, as having been "called authentically to the Divine Ministry of Healing."[3] A Roman Catholic priest and a bible-thumping fundamentalist preacher may seem strange bedfellows. But Father DiOrio is no ordinary Catholic priest; he is a charismatic Catholic. That seemed to me to be a contradiction in terms until I learned that the Charismatic Renewal Movement has in recent decades become at least marginally accepted by traditional Catholicism.

The root meaning of the ancient Greek word *charisma* is "gifts," the gift in this instance being the capacity to heal. But since Father DiOrio, like so many other religious healers, claims merely to be the channel for God's healing, the gift would have to be the capacity to serve as a channel for God's healing. Beyond etymology, however, members of the Charismatic Renewal Movement seek to correct what they perceive to be the errors of the orthodox Catholic church. According to DiOrio in his autobiography *The Man Be-*

neath the Gift, charismatics is a "temporary focal point of spiritual energy and love," a means of "reviving in today's church the fiery atmosphere of the Church's origins ... recreating the spiritual atmosphere of the early church community for whom the Holy Spirit was not just a theological abstraction, but was the source of life, energy, courage, enthusiasm ... restoring the true image of the church ..."[3]

Be that as it may, there is no doubt that Father DiOrio departs from ordinary church practice by practicing a healing ministry through individual consultation, by mail, and through public healings before thousands. These meetings include such familiar charismatic phenomena as "slaying," which means that the healee falls down to the ground as an external sign of internal experience, and speaking in tongues, a profusion of sounds purported to be a language which bypasses the intellect and thus "frees the spirit to rise to the Lord."

Father DiOrio's recounting of how he became charismatic resembles the familiar recounting of many psychotherapists and others in the '60s who in middle age thought they saw the light and deserted conventional careers for alternative occupations, beliefs, and lifestyles. An altar boy at eight, a seminarian at fourteen, and an orthodox priest for some 25 years, DiOrio found his order limiting, sought and got release from it, and discovered his healing charisma.

Around Christmas 1975, he felt his body to be aflame, with sparks occurring when he touched anything, and pains shot through his body. A couple of months later, one of the great mother figures of public faith healing, Kathryn Kuhlman, died. Though she was relatively unknown to him at the time, he later likened his work to hers, at one point writing that she "possessed one of the most exceptional and true Healing Gifts of our time." A couple of months after that, his mother fell ill, and he, seemingly unable to help her with his faith, flew into a rage. In response to her request, however, he prayed for her and laid hands on her head, and an hour later she was healed. History had thus repeated itself. For at age eight when he had decided to become an altar boy, he had done so in hopes that his decision would heal his sick mother, just then being carried away in an ambulance to the hospital — from which she returned healed.

At a charismatic service shortly after he believed that he had healed his mother, he accepted the reality of his healing powers. It was Mother's Day, May 9, 1976, which happened to be Kathryn Kuhlman's birthday. On that day, after conducting his own orthodox service, he attended a charismatic service where a child pressed upon him notepaper on which was written the request that DiOrio write a petition to God to be placed on the altar. As DiOrio describes it, he found himself petitioning God for a healing ministry in the Charismatic Renewal Movement. He then preached a sermon appropriate to the day, on the Blessed Mother. At its conclusion a woman begged him to pray over her husband who was bleeding internally from ulcers. The man fell over, "slain," and was cured. In quick succession he claimed to have cured a couple of mental disturbances and a crippled child by way of the laying on of hands. He now acknowledged that he had allowed his "natural gift of doctoring to emerge for the good of the people."

Kemper Arena in Kansas City, Missouri, is ordinarily the scene of lithe athletes and rocking bands — ironic counterpoint to the wheelchaired participants among the 10,000 on each of two afternoons who were there to hear, watch, and be healed by Father DiOrio under the auspices of the Kansas City Charismatic Renewal Society, Inc. Resplendent in a cream-colored habit, from a potted-plant dais, Father DiOrio preached, led songs and prayer as the tension and anticipation of healing miracles mounted. Then he performed one such apparent miracle, and then another and another. The sick fell over, "slain," and arose healed. One woman took off her neck brace and waved it joyfully to the clapping, exultant crowd. Another emerged from her wheelchair to dance with her husband. Later, the husband told me his wife had been incapable of dancing or anything close to it for many years. I tried to put myself in his position, a man who had yearned to dance with his wife suddenly being able to do so. I would have been dancing myself instead of laconically relating the story to a stranger as this man was doing. But then I probably would not have expected such an eventuality, as this man evidently had.

During the healing, Father DiOrio feels a great heat, first in his hands then throughout his body. He gets the knowledge of a person's illness by feeling the person's pain in miniature in the corresponding area of his own body, or by visual images of symbols translatable into illnesses. On this day in Kemper Arena, he left the dais to walk around the amphitheater pausing to call out, for example, "Is there a woman, named Ruth, dressed in brown, who has a shoulder problem? She is being healed." A woman stood up to the cheers of the crowd and acknowledged the correct diagnosis. James Randi in *The Faith Healers*[4] unmasked this sort of activity as chicanery rigged by placing accomplices in the audience — which, however, does not mean that nobody does it genuinely. After a good many of such remarkable feats, Father DiOrio and his fellow healers worked individually with those who requested healing. There was a lot of falling down, at first frightening to see, but apparently no one was injured in the fall, as Father DiOrio had promised.

One of these healing vignettes is unfortunately burned permanently into my brain. A putative healer demanded that a man get up from his wheelchair and walk, pitting his demands against the cripple's plaintive claims that he could not. Finally the cripple tried to raise himself and fell, not because he was "slain" as a sign of being immersed in healing power, but as if defiled by brute power. So far as I could tell, however, that scene was the exception to the beatific fallings and healings scattered over the convention hall floor.

As it happened, a woman with cancer with whom I had been working psychologically was there, unbeknownst to me until she reported it at our next meeting. She of course had hoped to be selected from the audience with the usual ringing diagnosis and presumably subsequent cure, but that had not been vouchsafed to her. And yet her condition showed improvement as documented by one of her laboratory tests, which however lasted only about a week, an all too familiar phenomenon in all kinds of healing that rely on suggestion. One person who was diagnosed publicly by Father DiOrio ("a woman in a yellow sweater has cancer") was an acquaintance of my patient and did indeed have cancer. Good diagnosis, but she was not healed, at least at this meeting.

After a while, such healings and phenomena as those of Father DiOrio and other faith healers take on the look of a gracefully ritualized ballet. Much less romantically I found myself, on this afternoon in a tarted-up basketball court, noticing the ones who were conspicuously not healed, at least not then and there. (Father DiOrio says healing may take place instantaneously, on the bus ride home, or anytime in the days ahead.) Before the meeting, people-watching at the door, I had noted a demanding gray-haired woman issuing orders from her wheelchair to her kindly-looking, wearily patient husband. But then in an unguarded moment between tirades she showed, for one vulnerable moment, the yearning and terrified expectation of disappointment that was driving her tempestuousness. It was an expression I saw, or thought I saw, throughout the afternoon, along with expressions of mournfully realized disappointment.

Well, nobody promised them a rose garden, least of all Father DiOrio. Indeed, in his written and spoken statements he presents healing as secondary to his avowed main purpose of giving others a "spiritual rebirth" which may or may not be manifested by physical healing. Like the psychic surgeons of the Philippines who claim healing is less important than demonstrating the power of God (and are thus justified in cheating if necessary), Father DiOrio adheres to the Charismatic tenet: to show miracles, "signs and wonders," in order to bring the people to Him. Father DiOrio is, in fact, sanguine about people's not being healed: "Paradoxical as it sounds, when a pain-wracked physical body has succumbed to the ravages of disease which God did not choose to heal, there was a complete and glorious victory over the affliction ... so the Great Healing, of course, is Death ... God will just give us the Big Healing into Eternity."

This chapter's title, "But Faith in What?", touches on an issue that is important to Father DiOrio. In his autobiography and from the pulpit, he ringingly declares himself a spiritual healer who practices Divine Healing, not a faith healer. He deplores the vision of a God who heals in exchange for the quantity of faith extended him. Yet he writes that healing comes about through "faith in Christ that *can* heal" and that "it is my faith in Christ that He *can* heal." Of a woman healed of a hemorrhage, "It was her faith, her faith not in herself, but her faith Jesus could heal her that mattered." If, as Father DiOrio says, he is not a faith healer, and healings are not due to faith in Jesus, then what are the healings due to? If they are faithless self-healings, as Unity and psychosomaticists and suggestion-placebo enthusiasts would claim, then how does the Divine enter into it all? Father DiOrio is (not unexpectedly) silent about the hypothesis that the healings could be due to the transmission of secular healing energy. But one could take his reports of heat and electricity as evidence for that possibility.

Father DiOrio excoriates those healers who maintain that faith in *them* rather than in God results in healing. There may be some such healers, but the closest that I know of is an occasional arrogant physician who demands that his patient have faith in him. The essence of faith healing as usually asserted is faith in God, however defined, and that seems to be Father DiOrio's position despite his disclaimers: "the cure, the deliverance have come because of man's simple faith ... Divine Healing brings forth a simple statement of faith — the simple call for a simple faith in God ..." and if you do not have faith, beware, for "it is substantiated in the Scriptures that Jesus could perform no miracles in His own town because His own townspeople would not accept Him" — as in Lourdes, where the townspeople also are not healed by the springs. Familiarity may not breed contempt, but it may well negate the effects of suggestion. And finally, DiOrio writes, "I believe that God answers prayer, I believe that God heals." Sounds like faith healing to me.

And who cares, so long as it works? Many need not care, least of all those who apparently derive genuine benefit from Father DiOrio's healing. But others would like to understand healing; some simply to ease scientific curiosity, and others in order to be able to bottle and prescribe healing for increasing numbers of people and kinds of illnesses. For those people, faith in *what* or *whom* is the central question — faith in God, in the healer-channel to God, in suggestion-placebo, in one's own power, in positive thinking, in unconscious motivation, in discarnate spirits, in electrical energy? We need faith in something, but faith in what? Perhaps faith in knowledge.

Chapter Seven

Dealing with a Dread Diagnosis

SOME PEOPLE REFUSE TO acknowledge their illness, to others or to themselves. They may believe, as Unity Church members or Christian Scientists or other positive thinkers do, that whatever reality one acknowledges is thereby created. Or they may sense illness as evidence of weakness of character or a harbinger of death. Most people, however, like to tell about their illnesses, and especially their operations. When Lyndon Johnson, while President, pulled up his shirt for photographers to show the scar from his recent operation, newspapers and magazines published the picture evidently believing that millions would be interested. People often think that there is something heroic about illness; they refer to an ill person as a fighter; survival becomes a matter of pride. Talking about one's illness compels attention by playing upon the listener's at least latent anxiety about bodies, sickness, and mortality. The listener feels sympathy, admires the survivor, and enjoys the tension — but only from a safe distance, as one enjoys pain, misery and fright in movies or plays. Such vicarious participation allows for morbid fascination, but with the reassurance that for now at least it is happening to someone else. Hence the old joke, "It could be worse, it could happen to me."

I am not impervious to trying to feel heroic, nor am I above enjoying sympathy. Yet I wish I had not had the experience reported here, and having had it, I have mixed feelings about reporting it publicly. It is a breach of privacy, I feel, and I sense the accusation of weakness at my (at least supposedly) being ill, with all of the implications of having done something to deserve to be sick, the primordial equation of illness with malfeasance — one reason for the rejecting behavior through history toward lepers, epileptics, mental defectives, the mentally ill, and the handicapped, barely seen by averted eyes. Further, many people take the recognition of motives playing a role in illness as an invitation to accuse the ill person of having done something (at least vaguely) wrong, even though the accuser may freely acknowledge motives for behaviors other than physical illness without such self-blame. Another source of my reluctance is that the episode was so anxiety-provoking that it may have tilted my balance between open-mindedness and gullibility — always in jeopardy — in the direction of gullibility. However, the following serendipitous events tell much about healing, healers, and patients.

IT BEGAN WITH THE appearance of a red spot in my throat — the soft palate, to be exact. To the tip of my tongue it felt sandpapery or furry. The first doctor I saw about it, at one of the new walk-in medical clinics that I had decided to try out, was as puzzled as I was, especially when his laboratory declared that the spot was not due to an infection. He recommended an ear, nose, and throat specialist, Dr. J. I knew Dr. J. from his having treated a previous minor medical problem of mine, at which time he seemed the soul of pleasantness. He seemed so this time also, at first, but then his demeanor and way of speaking became somewhat abrupt, and he seemed strangely reluctant to answer my questions. He wondered aloud whether or not he should have a biopsy done, or wait a while to see if the redness would go away by itself. He spewed forth a number of medically technical terms, of which only one was recognizable to me, namely, *carcinoma*. He mumbled that I would not like him very much if he did a biopsy unnecessarily, as it would be uncomfortable considering the area where it would be done. He finally concluded that I should wait a month and have a biopsy then if the spot was still there.

I left the office a little rocky, but not too much so. He had, after all, seen fit to wait the month, the danger in that evidently being less than the discomfort of a biopsy. I reflected, however, that what had always seemed to me to be the latent sadism of so many physicians had again surfaced. The rattling off of their esoteric language tends to increase anxiety as it introduces mystery and portent, not an inviting context in which to pick up words referring to cancer. Instead of laying out the facts, which in this instance at least could have been done encouragingly, he gave me a verbal ink blot from which I had to make out what I could — an ink blot whose ambiguity nonetheless carried the unambiguous word *carcinoma*.

As it happened, I was scheduled the following month for an annual physical with a physician, as well as another physical, undertaken as research for this book, to be done by a chiropractor. My annual physical was unremarkable, as it usually is. My physician did not comment after his routine visual inspection of my throat. I then brought the red spot to his attention, and with that cue he did see it. He did not show much interest in it, however, and at the end when we were going over the findings and I asked about it, he suggested that I see an ear, nose, and throat specialist. I then told him that I had seen one specialist already and about the proposal for a biopsy. "That's the way we make the diagnosis," he shrugged.

At that point in my life I had never seen a chiropractor. On a word association test, for *chiropractor* I would have said "bones" and "non-medical," and been hard put to associate further; this despite the fact that if one becomes aware of it, in many parts of the country there seems to be a chiropractic office on practically every block. As I made my rounds of research for this book, I had received more and more intimations that some chiropractors were in the forefront of alternative healing. So I was receptive when a patient happened to mention that a chiropractic holistic practitioner had just moved into my office building. I scheduled myself for a physical to see what a holistic practitioner would do and find, as contrasted to my medical physical the same month.

Back when physicians neither had nor relied so much upon diagnostic machines and extensive laboratory studies, they honed their observational skills. They knew that how the patient looked, felt, and smelled was to be a substantial proportion of their total diagnostic information. Such skills understandably have atrophied with the emergence of so many technological sources of information. The physician hardly has to look at you, since he knows he will soon have a dossier of presumably reliable and valid findings about you. Dr. Warren Novak, my neighborly chiropractor, also takes laboratory studies seriously, and in fact claims that his standards for what is normal are higher than the usual medical standards since he is interested in health and prevention rather than merely evidence of pathology. But in addition he believes in careful visual observation.

He claimed that I needed more Vitamin A on the basis of creases that he saw in the back of my neck. He did an iridology examination, a visual examination of the eye. By studying marks and spots in the iris, the iridologist can infer all sorts of things — clogged arteries, for example. From other marks in my eye he ascertained that I had difficulty producing hydrochloric acid, which he says can be found in all people over forty and needs to be dealt with through less heavy eating. From an examination of my skin he concluded that I had some vascular insufficiency. From the look of the enamel on my teeth he thought that I had a mild mineral deficiency which is found in more than half of all of the patients that he sees. He ascertained from my fuzzy tongue a need for B-complex vitamins, and from creases in the left lobe of my ear a closing of the coronary arteries. He judged a general inflammation in my ears and throat to be a possible result of insufficient adrenal strength. He thought that over-calcification of my toenails signified a minor osteoparetic change. And so it went, down a list of observations and associated physical difficulties that, if taken out of the context that they are found in most people to a greater or lesser degree, could make one feel like a walking textbook of pathology.

It was a welcome relief to be told that the results of his kinesiology and meridian examinations were negative. (The kinesiology evaluation consisted of my having to use specific muscles to push against him, and his calibrating how much force I was able to exert, as described in Chapter 12. The meridian examination was a mechanical measurement, yielding a reading, not unlike an EEG or EKG, of the status of various organs.) While my organs, as signified by measuring the meridians related to such organs, were in good condition, the pancreas reading was an exception, some 20 percent less healthy than the other organs. Since some holistic practitioners consider the pancreas to be the seat of cancer, my pleasure in the overall meridian findings was leavened by this blip of worry. The blip became a bit bigger when the results of the laboratory blood study contributed to a diagnosis of immunostatus deficiency. That meant certain of the blood readings implicating the immune system were outside normal limits — not by much, but it is a holistic article of faith that much pathology begins with a weakening of the immune system.

Dr. Novak also sent a sample of my hair to a laboratory that specializes in hair analysis. Those who believe in hair analysis assert that is the best way to ascertain the level of metals in the body. When metals are abnormally high, one tries to find the source of the contamination, which may be in what one eats, what one plays with, or where one works. If metals are abnormally low, they can be supplemented with pills. Even among holistic health practitioners there is considerable controversy over the validity of hair findings, whether they are in fact accurate, and if so, what the consequences are of high or low readings. (Of the essential elements, I was low in potassium, iron, manganese, chromium, silicon, and selenium, high in calcium and magnesium, and normal in sodium, copper, zinc, phosphorus, aluminum, cobalt, lithium, and nickel. Of the toxic elements I was happily normal with respect to arsenic, mercury, cadmium, and lead.)

The overall impression that I got from many of these procedures, particularly those that were unfamiliar to me, was a sense that if there was something "wrong" with me, Dr. Novak would find it. I thought this, particularly, because of his holistic orientation toward, and confidence in, finding incipient diseases. He and other holistic practitioners assert that conventional medicine only becomes aware of disease when it produces complaints, or easily noted symptoms. In the case of cancer, these are tumors or conspicuously aberrant laboratory findings. From the holistic point of view, people are ill long before such symptoms appear, and with their esoteric techniques such illnesses can be detected before becoming manifest. That was comforting with respect to the long-term efficiency of healing, but undermined such reassurance as I had gotten from my medical physical. Unfortunately, Dr. Novak speaks in a somewhat explosive way, high- rather than low-key, and every time he would make one of his uncharacteristically energetic observations, it would sound to me as if he had "found something." Moreover, any deviation from perfect health seemed to him an affront, something to be taken seriously, and reactions of seriousness to diagnostic probes were at that time something that I could do without.

In the midst of the several meetings that made up that chiropractic examination, I happened to run into an acquaintance who had for years been involved in holistic medicine and associated interests. He conspiratorially whispered — apropos of what, I cannot remember — that a fast was good for most anything that bothered anyone. Fasting, too, had been on my list of procedures to investigate, and so I thought that perhaps this might be an advantageous time.

Fasting enthusiasts claim that with fasting the body cleanses itself of all manner of toxins, and the digestive organs given rest become invigorated. I consulted one of many books on fasting, and settled on a juice fast designed for five days. Purists would claim that is not a fast at all; to them a fast means nothing but water. But it seemed to me that subsisting only on juices for five days was intrepid enough for a beginner. To serious fasters, of course, juice as found in the supermarket is not juice. Rather, they recognize that by the time commercial juice gets to the customer, it is a pale imitation of what comes from the tree or ground. Therefore, these people use juicers, machines that produce juice from fruits and vegetables fed into it. Just about any food or vegetable will go through the machine, and with the pulp removed, one can drink enormous quantities of, presumably, lifesaving juice, especially if one develops a taste for copious quantities of carrot juice, celery juice, greens of all kinds, in combinations limited only by imagination and kitchen storage capacity.

Such machines were not, at the time, mass-distributed. I got mine through reading advertisements in health food magazines and using the yellow pages. The lady who sold the machines, from her house, gave me a demonstration, during which her husband came in. He offered a testimonial to the great powers of drinking fresh juice by the quart. And then he told a story, complete with meaningful glances between husband and wife, about his disease that had been overcome through juice fasts. Whether out of concern for his anxiety or mine, I did not press him on what disease this was.

The fast was anticlimactic. I enjoyed saving the time that otherwise would have been devoted to eating. Except for a few scattered moments, the pleasure I took in being able to subsist only on juices and of doing something that I had wanted to do for some time made up for the deprivation of food. According to the books, after three days I was supposed to suffer malaise, indicating that poisons were, indeed, leaving my body. Disappointingly I remained, within limits, in blooming health, except for some slight weakness due to the weight loss. Most disappointing of all, however, was the lack of change in the red area of my throat.

At this point I checked with Grete Alexander, who at times had made apparently psychic, brilliantly successful diagnostic appraisals simply through talking to people or about people over the phone. Considering her track record for spookily accurate diagnoses, I called her with some trepidation. Her early remarks were none too reassuring. She began by saying she felt pains in her chest, that she wanted to take a deep breath. (Frequently, psychic diagnosticians feel in themselves representations of illness they are diagnosing.) "My hands feel funny, shaking, I feel really upset. No, I can't be, I can't be! There's a problem in the lower part of the body, it's coming through, interesting, to the back, down to the kidney, I'm concerned about that. *You don't know about that yet.* It feels in the lower part of the body. I'm concerned about a kidney, really concerned about it, really concerned about it." I then told her about the red spot. She said, "I'm more concerned about the elimination of urine. You should take garlic pills, one a day, and alfalfa six to eight a day. I see the redness going away. If you're concerned about it, I don't see malignancy." At that I began to relax, which relaxation lasted only until her next comment, "I see inherited quality of relatives." I have a number of relatives, and between them they have lots of qualities, but the two relatives and qualities that immediately jumped to my mind were my father and mother, both of whom had died of cancer. When I pressed her to be more specific about qualities and relatives, she said that she was referring only to a tendency to low-grade infections. That sounded avoidant. Psychic diagnosticians, whether from kindheartedness, fear of implanting toxic ideas, or the law, often pull back from making specific and serious medical diagnoses.

I began to lose track as to how much I was unraveling my own medical mystery and how much I was gathering material for this book, as I called yet another psychic, a local one named Jean Pease. I had seen her at spiritual and psychic gatherings, and at one such gathering at which I spoke, she had come up from the audience to open up the possibilities of future discussions with me. I had previously called her a couple of times to solve medical mysteries of friends, and she had then seemed fairly accurate. For example, she had said a friend had circulatory trouble, plugged-up veins; the friend was then being treated for phlebitis. It was difficult to detect what Jean *thought,* as compared to what she said when she visualized me during our phone consultation. She merely reported that I might have a touch of arthritis, and that there was something different about my hair. However, she then said she saw a spot of some kind below the ribs on the left side. She hastened to add that she wasn't getting anything too specific. Then, "you may be having problems and not know about it." So now both she and Grete had implied that they knew something pathological about me that I and no one else knew. When I asked what she meant by that, she said that people may complain about one part of themselves while the seed of the trouble may be elsewhere. At that point I told her about the red spot, to which she responded that it sounded to her like an allergy.

We were about to leave it at that when she made what turned out to be a portentous suggestion: Since, as she said, I was interested in alternative medicine and writing a book, I should learn about how one can diagnose with magnets. There was to be a demonstration of that approach in a few days, in a local hotel, for a meeting of mostly chiropractors. The presenter was Harry L. Pfeiffer, D.C., who over the phone invited me to attend as his guest. I let him know my usual investigatory procedure of being a subject, but not of my new personal motive, and he agreed to study me diagnostically at the meeting or some other time. I was apprised by him and those who knew him that "some other time" might be difficult to arrange as he lectures on weekends, and people wait months for appointments at his office. As I later learned, he occasionally lectures in Tokyo, where a coterie of practitioners use his approach; and people come from great distances to his office in his home in Kearney, Missouri, a tiny town 25 miles from Kansas City.

THE FIRST OF THE TWO days of meetings was held on a Saturday afternoon. I remember that I wore to it a navy blue blazer with tan gabardine trousers, an outfit in which I feel particularly sprightly, if not healthy. Despite the anxiety nibbling around the edges, I was looking forward to what sounded like a fascinating new healing excursion.

Some fifty chiropractors, with a smattering of other physical health workers, greeted Dr. Pfeiffer's arrival with cheers, obviously not for anything that he had said or done, since he had just walked into the room, and not as the result of some hyped-up introduction, but for his mere presence. As I soon learned, such appreciation was due to his work rather than his charisma. He is a pleasant, low-key, athletic-looking person in his forties, who got right down to business. He began with an idea dear to my heart: namely, that most people in the healing professions are successful, with respect to money, status, and acceptance. By virtue of that success they continue to do the same thing over and over regardless of the results. For example, he said that only five percent of cancer patients benefit from surgery, chemotherapy, and radiation, yet practitioners continue to use these treatments routinely. He, himself, had practiced only chiropractic adjustment for five years. Now he works with the lymph system, the inspiration and expiration of oxygen, the vascular system, the role of emotions in illness, energy transfer (which is sending energy by way of laying on of hands, or psychic healing), and nutrition. He similarly has seen errors in the ways of diagnosis, citing a Mayo Clinic study in which only 25 percent of dead people examined just after their death had been diagnosed correctly. As holistic practitioners say, by the time conventional medicine is able to make a diagnosis, the patient is often too ill to be helped. By contrast, using his diagnostic method, Pfeiffer is able to detect conditions such as diabetes, circulatory disturbances, and cancer *before* they become clinical. Not only that, but the diagnosis leads to methods of treatment that are also more effective and with fewer side effects and less expense than traditional medical treatment.

And what is his method? Here he held up two red and blue tubes that looked like ballpoint pens, but were actually magnets. The red one sent a positive flow of energy, and the blue one a negative flow. He explained that the protons in the atoms making up a cell carry a positive charge, and the electrons of the atoms carry a negative charge. In a healthy organism, he claimed, the overall total of these two charges equals an electrical neutral called a balance or polarity. In an unhealthy organism the charges are out of balance. He categorizes people according to how much imbalance there is, as follows: health, malfunction, disease, or death. An imbalance which is primarily positive indicates hyperactivity, an acid chemical level, swelling, irritation, hyperthermia, and inflammation. An imbalance that is primarily negative indicates hypoactivity, an alkaline chemical level, and hypothermia.

And how is the measurement of balance or imbalance made? The answer is perhaps best explained through the following statements: (1) Opposite poles (+ and −) attract, and like poles repel, or are subject to distortion. (2) In checking a bodily organ or other substance, one checks for possible positive imbalance by touching the area to be checked with the red magnet, and checks for negative imbalance by touching the area involved with the blue magnet. One learns whether the pull of the magnet and the pull of the item measured are in balance or equal, or whether they react positively or negatively out of balance, from the fact that an imbalance results in a mild but significant distortion of the body. (3) This distortion can be measured by having the patient lie on his back, with the examiner raising the patient's legs and seeing whether the heels match. If the heels match, the energy is in balance. If one leg becomes longer or shorter than the other, that bodily distortion reflects a positive or negative imbalance. In other words, the reaction of the body, as revealed in adjustments of the spine that lengthen or shorten legs, makes of the body a sensitive measuring instrument of cellular dysfunction. Not only can organs of the body be checked this way, but so can medicines, vitamins and minerals, and foods. One simply puts whatever substance is to be checked in a tray balanced on top of the subject's stomach and makes the heel measurement. In this way, for example, it was found that pasteurized milk is so toxic that it is considered to be carcinogenic. And, horror of horrors to many health food aficionados, some 20 percent of vitamin and mineral supplements and other products purchased at health food stores are toxic — which gives one some idea of just what percentage of ordinary, processed, mass-distributed products are toxic. By placing vitamins and minerals in the tray Dr. Pfeiffer could tell whether and how much the body required of that substance in order to achieve balance, again as measured by equality of the legs.

I had more than a little trouble assimilating some of these ideas, particularly that immediate changes in leg length would reflect energy patterns of cells. I thumbed through the booklet provided to me and the other participants in the hope of establishing some sense of validity merely from the surface presentation. Instead, I noticed a poor writing style, numerous misspellings, a format and style puffed up to appear pretentiously professional, and such bucolicisms as "barleycorn" to indicate disagreement. But, I asked myself, did such niceties matter for the purposes at hand? Chiropractors tend to be informal, often to the point of skipping over the niceties of professionalism; and writing good English is not necessarily relevant to their primary tasks any more than it is for medical physicians.

The first subject was a chiropractor whom I judged to be in his thirties. Dr. Pfeiffer began by making adjustments on the man's spine to bring his legs into alignment. This would provide a baseline against which to measure any changes in leg length. An assistant put the red and blue magnets on the subject's body at approximately where the internal organs being examined were, and at each resting of the magnet Dr. Pfeiffer would raise the legs, pull together the heels with a click (shoes were left on), and either call out "Okay" or note any deviation from equality in fractions of an inch or inches. It was hard for me to believe that in his swift movements of raising the legs and clicking the heels together he could spot a deviation as small as a quarter or even an eighth of an inch, as he claimed to be doing. I wondered if slight random movements on the subject's part could not be responsible for such deviations in leg length. One way to settle such questions is to see how reliable the measurements are with the same measurer at different times, and between measurers on the same person. I did have the opportunity later to make those comparisons and to be reasonably reassured that the measurements can be made reliably.

At the end of the examination Dr. Pfeiffer classified this subject in Category Two, malfunction. The subject might not know what was wrong with him now, said Dr. Pfeiffer, but unless he attended to the demonstrated subclinical malfunctions he would become clinically diseased. Despite my slightly nagging worries about my own health, I recall having a sympathetic, if not somewhat deprecating attitude toward the subject; in academic terms, Dr. Pfeiffer had only given him a "B" instead of an "A." By contrast, I pleasurably anticipated being told that I was in excellent health, just as I used to look forward to getting back examination papers in school with the expectation that I would receive a good grade.

Although obviously not perfect, Dr. Pfeiffer pointed out that a Category Two, malfunction, was a lot better than it could be. In particular he called attention to how a grouping of imbalances — pituitary, thyroid, adrenal, pancreas, and sex hormone glands (any or all of them) — required a further test as to whether the person would "accept," thus showing a need for, an apricot or peach seed pit. Each seed pit, he said, is the equivalent of one thousand milligrams of laetrile. If a person had such organ weaknesses and showed a need for the seed pit, then he would likely have a malignancy. "Patients who come into our office already diagnosed as clinically malignant all showed distortion of these categories and required seed pits of the apricot or peach to complete a balance ... Only people in pathology will accept the seed pit ..." This part of the discussion seemed of special interest to a young woman who I later learned was a cancer patient treated by Dr. Pfeiffer, who had come from Texas for the meeting and a checkup with him. Hers was the classic story, as I learned it second-hand from those in attendance: She had been given up as incurable by the medical profession, and Dr. Pfeiffer's therapeutic regime had saved her.

I was the next subject. I lay down on the chiropractic table, and was then given the spinal adjustments necessary so that my legs would start out equal in length. While I was on my back Dr. Pfeiffer's assistant alternately put red and blue magnets on various parts of my body, each one punctuated by the click of my heels as Dr. Pfeiffer snapped them together. Throughout, he mumbled various measurements — "... a quarter inch, a half inch, left, right." Something was happening to my expectation that each test would result in my getting an "A." I did not know what, exactly, was going on, but it didn't sound to me as if I was getting good, or maybe even passing, grades. Through the miasma of increasing anxiety and confusion, I heard, in the midst of comments to the audience, "Category Three." I tried to remember what Category Three was, and kept getting confused — maybe that was the wrong series of categories, maybe they were in reverse order so that Category Three was really Category Two. I only got the categories straight later, when I checked the blackboard and, still disbelieving, asked someone else whether Category Three referred to as "disease" was the category just above the death one.

Various pills were dropped into a tray on my chest, and I seemed to be accepting, or in need of, many of them. Instead of a pill, one of them was a seed pit. Dr. Pfeiffer called the audience's attention, particularly, to his test of me at this moment. A hush in the group provided the backdrop for his announcement that I had accepted the seed pit. He then ticked off the grouping of imbalanced organs, which when combined with the acceptance of seed pit, comprised his invariable findings in patients medically diagnosed as having cancer. Dr. Pfeiffer asked the group whether anybody noticed anything about my appearance. Dr. Linden Talcott, who I later learned had worked for some time in a hospital and was familiar with such matters, said that I was jaundiced. That was the answer that Dr. Pfeiffer was looking for. I did not know much about jaundice, then, nor do I now. What I always had vaguely heard was that jaundice represents liver involvement, and in the case of cancer that is a sign of imminent fatality. So now, I thought to myself as coherently as possible, I not only have been diagnosed as having cancer and that diagnosis is not merely a cancerous disposition, but I was in the group of patients with clinically manifest cancer, and finally was perhaps in the last stages even within that group, to judge from my alleged jaundice and presumed involvement of the liver. Swell!

When people are shocked seemingly beyond endurance by revelations, they often first try to deny those revelations. So I would intermittently register all of this information about my alleged cancer, and then think there must be some mistake, or I had been mistaken in putting the information together, or something.

Dr. Pfeiffer then demonstrated one of his healing techniques called "energy transfer." That turned out to be the name for, in effect, psychic healing. People were supposed to transfer healing energy through the laying on of hands, and according to Dr. Pfeiffer, the more hands the better. Thus, the procedure was for the whole group, or as many as could get a hand in, to grasp the subject or patient. There was some discussion as to who was going to be the demonstration subject for the energy transfer, but Dr. Pfeiffer settled that issue by saying that he was going to have me be that subject because of all the people there, he said I needed it most. What I did not need, at that moment, was to hear that. So it was that a dozen or so people gathered around my supine body and laid hands on whatever they could reach of me. For some minutes all were silent while concentrating on delivering healing energy to me.

As I got off the table, the group was given a brief intermission, and I tottered, still caught somewhere between belief and disbelief, into the bathroom. Here I met one of the participants, a chiropractor, who asked, or rather said, "Well, you do have cancer, don't you?" "No," I said, or at least I didn't according to the physician who gave me an annual physical last month. He looked knowingly at me, and said that anybody who accepts the seed pit and has the glandular imbalances that I showed had cancer. He meant this not only as a quotation from Dr. Pfeiffer's booklet, but as evidence gathered from his own experience.

As I now recreate this scene, I feel creeping fingers of anxiety, a sample of the surging tide of anxiety that I felt then. I went back to my seat, and during the ensuing demonstrations, read the book a lot more assiduously than when I had first meandered academically through it. There it was, in black and white, the criteria for clinical malignancy, which matched my readings. With a promise from Dr. Pfeiffer to meet with me at the end of the meetings I somehow staggered through attending the rest of it. As I waited for him amidst the group's leaving, the cancer patient from Texas came by and sweetly offered me good luck. She said, or maybe I just translated her look as, "you, too, can be cured." Well, there it was, I had entered a new category. I was now an object of sympathy, of "good lucks," in need of hope and inspiration.

Dr. Pfeiffer, who is taciturn and unruffled by nature, was, naturally, taciturn and unruffled, to the point that as I waited he was calmly passing the time of day with others, and even began to fool around with his colleagues at the chiropractic table. At the moment, I hated him. He had just told me my life was hanging in the balance (or so it seemed to me) and I was waiting to hear how the balance could be altered, and he was giggling and chattering while I was standing there waiting, exposed, awkward, and terrified.

When we finally began our interview, at the corner of the ballroom, he began with some ice-breaking questions, such as where did I live and for how long, all of which suggested to me that he was anxious about coming directly to my diagnosis. If he was anxious, then I had good reason to be, maybe even more than I was. Finally, he got around to uttering the words that so many people, justifiably from the standpoint of statistics, fear hearing one day. Yes, I had cancer. Like a fish on the hook, I struggled to get free of his pronouncement, pressing him on the validity of his approach, trying to pin him down on the issue of whether he was diagnosing a pre-cancerous or a clinical condition, and whether he really thought that I was jaundiced at the moment, He imperturbably nodded his head, dealt with each question with as few words as possible, reiterated the statements made in the booklet, and was not at all surprised by my recently having had an unremarkable annual physical or having just been on a juice fast. Indeed, he thought the fast had probably improved my readings.

What is clinically manifest does, of course, depend on who is doing the looking, and with what. Dr. Pfeiffer was sublimely confident that he could, with his magnets and clicking of heels, diagnose conditions before they showed themselves to ordinary medical inspection. So there I was with an alleged cancer that was either clinically manifest or not clinically manifest, depending on who was doing the judging and by what means, and with a jaundiced complexion seen by some observers and not others. Under other circumstances my view of these proceedings would have been, well, jaundiced. Dr. Pfeiffer was, however, (relatively speaking) most encouraging. He said that by following his treatment regime, people with findings such as mine changed those findings in a beneficial direction in a year to a year and a half. Ninety-five percent of such patients, he said, were cured. So now, I thought, we have not only a surefire diagnosis for cancer, but the cure for cancer! "Do you realize," I asked, "what you are claiming?" He merely nodded pleasantly. The cure consisted, mainly, of a stringent diet, supplementation with the vitamins and minerals which he ascertains that the body needs from the diagnostic procedure, and if possible, energy transfer or laying on of hands. He also recommended emotional health which, under the circumstances at the moment, was laughable.

In order to join the presumably happy 95 percent of cured cancer patients, I should eat a diet that consisted of 75 percent raw food, particularly vegetables and fruits. Meat in general was frowned upon, and pork was proscribed. So was head lettuce, to my surprise, because it registered inert or even toxic on the examination with magnets, while leaf lettuce was healthily in balance. A mainstay of the diet was to be three ten-ounce glasses of raw carrot juice and celery juice per day. Just buy carrots by the crate, he said. I should also drink lots of grape juice and cranberry juice. I should eat raw potatoes and a raw egg daily, never cooked eggs. Only unpasteurized dairy products were allowable, though how I was to get those was left vague, something about a local farmer who could be contacted. I should eat the pits and core of all fruits, as well as ten raw almonds per day, and so it went, all the standard health food diet regulations plus several from macrobiotic diets, the Kelly Anti-Cancer Diet, and a few suggestions that were new to me. The list of vitamin and mineral supplementations was a long one, corresponding as it did to the many instances of substances put on my body which my heels had indicated my body needed. I could get these supplements from Dr. Pfeiffer himself, or from his colleague who evidently prescribed and distributed them for the area. The quickest way, he thought, might be to order them from the colleague, and so several days later I received some twenty or so of such bottles, the contents of which I was to ingest daily, anywhere from one to four times per day. No matter how healthy the items that I was to put into my system, there was an accumulation of the residue of unhealthy items there already, which he recommended that I deal with by way of enemas using a mixture of freshly brewed coffee and water, and regular colonics, or professionally administered enemas that reach high up in the intestines. I was to walk a mile a day, to be followed later, when presumably I was less feeble, by jogging. For the energy transfer, he recommended that I visit Jean Pease, who he said had done remarkably good healing work with many of his patients.

I rather assumed that Dr. Pfeiffer would want to see me in his office, for what exact reason I was not sure; it just seemed that if he was going to treat me for a somewhat more than minor disease, he might do so on the basis of an office visit rather than a corner of a hotel ballroom. And anyway I was interested in a re-check of his findings, particularly after a few days more post-fast. However, the earliest appointment he had was not until some six weeks later. That kind of tolerance for anxiety I did not have, and so he recommended that I could have the re-check and advice and counsel with his colleague, the one who had joined him in seeing me as jaundiced, Dr. Linden Talcott.

I was later to learn that Dr. Pfeiffer knew my diagnosis just by looking at me, as he reads people's physical conditions from the light that he sees emanating from their bodies. The diagnoses with the magnets simply confirm his original findings. If I hadn't volunteered to be a subject, he later told me, he would have selected me anyway as someone in need of healing. Others in the group, too, claimed to make diagnoses by sight. One in particular was a naturopath from nearby Topeka who, at the next morning's meeting, confirmed Dr. Pfeiffer's diagnosis, having come to the same conclusion himself, psychically, as soon as I presented myself as a demonstration subject. He figured the primary site of my cancer to be in the colon, and was noncommittal about the red spot in my throat. He, too, offered a vitamin and mineral supplement regime which along with heat, hydrotherapy, exercise, and massage, was to release the natural healing properties of the body. He was his own best advertisement, once a sufferer from either cerebral palsy or multiple sclerosis (there having been no definitive diagnosis), and now in blooming health after learning and practicing naturopathy on himself. It seemed to me to be a bit unethical for him to be offering me a health plan in competition with that of Dr. Pfeiffer, whose meeting he was attending, and who had made me a customer in the first place. What the hell, I thought, people are people. The morning meeting passed in a blur, as I alternately listened for what I could learn and figured what I might do with these sudden and wondrous circumstances.

THE BEGINNING OF A treatment program presented itself almost immediately when I approached Jean Pease. It turned out that she is a member of a loosely organized healing group, made up mostly of five sisters, one a chiropractor, the others physical culturists. Physical culture rang a minuscule, muffled bell from my memory, a bell which nowadays is amplified through the old physical culture group being swept into holistic medicine on the basis of like beliefs in the advocacy of massage, manipulation, and especially probing points on the body with their fingers. There was to be a meeting of the healing group that afternoon at the rural home of one of them, and I was invited.

One of the members of the group remarked that her husband had had a diagnosis of cancer a year ago, had refused an operation (despite his son's being a medical student who became apoplectic at the decision), and was now in radiant health. They could show me, they said, some of the tricks of the diet, especially the bunches and bunches and bunches of carrots used to make quarts and quarts and quarts of juice. It was just as she said; her husband did claim to have had a medical diagnosis of colon cancer, had embarked on Dr. Pfeiffer's regime, never felt better, and was drowning in carrot juice.

The various members of the healing group worked on one another. They took turns lying on the table and being massaged and pressured on points that I gathered corresponded to the meridian points of acupuncture. I received my pressure-point treatment, following which the whole group gathered and again gave me an energy transfer. By then I should have been a bundle of energy, and maybe I was, though it was hard for me to separate energy from anxiety.

As I left the remote house in the fields of Missouri, I had some time to sift through these events. Belief, and action or inaction founded upon such belief, were now of more than academic and literary interest. I had hoped to formulate something in the way of answers to the questions of conflicting orthodox and holistic points of view about healing by the time all the material for this book was collected, but now I was forced, whether or not I had come to an academic decision, to act, one way or another.

One course would be to laugh the whole thing off, to focus on what easily could be cartooned and caricatured — the non-professional style, the unusual if not bizarre method of measuring by heel clicking, the extravagant claims. I could consign the whole thing to the old snake-oil gambit of convincing a patient he was ill only to "cure" him after selling him a useless product. Maybe what looked like jaundice to some was only a pallor from fasting, or my naturally somewhat sallow complexion caught in a pasty light. Hell, I didn't feel on my last legs, even after I removed my sprightly blue blazer. Maybe the whole thing was a money-making dodge; the supplements alone were to cost two or three hundred dollars. But it was difficult to sustain the conviction of outright chicanery. Dr. Pfeiffer seemed uninterested in where I got the supplements, and with his six weeks' wait for another appointment could hardly be accused of wanting to rush me into paying a fee. And his fee at the time for an office visit was under $20 anyway.

Any health procedure can be subject to wishful thinking, to sincere but misguided zealotry. Some scientific research would help on that score, though it does not fully take care of the problem. As is demonstrated in orthodox medicine, even when supported by scientific research, zealously held beliefs regularly fall into disfavor, to be replaced by the next discovery, which may also turn out to be a fad. Do saccharin or birth control pills cause cancer, does vasectomy raise blood pressure, should one take estrogen? Who at this writing really knows? Dr. Pfeiffer had no independent confirmation of his work, no basis generally agreed upon by the scientific community with which to support his claims, but did that mean in and of itself that his claims were false? Hardly. And suppose, just suppose, that he was right, both in his diagnosis and in his treatment. How would it look, to say nothing of how it would feel, to waste away into disease and death because I, in the course of what was supposed to be an open-minded study of alternative healings, turned up my nose at an alternative healing that might have saved my life? And anyway what was against it? — A few hundred dollars and the nuisance of taking supplements, following a diet which in its essentials I believed was healthful anyway, a regime that at the least had a reasonable chance of increasing the quality of my present health and preventing disease in the future. I thought I would delay a final decision until I saw whether Dr. Talcott would independently confirm the diagnosis as well as prescribe the same treatment. I knew, however, in a corner of my mind, that I was not simply going to dismiss the whole thing, that I was going to pursue the implications for my personal health.

Several days later Dr. Talcott came up with findings that were almost identical to Dr. Pfeiffer's. He prescribed the same therapeutic regime, along with a few additions. (It seems that practically all holistic practitioners have a few pet wrinkles, the natural consequence, I suppose, of their widely varying training, if not different grandmothers.) He had the same somewhat offhand, low-key attitude as Dr. Pfeiffer; yes, I had cancer; yes, I looked jaundiced; yes, I probably could be cured if I followed the regime to the point of turning orange with carrot juice.

I must have been doing my patient role quite well, as Dr. Talcott proceeded to show me the importance of mental health without any visible indication that he either knew or cared that I already had some acquaintance with the field. He had me extend my arm, then think of the most currently bedeviling conflict or situation troubling me at the moment, then cleanse my mind of that situation and think of something else either neutral or pleasant. When I was thinking of the difficult situation, he was able to pull my arm down with relative ease; when I was thinking of something neutral, he found it difficult to budge my arm. He then produced the famous smile picture, that adorns countless buttons and hangs in countless offices. When looking at the smile picture, my arm remained strong and rigid. When he showed me the same picture with the mouth reversed from a smile to a frown, my arm again became weak. Those people who tell one to smile and think only good thoughts may have something there.

It was 11:00 P.M. when Dr. Talcott and I finished; I stumbled off into the dark night, and into a dark night of the soul as well. Thenceforth, when I flipped on the radio, often the first word I would hear would be "cancer" — some message from the American Cancer Society, an interview with a researcher or a victim. Famous people suddenly seemed to be dying of cancer at epidemic rates; it seemed that the magazines reported on little else. The background murmur of my usual complement of aches, pains, itches, and twinges now suddenly burst piercing into awareness.

There was in this situation not only the irony of its occurrence in the midst of my writing a book on healing, but I had devoted a sizeable section in *Out In Inner Space* to the relationship between diet and cancer, and to the cancer work of the Simontons. Carl Simonton, a radiologist, and Stephanie Simonton, a psychologist, had developed a program and point of view in which people with cancer learned ways of dealing psychologically with their disease. I had taken several of their training courses in this approach, joined them in a week-long residential treatment program as an observer, and applied aspects of the Simonton work to some 25 cancer patients. In a nutshell, the Simonton approach can be divided in two parts: Patients are encouraged (1) to meditate three times a day, and during the course of that meditation to visualize their cancer, the treatment they are getting, and the treatment destroying and eliminating the cancer cells, in any form or with any symbols they choose; and (2) to think of the cancer as a last-ditch attempt to solve what seems to them life situations or conflicts insoluble by any other means. They then enter psychotherapy in order to find other solutions. Preparatory to joining the week-long residential program, I, masquerading as usual as a patient, had filled out several psychological tests and questionnaires. In the course of going over the results of these, Stephanie joked that to judge from my test responses, if I ever got cancer, I would get over it. She was basing her cheery prediction on the frequently reported formal and informal observation that the nicest patients get cancer and yield to it quicker than the fighting, more irascible patients. Hospital personnel frequently bemoan the fact that their most cooperative and pleasant patients are the ones who succumb, while the ones who make life miserable for them survive. Or, as baseball player and manager Leo Durocher is reputed to have said in defending his attacks on umpires, "Nice guys finish last." To what extent I was fueled by lifelong irascibility, my family, friends, and dogs could best say, but I did feel within me a gathering knot of resolve.

With respect to diet, on a scale of 1–10, with 10 the best, I would score about 7. As a result of my experiences, I already was observing the essentials of the dietary suggestions put forth by Drs. Pfeiffer and Talcott. I now became more stringent about them. Instead of occasional wine or beer, I switched to very occasional wine spritzers and even more occasional beer. I restricted further my low consumption of meat, already consisting only of poultry and seafood. I continued or instituted proscriptions against dairy products, white flour, caffeine, and sugar. Smoking was not a problem since I had never smoked. I never did get down all of that carrot juice, and I absolutely struck out when it came to eating raw potatoes. I started every day with a mixture of protein powder (a perhaps questionable move as I later found out), raw egg, fruit, and at first goat's milk, which is deemed preferable to cow's milk. Then I realized that juice would do just as well as milk. I met with Pat DeAngelis, a dietician at the American International Hospital in Zion, Illinois (discussed further below), who seemed to have sensibly analyzed and compared every dietary approach, and put together a dietary guide listing diets in five stages corresponding to five degrees of severity of illness. That organization and simplification created complexity for me. What stage diet should I follow, and could I really give up entirely — as required of the seriously ill — such delectables as shrimp, crab, and lobster, scavengers which Mrs. DeAngelis deemed to be toxic?

With respect to exercise, for the first six months I would have to give myself somewhere between a 0 and 2 on a scale of 10. I just walked a little bit more, and breathed more deeply, as had been recommended by several psychics along the way. I remember one pathetic day when I walked around my office building in the few minutes between patients, breathing deeply of the air, imagining that I was soaking up the sun, and wanly recognizing the basic absurdity of this little bit of exercise and air that I was introducing into my therapeutic regime. Months later I did finally join a health club and thereafter ran, bicycled, and did muscle exercises faithfully every other day, but still did not set any records for vigor. Let's say scale score 6.

The Simonton assertion that seemingly insoluble psychological conflicts dispose one to cancer is complicated by the fact that if we look at most lives at any given point, we are likely to find such conflicts. As the magician involved in the demonstration of Philippine psychic surgery said, if I tell you that you skinned your knee as a child and probably have a scar, you may think that I am prescient, until you realize that that applies to practically everybody. Yet some scars are more obvious and troublesome than others, infiltrate more dreams, stir up more anxiety, call for more difficult practical decisions. Scale score 7.

With respect to energy transfer, psychic healing, and the laying on of hands, I adhered at first to a weekly, then a biweekly schedule of meetings with Jean Pease. At our first tense meeting, she confirmed the diagnosis in three ways. (1) With her X-ray eyes, which get their power from a brief, meditative concentration, she "saw" the tumor. Where she saw it, she said, did not matter much, implying that maybe her image was only symbolic. (2) She also studied my organs with magnets and noted the same crucial imbalances as had Pfeiffer and Talcott. And (3) she can tell cancer by feeling the skin, which to her in a person with cancer has a peculiar quality of stickiness. She said that she had recognized my cancer when we first talked over the phone but had explained it away thinking that I was too young (though she well knew that young people also get cancer). As I have come to know her, she is too good-hearted a person not to fight off the recognition of unpleasant diagnoses. Especially at the beginning of our work, the treatment consisted of her laying on hands in order to give me energy, of which, according to her, I was badly in need. Where she would put her hands was guided at various times and at different sessions by an arcane intuition or by spiritual entities, doctor-helpers from the "other side" who would instruct her. From time to time she would complain of pain in her hands, presumably emanating from me with such force that she would have to stop and occasionally call upon her husband to substitute briefly. Increasingly, her ministrations shifted from merely transferring energy to a kind of acupressure; that is, again guided by who knows what, she would determine areas of the body that were out of whack, had "kernels" or "crystals" within them, and needed to be worked out through kneading them with her fingers. I can painfully attest that this woman, in her mid-seventies, so obese and seemingly weak that it was a struggle for her to get in and out of a chair, has fingers of steel. By the same token, at such times this woman who seems the soul of kindness had a heart of stone, pressing away irrespective of any of my moans or pleas for mercy. She seemed to believe, as is believed in many esoteric healing systems, that various points on the body correspond to internal organs, even though these are at a considerable distance from those points. The points may have been the familiar meridian or alternate nervous system points used in acupuncture or Shiatsu, but Jean claimed that she knew nothing of any systems, she just knew where to put her hands.

When apprised of the now infamous red area in my throat, Jean went to work on it. Her work consisted of laying on of hands in the throat area and then snapping her fingers and summoning the red spot. "Now come on, let's get out of there ..." The area did lighten greatly, as judged by an independent observer of the proceedings. "Thank you, Lord," Jean said. For my part, I thought that while He was at it, He could just as well have taken the whole thing. It remained definitely improved, but yellow and red alternated and changed shape in my throat off and on, and was furry to the touch of my tongue, for more than a year. During that time, I happened upon a brochure advising how to detect various cancers, including throat cancer. Warning signs of throat cancer included reddish areas in the throat that felt fuzzy or furry or sandpapery to the tongue's touch. Some nights sleep was scarce.

After the emotional pummeling I was taking from the cancer diagnosis and the physical pummeling that I was taking from Jean's attacks on parts of my body, it was especially gratifying to hear from Jean that I supposedly had a high tolerance for pain. That high tolerance for pain seemed an expression of what she considered a stoic, even impervious, body. Often I did not hear, sense, feel or react as she thought I should. She would often hear things in my body, feel things moving, and was always surprised when I reported that I was unaware of these internal events. Many times during our sessions she would say or do things that seemed contradictory to other things she had said or done. For example, she was constantly changing spots on my body to work on, each of which she would claim was connected to a particular internal organ. There are, in the lexicon of meridians in acupuncture, several spots which correspond to various bodily areas, but not as many as Jean seemed to find. Anyway she usually claimed not to be following the meridian points, just responding to her own sensations. At one point she claimed that a vision, or image, or sense of a medical guide was instructing her in how to deal with my health. I wondered with her that if such a guide was going to take the trouble to be interested in the matter, why hadn't it been done earlier in our series of treatments? Her reply: "Maybe the guide did, and I didn't know it." So much for that. She was not about to be shoehorned into the realm of logic and scientific method, or to be bothered by the strictures of conventional thought; and just to make sure that such issues are never joined, she almost never responds to a direct question with a direct answer. All of that, of course, says nothing about her alleged healing power. More to that point is Dr. Pfeiffer's observation that after a patient is treated by Jean, the patient's organs tend to read as normal, when days before and after her treatment they read as abnormal. Just as he instructs patients not to take supplements on the day of an examination because supplements obscure the cell imbalances, he instructs patients not to be treated by Jean for a few days before his examination.

Be that as it may, Jean was one of the many healers who failed to help my sore elbow. That offending part of my body had been making itself painfully known for years. Acupuncture is supposed to be highly effective with such disturbances, but failed completely to help me, as did chiropractic manipulations, and a dozen or so psychic healers. While one might leap to the idea that if such healings cannot take care of such a relatively minor matter as tennis elbow, how can one even consider that they could be helpful with serious diseases? — as usual, the healers have an answer, namely that there seems no rhyme or reason to what responds and what doesn't. Some patients do recover dramatically from, for example, life-threatening emphysema, as Jean claims one of her clients did, while the same patient may carry a minor arthritic pain in the knuckle to eternity.

Jean's psychic work was similarly variable and difficult to evaluate. Now and again she would take time out from the healing to do a psychic reading, sometimes in answer to my questions, and sometimes just because the spirit, so to speak, moved her. Often she was wrong. Often what she said remains to be seen, since it involves predictions. In one instance she spontaneously offered predictions that accurately reflected what happened to be on my mind at the time, though the predictions themselves turned out to be wrong. But how did she know that these were the thoughts and issues with which I was dealing at the moment? It may be that the reading, put in terms of prediction, was a reading of my current mind — telepathy rather than clairvoyance. On one occasion she was breathtakingly accurate. With no questions or priming on my part, she interrupted her healing ministrations with some thoughts arrived at psychically about my children, some accurate, some inaccurate, and some indeterminate. Then she "saw" one of my friends who at the moment was struggling with the question as to whether she and her husband should be divorced. She saw the friend with red eyes, weeping, with an umbrella, but being hit by bricks rather than raindrops. The patient was signing documents that she didn't want to sign. Not long after, she did reluctantly sign divorce documents. Jean then said, also correctly, that the patient had a narrow-band wedding ring which she favored, but another ring would also make her happy. Was Jean being telepathic, merely picking up thoughts and wishes of the friend, or was she making an accurate clairvoyant prediction? As it turned out, however much my friend mourned the first relationship, she eventually did happily accept another ring.

At the end of one of her readings, Jean offered a rare moment of introspection. She said that she knew she was finished with the reading when the vibrations slowed down, when she began to emerge from an otherworldly state. In that state she was only dimly aware of my presence, of the world around her; to come out of it was like waking up, She gave the example of doing a psychic reading on a husband, and remarking to the wife that she hadn't seen her for some time, only to learn that she had done a psychic reading on the wife just the day before; in her psychic state Jean had been too unaware of the woman to register her presence.

Patricia was another of the family of holistic health proponents who participated with her sisters in giving me energy on that awful afternoon in the isolated, rural house, the second day of the Pfeiffer workshop. For several months she worked on me once a week with a combination of massage and acupressure. She, as did all the others, took my diagnosis as a matter of course; she did not question it, and did not seem particularly upset or even interested in it. What she failed to understand was that I read every comment, facial expression, and reaction as a source of information about cancer. Thus, what may have been merely an idle comment about a weakness in this or that muscle, or a disproportionate amount of pain on one side or the other, stirred anxiety in me that she had *found something*. One antidote to the intermittent increases in anxiety was the massage which, whatever its medicinal value, felt good.

Patricia's place was where I experienced one of the strangest of all of the therapies, although the Chinese would not have considered it strange since the method is said to have been derived from them. How grandmothers got it from the Chinese is a mystery, but it is also said to be a remedy used by the American pioneers. It is a method of removing wax from the ears, not with your ordinary medical instrument or even a Q-tip, but by inserting a column of paper, called a candle, and setting it on fire. Wax is said to be produced by this procedure, sometimes in copious amounts, even after the ear has seemingly been cleaned of wax by usual methods. While the pioneers used brown paper and bacon grease, the candles are now said to be made solely by a woman in her mid-eighties who, unless she can be persuaded otherwise, will take the secret of their making with her to the grave. Apparently there *is* some kind of secret, as copies made by Patricia and another practitioner, Susan, who did the procedure on me, so far have not been successful. According to Susan, a copious production of wax is indicative of illness, since an ill body overreacts in most ways. I produced no more than an average amount. I reflected sourly that now I was reduced to getting reassurance about my health from wax spilling out of billowing smoke around my ears.

Every now and again I, and others, produce powder rather than wax, and this was said to be evidence of infection. The clearing of the wax is, as one may expect, good for hearing, but according to its proponents, it is good also for headaches, sinus trouble, and allergies. By enthusiastic implication, it is good for whatever ails you. My average amount of wax took three "treatments," a week apart. Having a flame tilted at what seemed to me a precarious angle from my hair and ear got no more familiar or seemingly safe with repetition. I was glad when it was over. The wax looked pretty much like one would expect, but the powder was a mystery among mysteries. I asked Susan whether the powder had ever been analyzed in a laboratory, and she said that was a marvelous idea, in a tone that suggested she had not thought about it before. The laboratory technician whom I consulted thought that the powder was alcoholic fats converted by heat to hydrocarbon compounds, as in charring. He believed that it had to have come from the outer ear, or at least beyond the tympanic membrane. I could hardly believe that so much debris could come from the ear drum outward, and yet if not, where did it come from, and how did it get there? Dr. Pfeiffer knew about the candle treatment and considered the powder a fungus. He had observed that upon burning the wax out of the ear, people's readings with the magnets became better; the energy in their cells became balanced.

In a study reported in *Laryngoscope* (1966; 106: 1126-1129), not only was cerumen (ear wax) not removed, but "candle wax was actually deposited in some ears." However, these findings were based on only eight pairs of ears. It is heartening that people are systematically studying esoteric methods, but using a sample of only eight cases hardly establishes confidence in whatever is found.

However, as a sign of the times, what was so esoteric to me at the time is far less so now. Andrew Weil recently wrote about it in *Self-Healing*. He and some of his Fellows in the University of Arizona Program in Integrative Medicine experimented with "ear candling" and found it pleasantly productive of ordinary ear wax (with no mention of mysterious white powder). Contrary to the hush-hush atmosphere and exotically quaint story of its provenance that I encountered, Weil reports that the candles are available at many neighborhood health food stores.

THE PHONE RINGS. Fred, a childhood friend, now a physician, is calling to invite me to a family affair. Fred has impeccable Establishment training credentials — the best places, with the best people, which dovetailed with what I knew of his personality. In college he practiced his saxophone until the notes shone, and studied until the A's tumbled around him. Later, if Grosse Pointe was the place to live, he lived there, and if Mercedes Benz and Rolls Royce were badges of Establishment success, then he had a couple of Mercedeses and a Rolls. We used to have moderately heated discussions about socialized medicine, and predictably Fred would have nothing of it. He was going to be the kingpin in a capitalistic establishment, untroubled by social consciousness, steering clear of the weak and lame except for the fee-paying ones who appeared at his office. He said it all, however, with a wry humor. And maybe that was the tip-off that his was not a seamless surface.

Now, he informed me, he had pretty much given up surgery, believing there were better ways of treating cancer than the strictly conventional ones. He had sought these out as a result of years of tragic inability to successfully treat cancer through surgery, radiation, and chemotherapy, or as the holistic people are inclined to say, cutting, burning, and poisoning. The better ways that he had found included low-dose chemotherapy, which carried fewer side effects and was at least as effective as high-dose chemotherapy; hyperthermia, which is raising body heat to a point where cancer cells were killed while healthy cells were uninjured; and plasmapharesis, a means of circulating blood outside the body through filters which remove its cancerous impurities, then returning it to the body. He believed, also, in stimulation of the immune system, and in specialized nutrition, including high doses of vitamins and minerals. He made himself aware of and, to the extent that he could, studied a variety of drugs that are used in Europe and elsewhere, but prohibited from use in the United States. Ironically, he was threatened with punishment by the medical establishment at the same time that he was declared "Man of the Year" by the Cancer Control Society. As a sign of the chaotic times, he was supposedly unfit to practice medicine according to some of his peers in one state, and anointed as a medical saint in another. One of his alleged malfeasances was said to be extending hope in excess of what he was able to deliver. Ironically, what he had to deliver was several years later delivered by many other members of the medical profession. He had been ahead of his time, apparently a dangerous thing to be. His story would have made a good movie about rugged individualists against the system, starring Gregory Peck or Robert Duvall.

Although Fred is a consultant to a chiropractic college, he was unaware of the magnet approach to diagnosis, and noncommittal about my alleged cancer. He did think a thorough medical study was in order, and since I was writing a book about healings, I ought to see American International Hospital (now renamed Midwest Research) anyway. Years back I had accompanied him on his rounds through the horrors of cancer wards (I shall literally never forget a man with a rubber face which took the place of the cancerous one that Fred had removed). When he briefly raised the possibility of doing the examination with me as a hospital patient, I negotiated myself into outpatient status.

In the meantime I had an appointment with Dr. Novak at which he delivered his summation and recommendations. He had me in reasonably good condition, though requiring some vitamin and mineral supplementation. My immune system, according to him, was moderately impaired, and that, of course, was an important issue as the immune system protects us not only from stray infections but from serious diseases and, according to many, from cancer. He knew of Dr. Pfeiffer's work second-hand, but had formed no opinion of it. He knew, also, of Dr. Pfeiffer's knack of making diagnoses psychically, and Dr. Novak is as willing to give him credit for that skill as he is willing to credit the magnets. When I told him of Dr. Pfeiffer's diagnosis of me, he was taken aback. He wondered whether he had missed something. Sometimes it happens, he said, though to him it simply did not fit. Of course, there was that peculiarly lowered efficiency in the pancreas, he mused, but still ... He said that he was disinclined to deal with cancer patients, and often sent them to Midwest Research and my friend Fred. Small world.

My examination at American International consisted of a physical done by one of Fred's surgeon colleagues. He thought the redness in my throat, by now alternating redness and whiteness, was nothing more than a pharyngeal infection. The rest of the examination consisted of standard blood studies and a couple of quasi-standard tests for specific kinds of cancer. Everything ascertainable at the moment offered no indications of cancer. Some of the specialized studies would take several days. In other words, I was to jump whenever the phone rang in my office for several days afterwards until getting the cheery news that those tests also revealed nothing remarkable. All of that certainly was better than the alternative, but was not much different from the results of my annual physical, which had not impressed Dr. Pfeiffer at all: He thought he knew what Establishment medicine was incapable of knowing.

At the same time that the studies of me were taking place at American International, I was making a study of it. Like a man without a country, I went back and forth: I would go from the public relations office after discussing advertising and the hospital's public image, to a laboratory for a blood study, from discussions of holistic medicine to observing plasmapharesis and other treatments for cancer. I lived in the half-world of academically collecting information, and wondering whether I would be on that table watching my blood leave and re-enter my body as in plasmapharesis, be under that knife, be heated to 108° for hours on end as in hyperthermia, or be instructed to follow Stage 1, the most austere and depriving of the diets.

I was eventually invited to become a consultant on psychological matters and a member of American International's Ethics and Review Board. From that vantage point, along with my other observations, I learned to make an important distinction between one kind of holistic medicine and another. American International Hospital advertised itself as a holistic health institution. Largely what it means by that is that it is more open than most medical institutions to new approaches, yet these approaches are within the established purview of medicine. That is surely understandable: the hospital and clinic are medical institutions, and subject to commensurate legalities and standards which make it, among other things, eligible for medical insurance payments. Being medical mavericks in some respects, yet professionals needing to remain within the system, its members have to be hyperconscientious and meticulous about following the rules. They feel themselves, for the most part correctly, as objects of suspicion from the establishment, whose members view them as unfair competition to most other practitioners and who would dearly like to find some way of discrediting them. Perhaps that is a partial explanation as to why its psychological services for patients and the implementation of its program of nutrition and vitamin and mineral supplementation lag behind its purely medical orientation. By contrast, Norman Shealy's Pain and Rehabilitation Clinic (see Chapter 10) exemplifies a holistic approach which not only strains traditional medical boundaries to their outer reaches, but happily spills across them into psychology, nutrition, spirituality, and psychic healing. Those who go now to Midwest Research expecting that kind of holism will be disappointed. Those who go expecting the outer legal limits of what medicine has to offer will be rewarded. Neither Shealy nor Midwest Research evidently were fully aware of this distinction when they briefly joined forces, only to separate when experience dramatized their different views and varieties of holistic medicine.

SOME FIVE WEEKS AFTER my diagnosis of cancer I set off for my first appointment at Dr. Pfeiffer's office, which is in his home in the tiny town of Kearney, Missouri. From the looks of the town, Dr. Pfeiffer may be the town's leading industry. That night, and every subsequent night that I was there, there were people waiting before my appointment and after my appointment. I tooled my way past the plastic animals on his lawn to find what looked like a safe place for my prized new car, wondering sourly if my concern for the car was merely a reflection of the damage that I feared with respect to my person.

Wild turkey was, to Dr. Pfeiffer, something that one shot at rather than drank; I was seated in his waiting room under what I took to be the understandably malevolent and injured gaze of the head and feathers of a turkey who had evidently succumbed to Dr. Pfeiffer's aim if not his diagnosis. In keeping with the turkey and the sayings and decorative art on the walls, a genial Dr. Pfeiffer greeted me rumpled and tieless. For all the reaction that he showed to his erstwhile dramatic demonstration subject, I could have been there for a routine spinal adjustment. Once again I lay down on his chiropractic table as he went through routine spinal adjustments, electrical massage, and manipulations to even out my legs. Once again, repeated clicking of the heels, snapped-out measurements, the placing of magnets, the dropping of supplements in the tray on my chest, and finally the thump of the seed pit in the tray. Only then did Dr. Pfeiffer's otherwise routine imperturbability give way to mild excitement. I had rejected the seed pit, I no longer needed it; I was on a page in the manual different from the one that described patients with malignancies. I was not, as they say, out of the woods yet, but I had made one of the fastest moves toward recovery in Dr. Pfeiffer's experience. I was to continue all of the supplements, the restricted diet, and, as he said, whatever else I might be doing. That damn turkey looked a lot friendlier on the way out than on the way in.

The vise was not, however, to be loosened for long. Anemia is not a prince of a word. In school yards it is readily translated as weak, puny, connoting a person who gets sand kicked in his face at the beach. In medicine it can be associated with serious disease, life-giving blood no longer being capable of sustaining life. On Dr. Novak's first study of my blood, I was not quite anemic, though as mentioned I did show a loss of efficiency in the immune system. A routine recheck of the immune system five days later revealed that it was now improved, but I had become anemic. Even one's basic desk dictionary reveals that anemia, among other things, is manifested by pallor or — in the eyes of some perhaps — jaundice.

Back to the laboratory for another blood study I went, my memory of Dr. Novak's furrowed forehead engraved just behind my own. The waves of relief that I had experienced after my visit to Dr. Pfeiffer had now turned to churning. The telephone's ring, which had begun to resume its usual probability of pleasantness, or at least a wrong number, was now once again a tolling harbinger. After many false alarms, it delivered Dr. Novak's directive to come upstairs, something was wrong. What was wrong was that my blood values had decreased again. For example, I had a 25 percent loss in hemoglobin, and a frighteningly substantial drop in hemocrit. Dr. Novak raised the question of internal bleeding, suggested a CAT scan, and admonished me to "do something immediately." On the other hand, he mused, maybe all of those supplements I was taking were depressing the bone marrow, much as he, a giver of supplements, hated to acknowledge that possibility. I stopped taking all supplements, with due concern that the supplements may have brought about my alleged recovery.

The Great Script Writer in the Sky, never missing an opportunity, delivered the news from one of my patients that she had been suffering dizzy spells, which her physician told her was due to severe anemia. For several weeks I listened to her reports, remedial measures, and sunny results with macabre as well as professional interest. She became convinced, maybe more than I was, that her readings were an expression of psychological distress (in its own way a comforting thought), when I, too, suffered a dizzy spell.

When next at the laboratory the technician, with whom by now I had a familiar relationship, asked whether I had internal bleeding. "Not that I know of," I replied weakly, musing about how sadism and omnipotence seem to have infiltrated the system. It wasn't much of a laugh, but I had it anyway, when the results of that blood study, though not exactly revealing a robust coursing of life-preserving fluid, did show a decided upswing on all measures. By then I had become something of an expert in comparing laboratory studies and had pasted alongside one another the results of all those done at my annual physical, at Midwest Research, and this series with Dr. Novak for easy comparison. I showed my paste-up to Dr. Pfeiffer. He thought it unlikely that his supplements had depressed the bone marrow, and mumbled something about the possibility of a virus. (Virus or allergy seem to be the court of last resort when healers of all kinds do not know what else to say.) Despite the blood finding, Dr. Pfeiffer's re-examination put me in the benign category of "malfunction," there poised to move up to that "A" in health. Nonetheless, I was to continue taking pretty much the same supplements at the same dosage, with the addition of what he called a blood builder.

Even with supplements resumed, the next blood test was the best yet —just a shade below normal in red blood count, hemoglobin, and hemocrit, but nobody's perfect. Anyway, Jean took a "look" at my blood and thought it was just fine.

Through the summer my health was judged by all involved to be improving. According to Jean, the feel of my skin was now so good that from it she would not think that I was at all ill, though, as she unnecessarily reminded me, the feel of my skin previously had revealed to her that I was "very serious." The markings in my throat were, by now, practically gone. I had not regained the 10–12 pounds I had lost on the fast, a mildly worrisome observation, but I was not losing weight either, and my specialized diet was not one that would necessarily encourage a gain in weight. At my next examination with Dr. Pfeiffer he opined that I had made an excellent recovery, still one of the fastest that he had ever observed, and that I was now close to the Number One, or "Health" category. Encouragingly, he slightly cut back on the program of supplements which he now considered to be more of a maintenance program than a therapeutic one. Just to keep me honest, however, he did suggest, when the subject came up, that I not do any laying on of hands since I still needed all of my energy for myself. Well, maybe they just didn't want competition. At any rate, it certainly was a pleasure to hear as an accompaniment to the heel clicking, "Okay," "okay," "okay."

I WAS NOW CALM ENOUGH to take a closer, more academic look, at Dr. Harry L. Pfeiffer, instigator of this strange and jolting experience.

At age nineteen, Dr. Pfeiffer received his first calling, to become a minister. He was educated by the Disciples of Christ and got his first pastorate in northern Missouri. Later he attended Vanderbilt Divinity School on a scholarship, and worked again as a preacher until he got his second calling which was to cure the physical body. He graduated from Palmer Chiropractic School, doing the four-year course in three years, and has now intermittently been a pastor as well as a full-time chiropractic physician. How he learned the approach with the magnets he reports as a mystery, something that was just given to him. However that may be, he had become open to healing possibilities other than traditional chiropractic ones since he was so troubled at the limitations of what he had been able to do for ill people. I later learned that a chiropractor in Kentucky claims that he invented the approach, which fact might supply an alternative explanation to Dr. Pfeiffer's claim that the information was mysteriously "given" to him.

The imbalance in length of legs resulting from magnetic imbalance is to Dr. Pfeiffer entirely understandable and expectable. The body reacts violently, as a whole, to such an imbalance, and measurements of such reactions could be made on the hands or head also, if one did not choose to use the length of legs.

Here, as elsewhere, from Dr. Pfeiffer's point of view and from that of holistic health in general, many problems disappear when one envisions the body as a whole, as a system. What may seem mysterious in and of itself becomes intelligible when one sees it in the larger context, in this instance the whole body reacting to an imbalance in one of its parts. Dr. Pfeiffer takes the same approach in treating, for example, a ballooning aneurysm. Instead of the segmented patchwork approach of operating on the aneurysm, he claims to be able to clear the blood flow that produced the aneurysm and to reverse the aneurysm with chiropractic adjustments of the clavicle and head and a prescription for as little time as a month of taking rutin, a nutritional supplement. In Dr. Pfeiffer's view, all difficulties related to blood supply — varicosities, phlebitis, diabetic circulatory disturbances — would be helped with such a program. By testing each supplement on the person he is able to avoid guesswork and wasteful broad-spectrum approaches. If the body needs the supplement, it will so register, and if not, it will register otherwise.

How much in my particular instance Dr. Pfeiffer was influenced by his reading of my aura, it is difficult to say. The feelings and impressions that he gets of illness, including what he reads in auras, he says just happen to him. He only became aware of this faculty when he started his chiropractic work, though he had been interested in and open to the possibilities of psychic phenomena for a couple of decades. While he himself did not need to be persuaded of the existence of healing energy, he cited Kirlian photography as evidence of the existence of such energy. He further believed in the capacity to manipulate such energy for healing purposes as is done in polarity therapy[1] (Gordon, 1978). In Gordon's how-to book, for sale along with other similar books at Dr. Pfeiffer's seminars, anyone can learn how to send healing energy. As Gordon writes, "Our hands are a gift. Through them we can channel the love in our hearts to relieve the suffering of those around us." So anyone who has love in the heart can relieve suffering through the laying on of hands. The energy, or life force, flows through an invisible circulatory system, charging every cell in its path, and becomes weakened and blocked as a result of stress or illness. As acupuncturists restore the flow of energy using needles, polarity therapists do the same through touch. If one is willing to grant the assumptions inherent in these beliefs, then the laying on of hands, far from being mysterious or occult, stems directly from a theory about the workings of the body. It therefore does not seem so cheeky to write, as Gordon does, in a paragraph headed "How To Stop A Headache" (apply your right hand to the back of the patient's neck, hold the palm of your left hand one-half inch away from the patient's forehead, and have the patient take deep breaths letting out a sigh after each one): "Within three to five minutes most headaches will be gone or greatly relieved."

The principles of polarity are the same as those underlying Pfeiffer's work: the top of the body and the right side have a positive charge, the feet and the left side have a negative charge. Just as positive and negative poles of magnets when in balance attract currents between them and repel one another if out of balance (some combination other than positive and negative), so it is with blocked areas in the body. Such blockages are the result of an imbalance of positive and negative charges, which can be corrected by the healer's connecting the "plus" of his right hand to the "minus" of the left side of the patient's body, and the "minus" of his left hand to the "plus" side of the patient's body.

The how-to books such as Gordon's and Kreiger's (1979)[2] are based on the belief that virtually anyone can be a healer, that all people possess healing power. That is what Dr. Pfeiffer says he believes. What then, I thought to myself, of the coherent picture that emerged from my psychological test study of healers which was different from my psychological test findings of other people (see Chapter 11)? Either some people's energy flows so much better than others and this goes along with the personality characteristics that I found, or those characteristics apply only to those who identify themselves conspicuously as healers, the rest of us modestly hiding our power often even from ourselves.

Dr. Pfeiffer says that he can tell the extent of the energy flow just by looking at a person, in the same way that he can diagnose their illnesses. While I, he said, might be a serviceable enough healer, I should not do any such healing, as I needed my energy. Healers lose their energy when doing healing, as blood donors lose blood. I can't say I liked the sound of that; after all, I was in Category Two and heading for Category One, and here he was telling me I was so low in life-preserving energy that if I used it to heal others, it would be only at my peril. When I pressed him on this score, he said that some 70 percent of the general population is in better condition than I am now. Well, at least he's consistent, I thought to myself. He really did have me diagnosed as terribly sick, and despite my remarkable gains he is none too sanguine about my health yet. He then went on to comment that the healing energy comes from God rather than from the healer. If it comes from the healer, then the healer becomes tired. When it comes from God, the healer can heal without being tired.

We have now, I believe, what is called in statistics a multi-factorial problem. Healing comes from God, or healing comes from people; if it comes from God, the healer is not drained, while if it comes from the healer, the healer is plumb tired. One implication from Dr. Pfeiffer's opinion about the danger to me from healing others is that he is assuming that any healing energy I have would come from me rather than God, and that is why it would deplete my supposedly slender resources. These issues began to crowd the tip of my tongue until I realized that what I would get for my trouble from Dr. Pfeiffer was a knowing, tolerant, slightly amused smile.

EVERY FIRSTHAND HEALING experience I entered into in the later course of research for this book was tainted by my cancer diagnosis experience; I still think of it once in a while, and so where to put an end to this chapter has to be somewhat arbitrary. Arbitrarily, then, I shall pick a healing session with Jean Pease that took place about fourteen months after the diagnosis. While I had been seeing her on the average of every two weeks, what with her being away and my being away, this session took place five weeks after the last one. She began by feeling my head, neck and upper chest and commented that my energy was low. She could tell this from the pain that she felt in her hands when she touched me. Overall, however, she thought me to be in excellent condition. I then proceeded to get energy from her at a rapid rate, and she remarked that I not only needed a lot of energy just then but I was now better able to absorb energy than I used to be, not only from her but from the world around me. (She believes that a major source of illness is a diminished capacity to pick up life-giving energy in the daily course of events, from other people or simply from the environment.) Sometime later in the session she worked on my feet, by which I mean she probed and pressed and held parts of my feet and pulled at my toes. She commented that she felt no pain in her hands when she held my left foot, but did feel some pain when she held my right foot. She concluded from this that my left side was stronger, and any physical difficulties I have would most likely occur on the right side. At any rate, it took only a few moments of work before she reported that she was free of pain from my energy-draining body. In between her working on my head and feet, she worked on the rest of me, and took time out to "look" into my body. She examined each organ in turn and concluded that each was in excellent condition. Even my bladder and prostate, which make themselves unpleasantly known to millions of middle-aged men, had shrunk and showed no signs of irritation. She said that I had the muscles and bones of a person fifteen years younger than I. She wondered aloud how I could have gotten into such a "run-down" condition as when I had first begun with her. Whether on theoretical or psychic grounds, she concluded that I must have had a difficult life problem, some kind of emotional stress, something that seemed to me insoluble. As so frequently is true, a case could be made for that.

Despite these glowing testimonials to my blooming health, she picked up her appointment book at the end of the session, and suggested that we meet in two or possibly three weeks. Why, I asked her, should we be meeting if I was in such excellent condition? "Dr. Appelbaum," she said, with an emotional tremor in her voice, "you were so sick." To put it more succinctly than she was able or willing to do, she concluded that once a person is "so sick," that person should always be sure to keep up their level of energy, and to work on their capacity to gather energy from the environment. One should not wait until their energy is depleted before building it up again, and, in effect, that person is potentially at greater risk than those who have never been so run-down.

In the course of a meandering conversation about travel, she said she would like to go to Japan and learn about Shiatsu. I pointed out that she was, in part at least, practicing Shiatsu at those times when she worked with her hands on points of the body that corresponded to organs which were at a distance from where she was working. "Oh," she said, "that must come from my Japanese doctor who guides me." She then told me about a group of doctors whom she "sees" and who are responsible for her deciding what to do with patients. "Don't you think," she asked me sweetly, "before civilization spoiled us, we had all kinds of abilities?" I suppose she meant that civilization had provided goods and services to the point that the skills necessary to provide them on one's own had atrophied. A good case can be made for psychic abilities having atrophied through lack of need for them, just as the sense of smell did. Some of us, such as Dr. Pfeiffer, she went on to say, have retained such capacities. However, they learned as children to keep quiet about their skills in order to avoid becoming considered peculiar or sick, and even in adulthood had to be careful when and where to reveal psychic capacities.

I had another firsthand opportunity to observe Dr. Pfeiffer's work and apparent results. As a preamble, here are some reflections on the anecdotal citations of single cases as done by Dr. Pfeiffer and others.

Most non-traditional healers try to make up for their lack of scientific buttressing of their healing activities with anecdotal citations of single cases. Seemingly oblivious of the need for control groups and blind studies, of the existence of uncontrolled variables, of the possibilities for inaccurate reporting and wishful thinking, and of the profit motive, they implicitly subscribe to the wisdom embedded in the aphorism that a thousand deaths is a statistic while a single death is a tragedy; or, in the instance of healing, a thousand cured patients is a statistic, while the report of a single healing, especially when it is reported dramatically, is an occasion for joy and belief. Characteristically, the proffering of the single case is offered dramatically, knowingly, and as proof sublime that the favorite remedy is effective. The typical anecdotal presentation has the rhythm, pattern, and inexorability of a Passion Play. The listener, never in doubt of the outcome, nonetheless is mesmerized by the familiar scenario — conventional medicine fails to help the sick person, brand X of non-traditional healing comes down from heaven as a *deux ex machina,* and now the erstwhile patient who used not to be able to walk can run, can hold two jobs while once unemployable, eats instead of starves, eliminates instead of constipates, or no longer exhibits any signs of the disease even on CAT scan or X-ray, much to the befuddlement of the traditional physician who originally gave up on the patient. And like the Passion Play, despite scientific or secular skepticism, the anecdotally presented single case can be persuasive; it can make the hopeful heart beat faster.

A friend of mine had urinary frequency and urgency to the point that she occasionally lost control of her urine. Both she and several physicians made the usual mistakes, some preventable, some simply inherent in the practice of empirical medicine. She used some old, perhaps outdated antibiotics on the assumption that she had an infection. A physician prescribed another antibiotic while waiting for the results of a test that her history suggested might reveal the source of her symptoms. He failed to learn about her susceptibility to side effects from that prescribed medicine; she developed symptoms from the medicine to go with the symptoms she was taking the medicine to cure. He prescribed another antibiotic which, while it did not produce side effects, did not do much for the original symptoms either. When the tests came back negative, she sought out a urologist who recommended other and more searching tests. He did a cystoscopy (insertion of a bulb through the urethra that makes possible a visual scan of the area), an intravenous pyelogram (ingestion of dye and a series of x-rays of the dyed area), a urinary stress test (learning the effect on the movement of urine of coughing or other bodily stress), and a cystometrogram (measuring bladder muscle tone by filling the bladder with water and having the patient push down). None of these fully clarified the situation. But he did learn that her bladder was squeezed as if, he said, something was pressing down on it thus reducing its effective size and interfering with collection and retention of urine. "I don't want to scare you," he said, "but we should do a pelvic sonogram to see whether a tumor or mass is pressing down on the bladder." At this point the patient was ready for a tranquilizer. Instead, she was, as physicians are wont to say candidly but disquietingly, "tried" on another medicine, again without ascertaining her susceptibility to side effects. And again she became ill from the medicine, or maybe it was from the fear engendered by his "I don't want to scare you ..." remark. Her symptoms worsened during the three days before the sonogram could be performed. The embarrassment that this fastidious lady endured with such symptoms can be easily imagined. It is less easy for most of us to imagine fully the terror that she felt upon being informed that she might have a tumor or mass. What a boon to medical consumers it would be if only in some eight years of medical school, internship, and residency the curriculum would include instructions about language and the mind so that such locutions as "I don't want to scare you ..." might be avoided. If someone says, "I don't want to interrupt you, but ..." you know you are going to be interrupted. As Freud said, there is no "no" in the unconscious. To the unconscious, "I don't" means, "I do." For example, "It's not that I don't like you" means "*I don't like you,*" and every unconscious knows it. How much more humane it would have been for the physician to say simply that we need another test to explain the symptom to figure out how best to help you, or something of the sort. It might have been necessary to frighten the patient if she had been reluctant to agree to such diagnostic procedures as were needed. Such was not the case here; the patient was willing to continue to submit to further procedures. There was nothing to be gained in talking about tumors and masses at that point,

The physician's ordering of tests raises the question of what and how many tests one should order to, on the one hand, protect the patient, and on the other not to over-diagnose with attendant risks, anxiety, and expense. It is an open secret that physicians in recent years have become increasingly frightened of making mistakes with their patients. To a point, they always have been frightened of that; after all, they chose work designed to help and not hurt people, and they administer an inexact, often largely empirical, science. (The penalty paid by patients for mistakes, however, is not relative, theoretical, abstract, or inexact.) Now, however, the gritty reality of the threat of malpractice suits forces physicians to leave precious few stones unturned, sometimes protecting themselves against error at the expense of protecting the patient against unnecessary tests. This patient could have an undetected cancer, as could anybody at any given time. All the physician needs to hear is a complaint that suggests that the patient might have cancer, and that physician then feels the malevolent judging eye of the law. Unfortunately, symptoms that could imply the presence of cancer are all too often symptoms that could eventuate from non-cancerous conditions: loss of appetite and weight, rash, cough, poor complexion, on and on. To neither over-order or under-order tests has now become the task for physicians who are artful as well as learned, and also brave.

The day before the scheduled sonogram I arranged that my friend be examined by Dr. Pfeiffer. I told myself that at the least I would have an opportunity to research his diagnostic skill, for presumably we would soon have a medical diagnosis to serve as a criterion. Or maybe I chose to think about this excursion that way while more or less realizing that I was seizing on this emotionally neutral and intellectual reason as a bulwark against what otherwise might have been terror.

Genial as always, and accommodatingly letting us come at 8:00 P.M. at the end of his long day, Dr. Pfeiffer glanced over a medical information form that my friend had filled out in his waiting room. From that he learned of her symptoms, and nothing else of relevance. As I could affirm, even with my untrained eye, her legs as measured at the heels were uneven. He made them even by manipulating her hip, remarking that the manipulation that he was using would affect bladder control and that the "outage" she demonstrated also causes bedwetting in children. As usual, his assistant placed the magnets on the skin above the organ he was assessing, and he compared leg lengths for each setting. He found, as he frequently does, a hiatal hernia which, he remarked, causes colitis among other things. He claimed that he fixed that hernia through further manipulations which took only a few minutes. He pronounced her lungs, pituitary gland, spleen, pancreas, and kidneys healthy, and said that she had good blood circulation with no sign of aneurysm. Only a slightly malfunctioning adrenal marred the picture of healthy organs. He told her that she need not worry about having cancer, though to this point he had no way of knowing that was on our minds. Perhaps he assumed that it is on everybody's mind. I asked why he deleted the seed pit test so crucial to his testing for cancer. He replied that there never is a malignancy in the presence of a good pancreas, and with the other key indicators such as the pituitary and spleen being healthy also, there was no point to giving the seed pit. He did, however, then put the infamous seed pit in the tray on her chest. He showed me how her suddenly unequal legs evidenced a rejection of the seed pit which, in the absence of cancer, he said, is poisonous. He gave as the reason for the bladder symptoms an abnormal placement of the bladder, perhaps as a result of a previous operation, which in fact she had had. Just as the urologist did, he offered a mechanical explanation for her symptoms. But he and the urologist would have no doubt diverged with regard to treatment. According to Dr. Pfeiffer, the bladder required lifting and tilting to the left, which he did through manipulation.

My friend tends somewhat toward uncritical believing, and under these circumstances understandably was willing to suspend any remnants of disbelief in favor of great relief at being told she did not have cancer. My relief was great, too, though it had to battle its way past my skepticism. While I was encouraged that Dr. Pfeiffer did not diagnose everyone as having cancer, where were the independent confirmations of the evidence and means of gathering evidence on the basis of which he made his pronouncements? Wasn't it too good to be true that he could come to *any* definitive diagnosis so quickly, painlessly, and inexpensively?

The next day, as fate would have it, my friend presented herself for the sonogram only to learn that it could not be given because she had eaten that day. Someone had forgotten to instruct her to fast. She decided against the sonogram. She did so perhaps partly because she took the mix-up on the instructions as a sign, linked with her happy diagnosis of the night before. But most of all, she was in no mood to undergo the sonogram because her symptoms had greatly diminished in severity beginning almost immediately after Dr. Pfeiffer's treatment. Unless one credited suggestion or other psychological factors, it looked as if Dr. Pfeiffer's manipulations had done the trick. Her symptoms continued to be greatly improved, and she is happily taking Dr. Pfeiffer's prescribed vitamins and minerals (only a small fraction of the many that he had prescribed for me), even more happily believing that she is free of malignancy. All this joy, relief, and physical improvement cost her $37, including examination, treatment, and several bottles of tablets.

Rationality cries out that a single case proves nothing — she may indeed have cancer, the remission of symptoms being a temporary fluke, and she may be in greater trouble for having lost possibly valuable treatment time; her symptoms may have been caused and cured through psychological means unrelated to the bladder anomaly and the treatment for it; the symptoms might have abated without Dr. Pfeiffer's intervention. Yes, in the absence of reasonable evidence, it is irrational to submit merely to the wish to believe. Yet that kind of irrationality is difficult to stave off when one glows with improved health and with the encouragement that healing is indeed available outside the expensive, often painful, official health care system. The theater, another crucible for teaching values and offering knowledge and beliefs, is also founded on the persuasive presentation of the single case. Perhaps good medicine is in part good theater.

How to think about these wondrous experiences with Dr. Pfeiffer? One way is to assume that Dr. Pfeiffer and his diagnostic and therapeutic approach are invalid. He and his followers may mean well, but they simply are a misguided, self-deluding lot. I was, therefore, unnecessarily put through the wringer. There is much about the situation, obviously, to compel that attitude. Is it true that each peach pit equals a thousand milligrams of laetrile, for example? Does the cancerous or pre-cancerous body crave laetrile, leaping to its presence with an extended leg? Who else in the scientific or therapeutic community says so, on the basis of what evidence?

Another possibility is that Dr. Pfeiffer's diagnostic acumen is invalid, but his dietary and vitamin and mineral supplements program are excellent contributions to health. As a result of his diagnosis of me, I followed that program; I was even more open than in the past to other therapeutic possibilities and cancer prevention programs; and I took more seriously than ever the challenge of preventing illness and maximizing health. I might have gotten the right medicine from the wrong diagnosis.

A third possibility is that his diagnosis was valid and his treatment based on it was effective; thus he had saved my life.

What being pre-cancerous means exactly is difficult to say. Some theorists declare that all of us are pre-cancerous, and in fact somewhere between one in three and one in two of us in the next couple of decades will demonstrate unmistakably that they were in a pre-cancerous state by becoming unmistakably cancerous. Or, I could have been pretty far along toward cancer, if not *in extremis*. Assuming that I was pre-cancerous or had a cancer, what could Dr. Pfeiffer have done differently or better with respect to how I was informed and the emotional consequences of that? If he had chosen not to tell me about it, and yet believed that I had cancer, that would have been wrong, even though I was only a demonstration subject. He did not necessarily have to tell me in front of the group as part of the demonstration, and therefore in such a way as to get me as confused and frightened as I was. He commented on that, somewhat sheepishly, suggesting that he had to do it because it was a demonstration, he had to let the people know the meaning of his findings. He could, however, put it in terms of probabilities; after all, he does not have a research basis for his inferences, only clinical experience with a limited number and possibly biased selection of subjects. He says that his grouping of signs — impaired organs and acceptance of the seed pit — are seen in patients with clinical malignancies. That does not necessarily mean that all people with the signs have clinical malignancies. He may see mainly the ones who come with clinical malignancies.

As to the setting, style, and manner of informing me, I resent having had to seek him out in that ballroom and wait for what seemed to me an interminable length of time while he played with his friends and chiropractic machines. When we did finally find a reasonably quiet corner of the ballroom to discuss it, he again chose to put his diagnosis flatly, with no suggestion of probabilities, no respect for any limitations of research and experience, no opening for exceptions. And as to having the procedure done over as a check on his results, I was asked to wait some six weeks to see him again, presumably taking my place behind those with chronic mild conditions and checkups. Would I have paid any attention if he had been less blunt? There are some people who in fear would dismiss out of hand any suggestion of having cancer. I would not have reacted that way, and he could have found that out, increasing his bluntness only as necessary.

I realize that I am suggesting here a high level of professionalism with respect to working with people psychologically and diplomatically. Many people say that medical physicians as a group do not function on that level either. While better organized, with better forms and structures to guide them than chiropractors, many medical physicians also seem strangely at a loss when it comes to dealing with patients as people. Holistic health practitioners have given organized voice to the criticisms that previously only family and friends have shared; especially in recent years, patients in the hands of conventional medicine feel that they are merely on an assembly line, their complaints objects of ever greater specialization. As people, rather than simply bearers of complaints, they feel lost to the coldness of physicians who are either openly rejecting or cover that attitude with a patina of forced and mechanical friendliness. And to judge from the many times that it has been brought informally to my attention, physicians frequently inform people that they or their relatives have a life-threatening disease in a way that could be greatly improved upon.

From one point of view, chiropractors might be expected to treat their patients with even less empathy than do physicians. They, themselves, are treated as second-class citizens, professionally, and may tend to treat others as they are treated. That is not to say that chiropractors are equal to physicians in terms of their training and overall therapeutic effectiveness. In some respects they clearly are not, while in other respects they may be a better source of health. Technical equality is less the issue than is the unempathetic, unfeeling lash with which people assault others. There is far too much of that in lots of professions. Within his own context, Dr. Pfeiffer is a highly respected leader. For him there is little precedent and few models for a humanitarian, psychological approach to patients. His perhaps maladroit treatment of me at that one point in our relationship is his fault only in a narrow sense. He is simply an instrument of a health-care system whose practitioners are more oriented towards technology than people, and who are rewarded for that orientation.

Reaching all the way to Japan there are coteries of professional adherents devoted to the theory and practice set forth by Dr. Pfeiffer. People's lives are being saved or lost by those coteries, people are being frightened necessarily or unnecessarily by them, people are expending money and often opportunities for other treatments wisely or foolishly when in their care. These practitioners charge along, parallel to other healing disciplines, not offering what of value they may have to other healers and the healing discipline at large, nor being subjected to the usual standards, however imperfect, of disinterested people employing the scientific method and amalgamating the experience of various practitioners with various groupings of patients. In a sensible, to say nothing of humanitarian, health care system, such confusedly unrestrained individualism would not be tolerated. My being terrified in the darkness of ignorance was an expression of all of us who are prey to illnesses without adequate knowledge of what to do about them. Dr. Pfeiffer told me that he had tried to interest the local chiropractic college in researching his work, but to no avail. To the extent that there is lack of interest in studying different approaches to diagnosis and treatment, medicine becomes increasingly a Bohemian art rather than an artistic application of science. Science, healing, practitioners, and patients all lose.

Chapter Eight
Affairs of the Heart: A Cardiovascular Adventure

PARTLY THROUGH THE INFLUENCE of holistic medicine, asking one's physician for a second opinion has become more and more respectable, and is taken less and less as an accusation of incompetence. Salutary as such a development is, it has only scratched the surface of the problem of how to decide what, if any, supposedly therapeutic procedure one should subject one's body to. Underneath the rock of homogeneity and monolithic *medical opinion* squirm the worms of the truth: there are many medical, and non-medical, opinions about diagnosis and treatment of the body. This is true even for those practitioners who fly the flag of science, supposedly grounded in scientific research, to say nothing of those practitioners who are avowedly unscientific.

Why such widely differing opinions? Note how often practitioners use such phrases as, "In my experience," "I have found …". What goes on here? On paper, therapeutic interventions are prescribed on the basis of research and accumulated experience from the field as codified and systematically taught. Yet one's local practitioner may make it seem that one is conducting one's own one-person research and accumulator of experience. And so, often, one is. The sad truth is that researches are regularly contradicted by other researches. (One major uncontrolled variable is the style, manner, or personality of the therapist.) Thus, practitioners who tell patients, "in my opinion," correctly cite the source of their evidence. Beyond the at least relatively well established remedies, practitioners prescribe according to their prejudices, whether they came by these prejudices by way of their personalities, or how they have been trained.

Again, in violation of the surface presentation of homogeneity, different modes of thought are purveyed by different schools. Variations in training, practices, and emphases can be found in different parts of the country and world. And all opinions are subject to how current the practitioner is and how much corrective contact is maintained with others in the profession. As a result of these realities of healing, once past the fantasy that doctor knows best, the patient has to recognize being on their own. As a small example of a large issue, take the following affair of the heart.

I have always enjoyed having my blood pressure taken and smugly predicting 120 systolic and 80 diastolic, which is roughly analogous to an "A" on a test in school. I was mortified, therefore, when during an annual physical I was told that my diastolic was up to 95. That meant that I had "mild hypertension," which put me in a group with millions of Americans who, among other things, are enjoined to leave salt out of their diet. There had to be some mistake, I said, and the physician agreed there might indeed be some mistake since I had just been subject to other stressful diagnostic procedures. I kept to myself the observation that blood pressures might better be taken *before* rather than after such procedures. But a repeat measurement yielded only a slight improvement. The internist told me that I could lower my blood pressure by taking a drink of alcohol a day or by exercising. Those were, he said in response to my pressing him on this point, my only options; my condition was not serious enough to warrant medicine. Since I tend to be comfortably sedentary, and under the influence of holistic nutrition not much of a drinker either, neither option entranced me. At an insurance physical some weeks later, however, undaunted I again predicted my usual sparklingly low blood pressure and was this time confirmed. A gold star, and this one rewarded me with an insurance policy also.

Despite my reservations about conventional medicine, some of my best friends, as they say, are doctors. One is a specialist in cardiovascular matters, especially blood lipids. According to him, cholesterol as measured routinely, "total cholesterol," yields little worthwhile information. Breakdowns of total cholesterol into LDL, or low-density lipids, and HDL, high-density lipids, tell the physician what he needs to know. These readings, and the ratio between them, may indicate a cholesterol disturbance, even when the total cholesterol is normal, or no such disturbance when total cholesterol is abnormal. One of my readings taken by him was aberrant, which meant little to my friend, much more to my pride. He smiled wryly at the option of taking a drink of alcohol each day, and urged me to exercise. I had, naturally, heard that before. Holistic health practitioners and devotees recommend exercise for the prevention and treatment of almost any illness. In the peculiar way that so many people have of resisting doing what even they agree is good for them, I had resisted that suggestion with the usual blather of being too busy. This time, under the goad of the cholesterol reading, I joined a health club where I worked out three times a week.

While gathering information about the activities of a holistic physician, I noted his new infrared thermography machine. He proudly reported that with this machine connected to a video camera he could instantly portray one's head on a television screen and tell by variations in light and dark the likelihood that that person would suffer a stroke. He made that prediction on the basis of how clogged or unclogged blood vessels appeared. Naturally, I had to try it, but I should have told him that I don't photograph well on the left side. Sure enough, in the midst of all that reassuring whiteness in my head indicating unobstructed flow of blood, there was some wash-day grey — 50 to 60 percent chance of stroke, he trumpeted. To a physician, holistic practitioner or no, that comment was all in a day's work, but such comments mean a good deal more to the receiver of such information. What was needed, he said, was the clearing out of plaque from the blood vessels. This, he said, could be accomplished through chelation.

Chelation was not entirely unknown to me. Another physician friend claimed that through chelation he had recovered from a severe heart attack which had left him, according to conventional medical practitioners, with very little time to live. Chelation is not entirely unknown to conventional medicine, either; it has traditionally been used for detoxifying lead poisoning or radiation, and is approved for these purposes by the Food and Drug Administration. However, a small number of physicians and a moderately large number of chiropractors maintain that the same cleansing mechanism that makes chelation a good antidote against heavy metal poisoning makes it equally beneficial against hardening of the arteries. My conventional internist made it clear that he neither knew nor cared about chelation. Patients are on their own.

The therapy consists of intravenous injections of a synthesized amino acid called ethylene diamine tetracetic acid, or EDTA. The substance locks onto, or chelates, the plaques and causes them to release their hold on the internal wall of the arteries. Calcium ions and cholesterol, among other debris, make up these plaques. EDTA also pulls calcium from other areas of the body where it is abnormally deposited, such as tendons, joints and ligaments, but supposedly does not remove calcium from the bones and teeth. Chelation enthusiasts claim that symptoms due to atherosclerosis improve with chelation — blood pressure becomes normal, hands and feet grow warm, kidney problems and the chances of stroke and heart attack are greatly reduced. Chelation injections are given over a period of months, some twenty to fifty, with each injection taking several hours. Alleged high gain at indisputably high cost: one spends several thousand dollars and lots of time, to say nothing of boredom, while sitting quietly for the necessary hours. According to its proponents, EDTA chelation is entirely safe, as demonstrated by more than two hundred thousand physicians who are members of the American Academy of Medical Preventics.[1,2]

There is, of course, another side to the story. Most of the medical profession is indifferent to chelation, and some physicians are openly contemptuous of it. Another of my physician acquaintances, who seems to me to be authoritative in many areas of medicine, warned me that chelation therapy is not only useless, but most likely dangerous. He cited recent research purporting to show that chelation washes out needed calcium along with harmful calcium.

Let us ponder our plight. This last physician friend said that he just happened to have seen that research report; he would probably have missed it, he said, if we had not recently discussed chelation. So what of the patients of the many practitioners who recommend chelation and who did not just happen to see the report? "Don't worry," one of them replied to this question, "it's only one research and has not been replicated; someone else will probably publish contradictory results." Other practitioners whom I know would dismiss the negative report with the dark suspicion that the A.M.A. or other Establishment group was behind the whole thing. Rational and resigned explanations for such an irrational state of affairs can be set forth. But in the meantime, patients are on their own.

Many practitioners of chelation insist on a diagnostic study to determine whether chelation is needed, and likely to be of value. Others, such as the physician who put me on his television receiver and predicted stroke, are sufficiently confident of the preventive powers of chelation therapy to recommend it not only to those with symptoms of atherosclerosis, but to anyone interested in preventing a long list of diseases. He makes such recommendations without a diagnostic work-up. In other words, debate, questionably substantiated beliefs, and idiosyncratic practices dictate what is done with the patient's health. The patients are on their own.

Maybe because I am skeptical about most material that appears on television, I found it difficult to get too worked up about my supposed 50 to 60 percent chance of having a stroke on any given day. But then there was that jumping-around blood pressure and the aberrant LDL reading. So I signed up for a plythesmograph and Doppler Study ($125 compared to another practitioner's $300. It pays to shop around). These two procedures give detailed measurements of the peripheral vascular system, and are recommended as ways to determine the advisability of chelation. They test the blood flow in different parts of the body and at different depths, which yields blood-pressure measurements from different arteries, and automatically records print-outs of blood flow.

Dr. Conley, the chiropractor in charge, was a cheery sort. I was in a good mood, and the whole procedure promised to be fun and productive of a gold star. Dr. Conley's first observation after scrutinizing my body: "You look jaundiced." Oh, no, I thought, images of Dr. Pfeiffer dancing in my head. Do chiropractors look at the world through yellow-colored glasses? We then decided that I might have the remnants of a suntan, or maybe, as a color expert has told me, I need red, pink, or blue to pep up my somewhat sallow complexion. I felt clammy clutches around my heart as he began to listen to it through his stethoscope. "Do you exercise?" he asked. What the hell did that mean, I wondered, as I murmured that I did a bit of exercise every two days at a fitness center, and wondered whether that qualified as exercise or whether he was talking about miles of daily running. "That's good," he said, "because with such a slow heart, if you didn't exercise, you would have big trouble." Jaundice and heart trouble! A number of measurements later, when he expostulated something or other, I wearily asked what he was responding to this time. "I have never," he said, "seen as good a set of measurements as you outside of a textbook." He later showed me how the squiggles and jiggles on the graph of my blood flow corresponded almost exactly to the ideal portrayal in the texts. He said that I had the cardiovascular system of a person in his twenties. When I told about the prediction of stroke, he could hardly believe it. "Your chances of having a stroke," he said, "are nil." I could hardly wait to take my report card home.

So, again, wildly conflicting opinions, sometimes from members of the same profession, sometimes from groups differing in their orientation, each one suggesting a different course of action, each one able to say, in hindsight, that the person should have followed his advice instead of the other advice. Some shrug off these discrepancies as the regrettable but unavoidable cost of specialization. To the whole person, with an illness embedded in, or expressing the total system, that argument is at best irrelevant, and at worst cruel sophistry. Such attitudes on the part of both conventional and unconventional healing serve to put the patient on notice. The fittest of the species survives in part by meeting and mastering the dangers of the healing jungle. Patients are on their own.

Chapter Nine
That Old Black Magic: Voodoo Healing in Haiti

AT THE MENTION OF voodoo, what comes to many people's minds is sticking pins in dolls in order to harm the people that the dolls represent, or deaths whose cause is inexplicable to Western medicine and is sometimes explained as a consequence of hopelessness, and in general an aura of mystery, fear, and spookiness. In addition to these conceptions (which are, surprisingly, based largely on fact), voodoo is also (1) a blend of Roman Catholicism and African tribal religions, with a strong admixture of magic and superstition; (2) an expression of the power of mind over body, in other words, psychosomatic medicine; (3) a community health system in Haiti; (4) a means of labor supply (zombies); and (5) an informal legal system.

Magic flourishes where people are most besieged with a feeling of powerlessness, which historically has been pronounced in terribly unequal struggles between people and nature. Living close to uncontrollable nature, Black Africans developed elaborate magical and superstitious religions. When these Africans were enslaved by the Europeans, they no doubt found even greater reason to feel controlled by external circumstances, and so held fast to their religion in order to sustain them in their new horrifying existence. Traditional practices also provided some measure of identity, some sense of self, in a system that was designed to reduce people to the impersonality of chattels. The slave owners, perhaps sensing in this a current which would work against their interests, tried to extirpate their slaves' traditional practices. When the owners were Catholic, their proselytizing tradition suggested conversion as a logical means of attempting to destroy the African identity. That task was facilitated, as it first appeared, by some similarities between Catholicism and African religions: both included a Supreme Being and a pantheon of deities or saints who were said to be available to help with immediate needs and accessible through daily prayer and rituals; both included malevolent devilish forces; both were highly ritualistic, the rosary beads, icons, and symbolic acts of the Catholics corresponding to the talismans and use of fetishes by the Africans. But unlike the Spanish South and Central American Indians, who converted to Catholicism, the African slaves stubbornly retained their native beliefs. They became only nominally and superficially Catholics. In some places, such as Haiti, going to church became a status symbol of the elite; in their hearts and in their practices the Africans worked out a blend of religions which became voodoo. In Haiti the Christian deity, Bondieu, heads the voodoo hierarchy, and Catholic services not infrequently begin with the voodoo prayer for the dead. The mecca of voodoo was and is Haiti, the Black republic sharing the island of Hispaniola with the white and Indian mestizo Dominican Republic. In Haiti, conditions for the development of voodoo were ideal: proselytizing French Catholics and Black slaves, the same mixture which produced voodoo in Louisiana.

In voodoo as in Black Africa and elsewhere, the line between religion and magical healing is blurred; illness is considered one of the great uncontrollable forces of nature that require divine intervention. I was intrigued, therefore, by a mailed flyer announcing an expedition to Haiti in order to study voodoo healing, to be guided by Stanley Krippner, a psychologist, author, and expert on folk healing with whom I was somewhat acquainted. The AIDS scare intervened; the tour was cancelled. But Stanley was willing to pass on to me the names of his voodoo connections.

Things are not what they seem in Haiti. Let us pass quickly over then-President-for-Life Duvalier's pretense of running a republic (one could not even walk near his palace without armed guards shooing one away); let us further pass briefly over the fact that the price of anything and everything in Haiti, at least to a foreigner, never turns out to be what it seemed at the start of the weary bargaining. It is as if every taxi driver is out to redress the wrongs of imperialism; every tourist finds himself the unwilling bearer of his own Marshall Plan.

Let us pass directly to the fiction that Haiti has a Western health care system. That is the official claim, to the point that the practitioners of alternative healing who make up the real health care system — voodoo — can be summarily thrown in jail for practicing medicine without a license. The fictitiousness of the government's position stands revealed by the fact that, at least a few years ago, there were only 513 licensed physicians in Haiti to treat 6 million people, 90 percent of the country was without electricity, and in the other 10 percent the supply of electricity was unreliable. Thus, there could not be, for example, penicillin and such other drugs that require storage at dependable, electrically-controlled temperatures; there was little X-ray equipment; in short, much of the medical edifice that requires electricity is unsupportable in Haiti. The fact is that, in a grand change of perspective, the term "traditional medicine" in Haiti should refer not to Western traditional medicine but to voodoo, the traditional medicine for centuries which continues to this day to minister to the health care needs of Haitians despite the claims of the "progressive" state apparatus.

Whether Western medicine is actually progressive, as compared to voodoo, is worthy of debate. As a mixture of religion and magic, with ancient roots in Black Africa, voodoo can be considered "not progressive" when progress refers to modern and technological progress. But progress can refer to possible effectiveness, minimal side effects, low cost, easy availability, and the taking into account of mind and spirit as well as body. From that point of view, voodoo can be considered progressive, possibly even more so than Western medicine.

Things turn out not to be what they seem in Haiti with regard to the task of finding authentic voodoo rather than the watered-down versions retailed to tourists. The guidebook authors that I read recommended touristy nightclub voodoo shows, with the understanding that the real thing — the sacrifice of live animals, for example — is available only to indigenous Haitians, particularly in rural areas. According to the guidebooks and others, genuine voodoo is semi-secret. Why? Because it is a religion, and thus should not be made available for a price to casual onlookers with cameras and a taste for the exotic, people uninterested in the faith or the needs of a people. Moreover, as with psychotherapy, voodoo healing may include personal confession, and be dependent upon an intensely emotional relationship with the therapist, the *hougan*, which is the name for the voodoo priest or healer or witch doctor or medicine man. Such a personal interaction should no more be made public than should a psychoanalytic session. Finally, voodoo includes the capacity to do harm, and some of its activities are blatantly illegal. Its practitioners claim that they can work against targeted people, whether in seeing to it that a lawsuit is declared in favor of the client employing voodoo services, or in seeing to it that someone is killed. It works in some respects like Murder Incorporated used to do: for a price, anyone can be expunged. The major difference, at least as explained to me by one of its practitioners, is that he and other hougans first must satisfy themselves as to the justice of their client's cause. In that way voodoo is a quasi-legal system, albeit a questionable one in that the hougan hears only the client's side of the case. Still, the ethical hougan insists that he will do no evil.

Thus apprised of its elusiveness, I assumed that in order to learn about real voodoo in Haiti I would need special contacts. Since things are never what they seem to be in Haiti, these contacts produced only a semi-authentic and limited experience fit for tourists. I found what at least seemed to me to be the real thing from a taxi driver.

The friend of a friend on the telephone who arranged my meeting with Madame C assured me that Madame C was an authentic *mambo*, or voodoo priestess. She certainly lived in an authentic Haitian slum; though perhaps it was a slum only by American standards — most of Port-au-Prince looked as it did. The inevitable grasping and surly taxi driver dropped me and my interpreter off on a torn-up side street at a door to a tiny courtyard packed with lots of furniture, food, and plants in disarray. The old woman seated there nodded toward a half-outside, half-inside hovel. There Madame C was conducting what appeared to be a counseling session with a middle-aged woman who evidently had stopped in on her way home from work for her session. Madame C looked like Aunt Jemima and had some of the charm and implicit stature and wisdom of a Hollywood mammy. She resembled many of the other healers I had studied in that she was overweight and loquacious, her speech revolving peripherally and tangentially around the flickering point.

Madame C spoke French. My French is not worth speaking of, so what I learned from her was filtered through my interpreter. Some of it, according to Madame C, was from the spirits, filtered in turn through her as a medium. As we took off our shoes, according to instructions, preparatory to entering one of several rooms made up like shrines surrounding the center of the house, Madame C sprinkled us with a few drops of water. "Only the

Eternal can make water," she explained. The room in which we settled was so packed with tiers of religious artifacts, icons, pictures and statues of Jesus, there was only just about enough room for us to sit down. My interpreter and I were almost immediately told that we were mystics, had "strong forces," and were clairvoyant; Madame C could see that I had "a sign" — we were special people. I thought sorrowfully about how often I had been told such things by psychics. Of course, it could be true about me, I like to think, but my companion and friends of friends who visit psychics all seem to be, in the view of the psychics, worthy of the same commendation. Unless we are all saints, such remarks seem designed to make us feel good and receptive to parting with money. All of which does not mean that the purveyors of such business practices do not also heal. Indeed, healing may be abetted by such compliments; compliments may have the power of any other of the ingredients of a good bedside manner.

Madame C let us know straightaway that there was a hierarchy of mediums, priests and priestesses, not unlike that of psychoanalytic candidates, graduate analysts, and training and supervising analysts. Only at the end of the training, at its topmost tier, did the priest become privy to all of the secrets. Madame C herself was so special that the spirits, called *loas*, had inflicted bruises on her legs, which she showed us, as punishment for at one time not practicing voodoo.

She gave credit to one spirit, named Ghede, in particular as being responsible for her healing. She took us to a room in the cellar that housed his clothing, a wooden phallus and baby bottle that he liked to play with, and she offered us a drink — something on the order of tequila — that he particularly enjoyed. She took a drink herself to show me that it was harmless, but down there in that dank basement, I just wasn't thirsty. Apparently, Ghede is a card, addicted to playing with these toys, eating and drinking, singing, dancing, and joking around at the party Madame C gives for his annual November visit.

Ghede and Madame C spend a good deal of time healing infirmities brought about by evil spirits at the behest of evil voodoo practitioners. Evidently, much of the voodoo health care system is devoted to undoing illnesses brought about by members of that same system. Madame C cast herself on the side of the angels. She claimed that she would paralyze only wrongdoers in order to stop them from hurting her patients. In other words, her voodoo weapons were for defensive purposes only. She would not cast an evil spell and would have nothing to do with zombies either. She explained that zombies were possessed by evil spirits. They were buried at midday and released from the grave by the spirits at midnight, and were thus alive, but with something missing in their makeup that renders them without will so that they become virtual slaves. Thus, descendents of slaves have incorporated in their practices the creating of slaves. In psychoanalysis this is called identifying with the aggressor — a way of reassuring oneself, by becoming the victimizer, that one is not a victim.

Madame C said that she had merely to look in my eyes to see whether any illness I might have was the work of evil spirits. She would diagnose illnesses not caused by evil spirits by feeling my pulse. How, I wondered, had pulse diagnosis, the traditional means of diagnosis in Chinese medicine for thousands of years, found its way into voodoo healing? My pulse revealed to Madame C that I sometimes feel uneasy, especially after eating. She said that I felt bad and tired from small annoyances in my life, one of these being that many people love me but at the same time are envious of me. From the last, she said, stems my "anguish."

She several times repeated that I was the unhappy object of envy, and this envy was supposed to be sapping what she said was my great strength. All of this was on the basis of her reading of me through the use of Tarot cards. This reading entailed my cutting the cards into stacks of three, which she turned over so the pictures could be seen. The pictures thus revealed were supposed to be revealing. What was initially revealed to Madame C was that I was not "purely American; I had mixed blood" — like the rest of my 250 million fellow citizens, excepting some Native Americans. I was, according to her, helpful to a lot of people (she had heard me addressed as Doctor). But some people who claimed to love me were just hypocritical. (Probably so, but hardly exclusive to me.) Was I a widower, she asked. (No.) Did I have two children? (Yes.) Perhaps Madame C should not be judged too harshly; she said the spirits were having trouble getting close to me because of what she assured me was my vigorous sex life. She advised me to forego sex, especially on Thursday and Saturday (TGIF immediately took on added significance). She said that I was involved in legal matters with two men; this information was precisely correct. According to her they had taken advantage of me because I was truthful, which I believe is a good approximation of the facts. Because of the imminent danger from the men, she suggested that I keep on my person a perfume, a precious metal chain, and a particular handkerchief, that I take a potion and have a candle burning for me. The whole campaign was to be launched with a "lucky bath" given by herself which was to include Coca-Cola and flowers. "It is becoming very expensive to do voodoo," she said, as she quoted me $400 for the works, one-half now and one-half when I was sure she was successful. If that was too much, she said, she could give me the perfume and the bath for $140.

We were suddenly in a buying-an-automobile mode. When I did not accept her offer, she thought I was just temporizing instead of beating a retreat, and admonished me that I must make up my mind now; evidently, this was a one-day sale. My interpreter, having experienced many fewer of these readings than I, took a less jaundiced position toward the salesmanship aspect of Madame C's readings. Indeed, to the extent that her presentation is persuasive by way of suggestion, it may even be helpful with some people's difficulties. I had to remind myself that style might not be substance. Blatantly offensive or misleading advertising need not necessarily signal a poor product. That requires far different evidence. So much for the private information, the contacts, the assurances of authentic voodoo. While Madame C might be authentic in various ways, she did not epitomize the authentic voodoo about which I had heard and read.

Public information about voodoo came to me from a taxi driver, and from Aubelin Jolicouer, man-about-Port-au-Prince. When this boulevardier is not selling paintings in his gallery or jauntily twirling his stick, he hangs out in the lobby of the Grand Oloffson Hotel, a mecca for artists and show people. (The hotel bills itself as the Raffles of the Caribbean. I was put in the Budd Shulberg Room, by coincidence or psychic predestination, since Shulberg has for years been one of my favorite contemporary authors.) When Jolicouer learned of my healing interests, he regaled me with stories of his grandmother who was, in effect, the doctor for her area. She healed with prayer, roots, herbs, tree bark — and belief. Jolicouer said that he heals himself in these ways; he is convinced that his being convinced is the *sine qua non*. He put me in telephone touch with one of Haiti's few psychiatrists, who, it turned out, had been in his residency training program at the Menninger Foundation when I was there. I gathered from him that a cold war exists between the Western and voodoo health care systems. He said that voodoo practitioners do not like medical doctors to observe their work. For his part, he declared voodoo to be a form of psychodrama, with the implication that it was unworthy of the sustained interest of Western physicians.

Aubelin Jolicouer urged me to visit Le Peristyle, an outdoor theater, where voodoo ceremonies are put on nightly for tourists. I should, he said, talk privately with its owner, Max Beauvoir, who he said was an authentic intellectual and healer himself, not just a nightclub owner.

For once, something in Haiti seemed to be what it was supposed to be. Max Beauvoir is a Haitian, probably somewhere in his fifties. I met him in the gathering darkness of his outdoor nightclub–exhibition hall where his white clothing stood out from the darkness of his color and the night. He is built like a fullback, and has heavyweight intelligence also. He told me that he has a Bachelor of Arts in Chemistry from City College of New York, studied at the Sorbonne, worked as a biochemist at Cornell Medical Center in New York City, and holds a patent on a method for extracting cortisone from plants. He has been a hougan for thirteen years. He comes from a long line of mambos and hougans; his grandfather requested on his deathbed that Max carry on the family tradition. Symbolic of his shift from modern technology to indigenous methods, Beauvoir discovered that he can use the whole leaf from which he derived cortisone to better effect than he could the derivative, so he has replaced his new patented invention with old wisdom. Though modern in his outlook on medicine and psychology ("all diseases are psychosomatic"), he practices only voodoo medicine. He does so as a private practitioner, with patients coming from around the world as well as from Haiti. Joining in our conversation was his daughter, a student of anthropology at Tufts University, who is as knowledgeable and culturally sophisticated as her father. Before and after the evening's performance, the two of them oriented me toward an understanding of voodoo and its place in Haiti as a religion, health care system, provider of labor, and means of achieving justice. As a medical system, pressed into service through the unavailability of Western medical personnel and lack of electricity, voodoo was, according to the Beauvoirs, highly effective. Max Beauvoir believes that the thousands of leaves, roots, and barks, often mixed into potions, are specific remedies for the various ailments. They constitute a pharmacopeia derived from thousands of years' experience; indeed, many Western medicines are derived from such natural substances (e.g., quinine from bark). While as with any medical care system, some medicines are more effective with some ailments than others, there is little in the catalog of human ailments that voodoo practitioners believe is beyond them. For example, Beauvoir described how voodoo healers set bones without the use of conventional casts.

Beauvoir laid to rest the romantic notion of zombies as people raised, like Lazarus, from the dead. What really happens is that a supposed wrongdoer is slipped a substance made from fish testicles that is 160,000 times more powerful than cocaine and second only to botulin in its dangerousness to humans. Within five days from the supposed death and burial, the person is dug up, alive, but without their erstwhile capacity for willpower. The person is now a zombie, capable of performing labor at the behest of others, but of not much beyond what is necessary for survival. (For an account of this phenomenon, see *The Serpent and the Rainbow* by Wade Davis,[1] who reports that the toxin includes extract of toad skin.) As if anticipating my disapproval, Beauvoir pointed out that in so-called enlightened societies, wrongdoers are killed or caged for long periods of time. In voodoo justice, the taboo against killing is observed (never mind the Murder Incorporated aspects of voodoo; see below). The zombie may eventually be forgiven and freed, though I gather the loss of will, presumably reflecting neurological damage, is permanent. The problem with all this as a system of justice is, of course, the capricious, if not self-serving, manner of deciding who is a wrongdoer.

The same issue surfaces with regard to some of the services offered by voodoo practitioners, Beauvoir among them. For a price, people can be injured or killed from a distance, with or without the sticking of pins in the famous doll or other representation of the victim. Apart from assault and homicide, Beauvoir offers such services as seeing to it that one wins a lawsuit or, as in a recent case of his, that a natural mother should go ahead with her promise to give her baby up for adoption to Beauvoir's clients. Again, Beauvoir emphasized that what might seem unlawful and cruel was in the interests of justice. He said that he would not undertake any of these activities until he satisfied himself that he and his clients were in the right. Again, the obvious problem with that is that he hears only his clients' side of the story, to say nothing of the complexities of justice and moral relativism. But then, this may be only irrelevant carping. All these matters, Beauvoir said, are masterminded by the spirits; each individual has approximately seven of them, according to him. With the aid of such spirits, Beauvoir claimed to be able to tell the future, make physical diagnoses, and divine unconscious motivations. Unlike Madame C, he did not need Tarot cards for such purposes. Beauvoir believes in both the direct intervention of spirits and the effects of a patient's personality on his physical illness. The question of where one leaves off and the other begins is as foggy as the boundary between the physiological and psychological in Western medical diagnosis.

Beauvoir is a private practitioner of voodoo healing, much as I am a private practitioner of clinical psychology and psychoanalysis (his cards read "By Appointment Only"). He treats patients for a wide variety of physical and psychological complaints, and for legal and marital problems having ostensibly less to do with their health problems than with the difficult behavior of others. Beauvoir is nothing if not confident. He claims, for example, to have cured cancer, anorexia nervosa, and lupus erythematosus. When I asked what he could do with a variety of symptoms that I had from an internal disorder, he claimed that I would be relieved of the symptoms in six days without question. The treatment would consist of several baths and a medication in the form of a potion prepared especially for me. The cost would be $450, one-half payable at the start, the second half payable by mail as soon as I was completely satisfied. I thought, gloomily, of what measures he might take to enforce collection. The terms were similar to those of Madame C, but coming from this erudite, Western-educated, prepossessing man, they seemed more like a reasonable arrangement than car salesperson hype. Anyway, I was only making my cautious inquiries to him through force of habit and general interest. I knew that I could hardly pass up this chance to experience what gave promise of being an authentic voodoo healing ceremony. The time for the healing was set for the next morning, late in order for Beauvoir to get supplies that he said were selected especially for me.

That evening's nightclub ceremony was performed by a dozen or so men and women, with Beauvoir himself joining in from time to time. All the activities were propelled along by the practically nonstop beating of drums and rhythmic chanting. The ceremony began quietly and politely, and what with the white costumes accented with red decorations, reminded me of a Broadway musical. Gradually, however, the ceremony gathered momentum — the drums were louder, the dancing more abandoned, the chanting more insistent, until the participants had apparently put themselves into a trance. That trance state was the explanation given to me for the following event: Two of the participants held aloft a burning ember so that one could see them take bites out of it, clearly leaving behind in the embers the curved opening from which the embers burning in their mouths were taken. Seemingly unbelievable as the sight was, the explanation that they could do this because of being in a hypnotic trance could be accepted. Under hypnosis people perform a variety of seemingly impossible feats. For example, dentists reverse the flow of blood from patients' gums so that teeth can be extracted more easily; under hypnosis some subjects are impervious to heat and cold. However, Beauvoir further commented that the participants could pass along the power to withstand the heat of the flames to others who were not hypnotized. That was a lot harder for me to take. As if sensing my skepticism, a German doctor sitting next to me, who, he said, had been studying voodoo for over a month told me it was true, strange as it seemed. He himself had, after summoning his courage, been able to hold flame in his hands without ill effects while under the influence of a fire-eater.

In one of the dance rituals, a participant waved a chicken at the head of a commandeered member of the audience, who fled in horror at the flapping of wings around her face. Being busy with my camera, or unwilling to look, or some combination of the two, I failed to see what happened to the chicken. I was later to learn firsthand, but now it was just another detail in the phantasmagorical scene: the fire and fiery red bits of clothing set against white background and the black of skins and night. It was internally phantasmagorical for me as well; tilts in familiar reality do it every time.

The next morning, once past the gates, I saw that the voodoo theater was but one element in Beauvoir's compound. Here and there through his private jungle I saw his round, remarkably contemporary house, several buildings which he later identified as shrines, and then his consulting room. Except for the outside environment, Beauvoir, in front of his bookshelves and over his desk, could have been a mental health practitioner in his private office anywhere in the industrial world. Our initial conversation could have taken place in any such office anywhere as well: how business was, where his referrals came from, recent cases, the variety of services offered. Collecting the half-payment in advance was, of course, a difference; as was my dropping my American Express checks into a ceremonial bowl.

Another of Beauvoir's daughters appeared, this one dressed in typical Haitian white, to assist in my healing. We walked through the greenery to a submarine-like building, and entered through a tiny half-door. Inside there was a dais cluttered with religious artifacts and a couple of sheet-covered pallets. Beauvoir told me to stretch out on a pallet and relax, warning me, however, that what looked like a pillow under the sheet was really a stone.

He asked me to replace all of my clothing with a proffered hospital gown. He left me to muse about whatever one muses about in such circumstances: I chose to review the steps that got me here and ways of getting others here should I be convinced of voodoo's healing power. His daughter and a wizened woman, also dressed in typical white robes and bandanna, escorted me outside to an iron tub set on the ground. The tub was filled with brownish liquid with a mat of leaves floating on the surface. At the gestured instructions of Beauvoir's daughter, I took off my gown and climbed into the tub. The wizened lady dipped a gourd into my bath water and poured it over my head. The sun and air were warm, but the water cascading over my head and shoulders was cold enough to make me suck in my breath, thereby forcing me to swallow some of the bath water. Thus, huffing and puffing away, I was thoroughly watered, and leafed as well, since the sticky leaves soon covered my body. The two of them rubbed water over me and massaged my muscles with it. This went on for maybe ten minutes. All the while they were chanting. My camera was within grasping range, and I would have liked to have had photographs of the scene. But I realized that I had to decide how much psychological distance I wanted to take from this religious healing ceremony; to have photographed it seemed to me a travesty of the experience that I wanted to have. The distance that I could not but maintain was a wry inner photograph of what the outer picture looked like. I remember at one point thinking of my stiffly conventional bourgeois childhood — I think I was nine years old in the fantasy — and contrasting its right-angled polished forms with the present jungle scene. I enjoyed the contrast; a nice guy like me gets into places like that partly in order to flee the always-threatening remnants of upbringing.

Following this first bath, I was led back to my pallet for more relaxation until it was time for my second bath — the same procedure, except that this time I was bathed in warm oil.

Beauvoir visited me back on my pallet, checked my eyes and pronounced me all right, by which I assumed he meant we could proceed. He soon reappeared with a chicken which gently clucked through the next step in the healing which was a religious service. Beauvoir and the two women shook gourds, rang bells, lit candles, and chanted at the shrine in front of me. When what appeared to be a suitable amount of religious heat had been achieved, Beauvoir picked up the chicken and waved it at my head, its wings flapping through my hair and across my forehead. Then he ripped its head off and threw the head on the floor where I could see the presumably reproachful complaint of its still-moving beak. He then held the body of the chicken over my head so that its blood and other internal fluids and debris poured down on my head, neck and shoulders. I remembered his previously saying with regard to animal sacrifice that sacrifice, in fact or symbolically, has always been a part of religion. At the moment, I found it difficult to be philosophical.

My third and last outdoor bath was partly to remove the chicken's blood and debris from my body. It included also the spraying of a burning liquid on my neck and on my back, a liquid which I later learned was extracted from a leaf. Finally, I was treated to a gentle but probing massage of my feet by Beauvoir's daughter, which seemed to me like reflexology, a standard treatment in the non-standard armamentarium. Whatever its healing properties, it felt good, as if in reward for my efforts, although I, of course, had done nothing more than show up and submit.

Back in Beauvoir's office I received my first demitasse cup of healing potion. It was, Beauvoir said, laced with sugar for taste. (I suppressed my indignation that a purported healing agent should contain sugar, a substance held by many to be injurious to one's health.) Rx: Twice a day for thirteen days even though the symptoms will be gone in six days; the full course was necessary in order to prevent a relapse. On that bittersweet note we parted.

I took the potion as directed. On the sixth day after the healing ceremony, my symptoms vanished. On the seventh day they returned with a violence, as if to make up for the hiatus, and have continued just about the same as before. It looks as if the chicken died in vain. How to explain the vanishing of symptoms on the day predicted? It could be that I was in the grip of a massive suggestion. I did have a good feeling about Beauvoir and his healing ceremony, esoteric as it was, and even now I would not be surprised if, in fact, he healed a good many people. That the potion was supposedly derived from years of trial and error and from natural substances, just as many conventional medicines have been derived, created confidence. As always, in my healing explorations, I at first hope that each modality will turn out to be useful. I then bring to bear my evaluative, skeptical point of view. Such a point of view makes for good science but poor healing by suggestion. Finally, as I was looking over my notes of my voodoo healing experience, I saw that Beauvoir had instructed me to refrigerate the potion, which I had forgotten to do. Investigating my motive for that forgetting would take us afield from the now still intriguing question about the efficacy of voodoo healing.

Something can be learned from my preference for Mr. Beauvoir over Madame C. Actually, they both did a sales job on me, including the same half now/half later terms, and they both promised success on the basis of a set of beliefs foreign to mine. The difference was in their respective trappings and styles. Beauvoir's were similar to mine — his education, his office practice; we spoke the same language, literally and figuratively. So here I was, searching for unconventional ways of healing yet being persuaded by conventional characteristics; in the absence of factual information, I was thrown back upon prejudice. In that sense I was like most medical patients, ignorant of facts and persuaded by bedside manner, degrees, and word-of-mouth from often equally uninformed others. It could well be that Madame C's healing is as effective as that of Beauvoir; her healing could be more effective for those who respond to the suggestion inherent in her primitive presentation; it could be less effective for those disposed as I was to his erudition and smoothness. Or, to put it another way, what each of them does may be effective or may not be effective, or their varying effectiveness might result only from the kind of suggestions they purvey. While Madame C might in theory have cured me more effectively than Mr. Beauvoir, she would not have done so to the degree that her cure was dependent upon similarity between herself and her patients. One person's healing reality need not be another's. I simply was not one of her kind of patients. Perhaps that was too bad for me rather than an indictment of her.

Chapter Ten
C. Norman Shealy and Friends: A Holistic Healing Center

WHETHER EVENTS CREATE HEROES or heroes create events is a matter debated in countless historical texts. The question applies to Dr. C. Norman Shealy, a major figure in non-traditional healing. He could not have achieved his eminence and influence in a time that was less open to unconventional approaches to healing, and unconventional healing would not be the same without his protean efforts as physician, founder of a pain clinic, nutritionist, author, columnist, speaker, researcher and proponent of psychic healing. Indeed, united in him are the three major strands of contemporary healing: conventional medicine, unconventional or fringe medicine, and psychic healing. It *may* well be that the way that Shealy organizes and implements these strands within himself will provide a model for how the healing culture at large will one day accommodate these trends.

Shealy decided as early as high school that he wanted to be a neurosurgeon. He attended Duke University, then Duke Medical School; the college was only a short distance from the family farm in his small Bible Belt home town. He left North Carolina to take a general surgical residency in St. Louis, and then went to Massachusetts General Hospital for his neurosurgical residency. Then he flew the coop in earnest, spending eight months in Australia under Sir John Eccles, a 1963 Nobel Prize winner. He left Australia to become professor of neurosurgery at Cleveland's Case Western Reserve University, where he stayed until opening his Pain and Rehabilitation Institute in La Crosse, Wisconsin, in 1971. He has since moved the Institute to Springfield, Missouri. Despite his coltish leaping from place to place, tradition remains important to him. A descendant of Lutheran and Baptist farmers, he still lives on a working farm, though it is hard to see how he has much time for farming himself; he wears a string tie, and never lets you forget that he is a conventionally trained physician who is loyal to conventional medicine. When he writes that before embarking on unconventional or occult healing practices, you should FIRST SEEK COMPETENT MEDICAL CARE, he puts it in capital letters. His is a bourgeois revolution. He moved toward unconventional medicine and to the occult in slow stages, drawing on his traditional conservative beliefs as these connected themselves to modern trends and practical problems.

Indeed, it is not always easy to draw a line between conventional healing and unconventional healing. How, for example, does one categorize putting electrodes on the spinal cord to control pain, as Shealy did in 1965? At the time, the use of this "dorsal column stimulator" was considered unconventional. Now many physicians recommend a similar device placed on the skin over the nerve involved, which the patient controls. Shealy's work with needle electrodes for the control of pain in local nerves was once considered daring, though now conventional medicine accepts it; many physicians may not realize that it is a Western equivalent to acupuncture. Dr. Paul Dudley White, prestigious physician to Presidents and one of the first American physicians to visit Red China and observe the modern use of acupuncture, apprised Shealy of the similarity. Shealy then largely taught himself acupuncture.

Shealy's next step was a decisive one away from medicine's traditional core and came about by way of apparent happenstance: Shealy substituted for Dr. White as a speaker at the Academy of Parapsychology and Medicine. There, stimulated by the discussion of psychic phenomena, he remembered the times at Duke University when he had observed the much publicized work of Dr. J.B. Rhine. Rhine's experiments had convinced him that some people had the ability to guess symbols on cards (clairvoyance), to receive knowledge from a person in another room (telepathy), and to will dice to come up in desired ways (psychokinesis). At the time Shealy was unable or unwilling to see the practical use of such abilities; caught up in his medical education, he relegated Rhine's work to a corner of his mind. Now he brought it to the forefront of his mind and added it to the healing armamentarium in his Pain and Rehabilitation Clinic. The happenstance of his becoming enthusiastic at the Academy Meeting was probably not really happenstance. Presumably, the Rhine experience had touched a responsive chord in Shealy's personality, whose reverberations he had stilled at the time.

Shealy left one explanation for his apparently belated but enthusiastic response to psychic phenomena and healing out of his book, *Occult Medicine Can Save Your Life*.[1] Whatever the reason for that omission, he was not reluctant to tell me about it and to send me the excerpt from a book where it is described. The book is *Americans Who Have Been Reincarnated*.[2] The publisher is no obscure California back room operation, of which there are many, but the estimable Macmillan Publishing Company, Inc. The author, H.N. Banerjee, Ph.D., details the evidence for his and Shealy's belief that Shealy is a reincarnation of John Elliotson, a British physician who pioneered the use of hypnosis for surgery and other medical purposes.

The evidence: when Shealy first heard Elliotson's name, during a lecture on hypnosis, he felt a physical shock accompany the felt recognition that Shealy himself was being referred to in the person of John Elliotson. He experienced a similar eerie feeling when, on a visit to London, his taxi passed a small brick Victorian house which turned out to be a house where Elliotson had practiced medicine. There is, in fact, a physical resemblance between Shealy and Elliotson. Elliotson had a congenital limp, while Shealy for a time limped from osteomyelitis of a knee. Elliotson showed that hypnotized patients could clairvoyantly diagnose correctly the illness of other patients. About a month before he heard of Elliotson for the first time, Shealy had initiated a project to study the ability of psychics to use their powers to diagnose illnesses.

Banerjee writes, "In order to verify that he was Elliotson, Shealy consulted more than twenty psychics throughout the United States. Interestingly, all of them said that he was Elliotson." Stanley Krippner remembers Shealy telling him the number was closer to a half-dozen than twenty. Even so, that is some remarkable finding. But did it happen as is implied? Did the psychics come up with Elliotson's name without being primed? Or were they asked whether Shealy was Elliotson, or, for example, what English physician he might have been, or were they given a choice between Elliotson and others? If all of them had identified Shealy as Elliotson without any priming whatsoever, such a finding should be written in neon lights, should present itself as a candidate for white crowism. Be that as it may, as far as

Shealy is concerned — in the same tone of voice and sober demeanor, and surrounded by the practical evidence of his accomplishments — Norman Shealy is John Elliotson, or vice versa. Well, it's an interesting story. The evidence would hardly pass muster in a court of law or in the halls of science, and as such is on par with most of the evidence for reincarnation.

I FIRST MET DR. SHEALY at a plastic coffee shop in a plastic hotel where we were both attending a conference on holistic medicine. While breakfasting on an experimental macrobiotic diet, I discussed with the waitress the relative merits of margarine and butter. Shealy, himself bored and troubled by the food available to us under the circumstances, intervened from a nearby table with the advice that I have the butter. Margarine, he said, was bad for one's health under any circumstances, while under some conditions butter not only does not raise cholesterol but can reduce it. So our relationship immediately started out with my being grateful to him. And that has continued through the years as I have corresponded with him and read his books, *Occult Medicine Can Save Your Life*, *The Pain Game*,[3] *Ninety Days to Self Health*,[4] and his regular column on holistic health in *New Realities*. He recommended many of the healers that I studied.

In 1971, when Shealy started his Center, there were twenty "pain clinics" in the U.S., usually in hospitals. Now there are approximately five hundred, some having taken their cue from Shealy's. Most orthodox pain clinics tend to restrict themselves to relieving pain from specific diseases or injuries. Shealy broadened his approach for at least these two reasons: (1) Pain is not an isolated phenomena, but the subjective reaction of a whole person to some interference in usual functioning, an interference whose source can range all the way from a spasm of particular muscles to spasm of the whole personality. (2) Most people, in pain or not, can benefit from learning a healthy way of life, which can range all the way from healthy diet to physical exercise to thinking healthy thoughts. Thus, his list of treatments includes those directly related to relief of pain — such as electrical stimulation of nerves, the application of ice, acupuncture, local nerve blocks, facet rhizotomy (destruction of the nerve supply to joints in the spine), and other drug injections — and measures suitable not only for relief of current distress but designed to prevent later distress and to improve the quality of life. These measures include physical exercise, nutrition, drug detoxification (including alcohol and cigarettes), and consultations with specialists in a variety of fields. Some modalities are good both for relieving specific pain and encouraging overall prevention and health. These include biofeedback training, and Shealy's more wide-ranging system based in biofeedback trademarked "Biogenics," which includes massage and electro-sleep therapy (an electrical stimulation designed to establish sound sleep patterns). Though some people come to Shealy's clinic on their own in order to improve their present and future health, most come after being dissatisfied with help from more conventional medical interventions. Thus, Shealy tends to get the hard cases.

These hard cases should be prepared for an approach quite different from their previous medical experience. Before coming they will spend several hours filling out questionnaires which not only cover a detailed history and description of their pain and medical histories but ascertain whether they like X-rated movies, giving parties, and being told whether they are loved or needed. The latter questions are included among the 147 items which comprise a "pleasure scale," a measure of how much patients may be enhancing their own physical well-being by pursuing pleasure. The hard cases also had better realize that while previous treaters had dulled their axes through unsuccessfully doing something *to* them, the main axe that would be dulled at Shealy's place would be the patient's. In conformance with a major tenet of holistic medicine, the patients are put in charge of their health, both through the way many of the exercises are designed, and the need to continue the program on their own after leaving. The twelve days (and thousands of dollars) invested in the treatment itself is only the beginning. While some 90 percent of patients show significant improvement at the end of the twelve days, that improvement diminishes sharply for those who fail to continue the programs after they leave. Shealy can cite the statistics for this assertion through his follow-up of patients months and years afterwards, usually through telephone interviews. Here is another, and most welcome, departure from conventional clinical practice. Both with physical medicine and psychotherapy, improvement or cure tends to be judged at the end of the treatment. That may be a reasonable time for such a measurement when all one is interested in is getting rid of a crystallized symptom and returning the patient to how he was before. But when one hopes to bring about better health throughout life, then measurements should be made not only at termination of treatment but later in life.

Springfield, Missouri, rises up out of miles and miles of farmland, a metropolis by contrast with its surroundings. It has a remarkable number of Chinese and other Oriental restaurants, mostly of the plastic and takeout variety. The story goes that a Chinese emigre to the area had a large family in the old country whom he also encouraged to emigrate; they in turn had large families, all of whom were, or shortly became, cooks. At any rate, here in the toxic red meat beeflands, complete with the obligatory, dreadful fast food valley, one can gorge fast-foodly on healthy vegetables cooked Oriental-style. Springfield is also noted for its federal prison and hospital, other centers of toxicity. It is a nice metaphor: amidst the toxicity of social ills and bad diet leading to physical disease and questionable medicine is Shealy's assertion of a new and better treatment for a new and better life.

The Institute is a collection of rooms in a free standing building administratively attached to a general hospital next door. Patients live in the city and come there for the 12-day program. The first two days of the program are largely spent evaluating the patient. Based on this evaluation, the staff tailors individual programs, or one or both parties decides that the best program would be no program. Few people choose the latter option. Despite this being a gathering place for medical failures and intractable pain, the atmosphere is upbeat, redolent with much to offer in exchange for participation.

I came a bit late to my first large-group meeting and was at first shocked. Sixteen people, looking only partly conscious, were stretched out in recliner chairs with white bands around their heads, splashes of white tapes here and there, wires protruding. Thoughts of dread diseases raced through my mind — for the most part needlessly, as it turned out; the gadgetry was simply part of the feedback mechanisms. Patients were partly conscious because that is the way it is with feedback techniques. Some people were there merely because it was a stressful time in their life, following such events as a divorce or death in the family. Others had pain in various stages of remission, including merely a nuisance stage. Still, there were stories of people who had limbs amputated, and one whose leg had turned black was saved from amputation by the Shealy program. Soon I, too, was settled in with a white band holding electrodes to my head, stretched out on a recliner and alternating between taking notes and drifting off.

The activities in the large-group meeting — indeed, the program as a whole — might best be discussed by way of the following, sometimes overlapping, categories: Biogenics, psychological-spiritual, and psychic healing.

Biogenics is the name that Shealy gives to his collection of self-help relaxation exercises. These include the autogenic training of J.H. Schultz. This approach is known to many people who might not be able to name it; it is an old wives' remedy to induce sleep and tranquility. The subject, or patient, is asked mentally to go up and down his body relaxing each set of muscles in turn. Remarkably, while one may think that one is relaxed, concentrating on each set of muscles allows one to see how a low level of tension has muscles partially spastic almost all the time. Autogenic training includes such statements, to be repeated by the person and concentrated on by him, as, "My whole body feels quiet, heavy, comfortable, and relaxed," "I withdraw my thoughts from the surroundings and I feel serene and still," "My mind is calm and quiet."

Another exercise in Biogenics was developed by Emil Coue, whose work has also through the years been included in many mental medicine cabinets. Coue contended that if a person were persuaded that he could do various things, he would be able to. And if individuals imagine that they cannot do something, then that thing becomes impossible for them. So he would have patients, preferably in states of reverie or when hypnotized by themselves or others, say such things as, "Every day and in every way I am getting better and better," "I am going to be cured," or in the case of physical pain, "It is going away." He had specific directions for specific diseases, for example, asthma: "From this day forward, my breathing will become rapidly easier. My organism will do all that is necessary to restore perfect health to my lungs and bronchial passages."

Edmond Jacobson, while agreeing with Coue on the importance of relaxation, contended that such relaxation could be actively taught rather than relying upon the person to use his imagination, willpower, or self-suggestion. Jacobson would teach patients that the tensing of their muscles requires effort, while relaxation requires none. So he would have patients make their muscles tense, and then relax them. That procedure, too, is part of Shealy's Biogenics.

Biofeedback, another Biogenics constituent, teaches the patient how to control physiologic functions. It combines the old and the new; a variety of meditation, used with machines that "feed back" information from the body as to how relaxed it has become. On the basis of this information, one can train oneself to achieve the desired state. So, in biofeedback, East meets West; the ancient wisdoms of Yoga and Zen, captured in the various relaxation techniques, are combined with the glitter of Western machinery.

Shealy offers the essentials of his Biogenics in a three-hundred-page booklet describing relaxation techniques in detail, instructions in their use, and their place in total health care. In the midst of the largely technological approaches of Biogenics, as described in the booklet, Shealy throws in without comment a couple of pages about the ideas of Robert Assagioli, the creator of "psychosynthesis," one of the human potential movement's "new therapies." Assagioli may be his own worst enemy in that in the midst of his fairly original and seminal ideas he offers so many staggeringly elemental ones, such as "Each individual is unique." These create a glaze over the reader's eyes to the point that the central issues may be obscured. Yet central to Assagioli's approach is his assertion that a systematic and vigorous employment of conscious aspects of the personality can bring about desired aims, and that there is available to each individual a reservoir of "superconscious spiritual energy" for this and other purposes. Shealy believes in psychosynthesis, and it provides the theoretical substrate for many of his healing practices. He also underlines a quality that is usually at least latent in psychosynthesis and similar approaches to personality, namely anti-Freudianism. Thus, Shealy says, "A prominent part of my philosophy is that emotional distress does not have to be deeply re-experienced, discussed, or analyzed." Assagioli, too, rather coyly asserts, "The future and the active role of the future in the present are emphasized." In other words, there is no need to go mucking around in the past, which Freudians are caricatured as doing exclusively. Assagioli also writes, "There is a need for awareness of *motivations* which determine choices and decisions." If he really believed that, and was able to recognize the depth and complexity of motivations, he has not left the Freudian camp at all; the elucidation of motives and meanings is what the clinical practice of psychoanalysis is all about. In the individual counseling sessions that I observed at Shealy's, in my interviews with staff members, and in the large-group discussions, staff members repeatedly emphasized the following psychoanalytic beliefs: (1) Thoughts and feelings can express themselves in physical terms, and if such thoughts and feelings are stressful, bodily disturbances or symptoms result. (2) Stressful thoughts and feelings tend to issue from conflicts beginning in early life and are expressed in troubled ways of living as well as in bodily symptoms.

Shealy and his group lavishly honor Jung while they make much less use of his ideas practically. Shealy cites his agreement with Jung, for example, that there is an inextinguishable soul and thus life after death. The existence of a soul implies a purpose to life. Here Shealy cites Jung's concept of synchronicity, the word given to the existence of things working out the way they were meant to be; not through coincidence, but because that is the preordained purposeful fate of events. Shealy asserts the existence of God, and opines that Christianity merely puts a face on the God who is everywhere in various manifestations. Another of Shealy's major beliefs is in the Golden Rule, which he considers simply logical: it is in one's own interest to do good for others. Shealy's staff members echoed his philosophy: "A person who is whole, loves oneself and loves others, has a God-given unearned right to 'be'," and "Positive thinking invokes God's power." Just as there may be no atheists in foxholes, there may be no atheists who get cured of physical ills. Or if they do, they do it the hard way, relying solely on materialistic and secular interventions, missing out on the beneficial effects of believing. Or at least that is one way to look at it.

But there may be more to it than that. One does not necessarily have to believe in each and every idea, perhaps even in the main idea of God, to notice the relaxation possible during church services, for example, and at times Shealy's meetings create a feeling of being in a church. The very discussion of matters transcending the workaday world, especially the grubby world of pain and diseases, has a tranquilizing effect on many people. It is a kind of meditation, a change in consciousness, a heightened perspective an awareness of oneself in relation to others. During the Shealy group meetings I found that often, when I listened hard and critically, I became impatient. When I let the words flow and experienced the sweep of the objectives, I felt more accepting and tranquil. Whatever its source, healing has awesome, perhaps religious, overtones.

Recognizing that people are in pain from their lives as well as from their diseases, Shealy provides individual psychological counseling.* Shealy's coun-

---

* This may be as good a time as any to rid myself of a peeve; namely, substituting the pallid and misleading *counseling* for *psychotherapy*. "Counseling," after all, refers to giving people counsel or advice. Thus, school *counselors* tell students how to fill out applications to college and how to prepare for tests. In the majority of psychological interventions, however, the client or patient learns about himself in order to make new and informed decisions, to behave differently. Indeed, simply giving advice — counseling in its transitive sense — shuts down the process of self-discovery and self-determination. Calling psychotherapy "counseling" seems to me an arch way of attempting to smooth over the medical or therapeutic implications that many people attach to psychotherapy, and thus is in the prevalent mode of nonspeak, circumlocution, failing to call a spade a spade.

selors affirm the Institute's ambience of positive thinking. As one counselor put it, "We are what we think and so we need to think differently about ourselves." Another way that Shealy uses to change the way people think is hypnosis, and he has a hypnotist-counselor on the staff who describes his work as "dehypnotizing people of old beliefs." The piece of wisdom that I got from that phrase is that we tend to form our beliefs through life under sway of a more powerful Other (be it specific people or the culture at large), which could be considered a form of hypnosis to be undone by the hypnotherapy.

Despite the ministrations of these new, counterculture, and anti-Freudian therapies, many patients have a stubborn way of being Freudian. When given the opportunity to tell about themselves, they tell of stressful situations that seem to issue from conflicts whose sources, not immediately apparent, are unconscious. For example, in the midst of the glowing testimonials of improvement and cure prevalent in the group sessions, one patient remained dourly skeptical and reported either no beneficial change or worsening. The zealous and unsophisticated counselor urged her to have faith, hope, trust, and to love. A psychologically sophisticated psychotherapist would, after drawing her attention to her stance, reflect with her on such possibilities as that she needs to remain ill, perhaps out of an angry wish to defeat others, or a fear of having things better than important people in her past life, or to pursue the fantasy that nurturing can only come to her if she presents herself as sick and helpless. On the other hand, a psychologist sophisticated in the ways of the unconscious might overlook the beneficial possibilities of Shealy's appeals to consciousness, the summoning of will, inspiration, determination. Indeed, all therapists would do well to consider also the effects of people's living together in an environment removed from their ordinary one and imbued with an atmosphere of healing. Such conditions obtain in most of the new therapies. Extended meetings characteristically generate feelings of commonality, love, hope, and inspiration; and not infrequently they produce healings of various kinds, though unfortunately these phenomena may not last for too long after the meetings.

Not only is the boundary between spirituality and psychology in Shealy's program vague, but so too is the boundary between psychology and psychic healing. That issue is epitomized in the person of the remarkable Henry E. Rucker. This imposing black man in his seventies compellingly captures spiritual and psychological ideas in hipster language; e.g., "God is up there with a big stick waiting to whack you on the head when you make a boo-boo." "Sally, you're not guilty, you're beautiful." (The latter example probably comes to mind because Rucker frequently wears a button emblazoned with the words "NOT GUILTY.") He is given, also, to such poor man's Oscar Wildeisms as "Humanity can't evolve faster than itself." He leaps from subject to subject, image to image; a direct question merely sends him off at right angles spinning out stories, homilies, and wisdoms. If one doesn't listen to him carefully, one can easily be caught up by his infectiousness and believe anything he says. If one listens more closely, one begins to notice his style, mannerisms, and vaudevillian effects, and consider that he might be merely a con artist. But if one listens very carefully, observes him at work, takes note of the testimonials and some research studies of his remarkable abilities, then one considers seriously the possibility that he is a gifted person psychically and secularly.

For more than a decade Rucker has come to Shealy's Institute to spend several of each patient group's twelve days giving lectures and meeting with individuals in counseling sessions. His smooth blend of psychic powers and psychological savvy was illustrated in Shealy's comment about him in a letter to me: "Actually, we minimize the fact that he is psychic or a healer, but I think by the time most people leave, they are aware of his role in that regard." Indeed, during the individual interviews that I observed, he blended inspirational remarks, cracker-barrel philosophy, and descriptions of God's role in the healing — "Sometimes He puts you in a holding pattern ..." — with sudden flashes of intuition or clairvoyance. For example, to a woman whom he barely knew, "You have trouble sleeping. You programmed yourself to get men that you could reject. That way you would never again suffer the pain of loving and losing."

There is little in the realm of psychic healing and the paranormal that Rucker does not do. Since the age of eight he has been able to go "out of his body"; he sees auras; he does "psychic surgery"; he is clairvoyant, a palmist, and a reader of Tarot cards.

Rucker initially impressed Shealy by giving a remarkably perceptive reading of Shealy himself. Shealy then included Rucker with eight other psychics who, knowing only the patients' birthdates, and given a few minute's look at the patients and a sample of their handwriting, were remarkably accurate in their diagnoses of physical ills. Rucker by himself has been (according to Shealy) 80 percent accurate in diagnosing physical ailments, sometimes using just a photograph, palm print, or handwriting sample. Oh, the comforting percentage so easy to let roll trippingly and portentously off the tongue. Was it exactly 80 percent? And 80 percent of which ailments? Does the percentage vary with the prediction and diagnosis of cancer or measles?

Shealy estimates that Henry Rucker has treated approximately fifteen hundred people through psychic means, and that many hundreds of them have gotten rid of pain, though whether they maintain that improvement is questionable. Rucker may lay his hands on some people, or simply send healing energy across the room, as I saw him do in a workshop at a private home in Kansas City with a patient with leukemia. She reported feeling great warmth in her abdomen. Rucker says that people with serious illnesses may get great benefit from healing, as might people with trivial illnesses. He believes that his healing from a distance is likely to be as helpful as the laying on of hands. By distance, he really means distance. He asked that a patient/friend of mine merely send a photograph and be ready for a collect call; Rucker would arrange a time when he would send the healing. It would be better, he said, if the patient were in bed at the time, since many people report becoming tranquil during the healing, perhaps too much so to drive a car safely or do other daily tasks. Rucker judges that his healings are successful when in their wake he gets requests for work on other physical or emotional symptoms, from the patient or from friends and relatives of the patient. People are inclined, he says, to send him long lists of symptoms, which he says are unnecessary. He believes he can tell what is wrong with them without the symptoms, and even tell ills they have of which they are unaware.

As far as my tennis elbow is concerned, Rucker joined the long list of healers who failed to heal it. Rucker was, however, impressive in his first reading of me using Tarot cards; at least that is the way I remember the first reading. Much to my dismay, the tape which could have substantiated my memorial impression and filled in the gaps in my memory when I rechecked the reading some years afterward, was suffused with noise. That noise resisted the efforts of sound technicians who tried to filter it out. I do remember, however, that he placed my past life, or at least one of my past lives, in France at the time of the Revolution. According to Rucker I was something of a rogue, a free spirit who even preferred the guillotine to internment, and I got my wish. During a second reading, he placed me in Europe, at about the same time as the French Revolution, and having the same need for freedom. I suppose he could have remembered the first reading, though that is unlikely. For what it is worth, other readers of past lives have placed me in France at the same time. Rucker's readings of my palms on both occasions resulted mostly in comments that one could have guessed simply from seeing me or knowing a little about me, or were so general as to apply pretty much to anyone. His readings of the Tarot cards, however, resulted in some highly specific predictions of eventualities and when they were to occur. He is ordinarily able, he says, to predict up to a year, in six-month segments. I awaited the fruition of one of his predictions with great anticipation: I was to achieve great financial gain around the first of that year. (It didn't happen.)

I can hear Rucker with my mind's ear now, cracking wise, trying to be intellectual (and in the process being wiser than many intellectuals I have known), provocatively dazzling people into a healthy frame of mind, and I dare say, whether through his dazzling or through transferring healing energy, making a healthy difference in many lives.

I began this chapter with the observation that Shealy's organization and implementation of conventional medicine, unconventional medicine, and psychic healing, offers a model for how the healing culture at large may one day accommodate these trends. I had an excellent opportunity to observe and experience Shealy organizing and implementing these trends at the end of my stay at his Center. It was Sunday noon, at the end of what I had observed as a nonstop, grueling week for him, directly following his leadership of the last large-group meeting, and fresh from attending to a variety of last-minute needs of the departing patient group. I half expected him to heave a sigh and collapse, to deal politely, efficiently, but feebly with my collected questions, and to hurry home to rescue what he could of the Day of Rest. Not so. As befits a man who practices what he preaches about holistic medicine and healthy living, and reaps the rewards of it, he had the energy to complement my patient role with his doctor role, and my observing journalistic role with his being the giver of information and explanation. Whether through his devotion to holistic medicine or through some identity as a small-town family doctor, his patience and encompassing store of information set a standard that conventional medicine's modern specialists could well emulate.

On our last day together I was provided with a sort of coda to the week's immersion in Shealy's brand of holistic medicine. Fifteen acupuncture needles protruded from my body while I did a healing meditation, an electromagnetic generator ran below my cot, seemingly Oriental music was in the background, and I was stuffed with Tryptophane. During the previous days, I had electromagnetic charges to the temples designed to release serotonin for a restful sleep, attended lectures on healing, did relaxation and physical exercises, had Rucker's healing ministrations, was hypnotized, used a portable machine which delivered electrical charges and a non-portable machine which did the same, and did meditation and biofeedback. Still to come from Shealy's cornucopia on the final Sunday was an injection and spray of pain-killing chemicals.

There not being much more physical area of me left to work on, we merely discussed such therapeutic interventions as treatment with DMSO, castor oil packs, the areas where various acupuncture practitioners might recommend the insertion of needles, the "brain equalizer" (a machine designed to bring the left and right sides of the brain into harmony), and a variety of vitamin and mineral combinations for a variety of purposes. The list came up in response to my shopping list of questions from friends and associates who knew about Shealy's encyclopedic knowledge. I merely pressed the question button, and the words were barely out of my mouth before he responded with therapeutic suggestions and mini-lectures on information relevant to their use; it was a bravura performance. I was reassured that he was not simply making all this up on the spot when one question finally stumped him, and he straightaway said so. While experts have been described as "people who know more and more about less and less," Shealy as a holistic expert knows more and more about more and more.

He ought, however, to get some consultation from an empathic typesetter. He offers a booklet entitled "Health Maintenance," which in eleven of its tiny pages lays out the bases of healthy living from heredity to regular medical checkups. The booklet is about the same size as those used as programs at funerals, and "Health Maintenance" is set in the same austere, medieval, serif-laden type used at such lugubrious events. Typesetting and inherent wisdom are much more congruent in a large plastic card written by Shealy entitled "The 10 Commandments of Health." The card is reproduced on the next page.

Shealy may or may not turn out to be the Moses of holistic medicine. But I am inclined to believe that his holistic approach as made concrete in his Institute is the wave of the future, or ought to be. Under one physical

The 10 Commandments of Health
by C. Norman Shealy, M.D., Ph.D.

Disease is expensive, but Health is the least expensive commodity you can obtain. If you really want to live and Be Healthy, the following 10 Commandments of Health will do more for you than medicine or surgery. Don't ignore illnesses, but Do Choose To Be Healthy.

1. Eat 3 meals a day.
   Eat a wide variety of foods; avoid caffeine and table sugar
2. Eat breakfast every day.
   Be sure you have adequate protein to start the day
3. Do not smoke
4. Do not drink alcohol, or be very moderate
5. Exercise regularly.
   Start slowly and build up to 3 or 4 sessions per week of exercise which doubles heart rate for at least 20 minutes[a]
6. Sleep 7 or 8 hours in each 24
7. Keep your weight within 10% of your ideal
8. Relax and rebalance regularly at least 10 minutes three times a day[b]
9. Have a positive attitude and belief that you Can Be Healthy
10. Resolve your anger and fear daily through prayer, counseling, or Biogenics

References:

a. *New Aerobics* by Kenneth Cooper, M. Evans & Co., Inc., 1970.
b. *90 Days to Self-Health* by C. Norman Shealy, Dial Press, 1977.
c. *Mind as Healer, Mind as Slayer* by Kenneth R. Pelletier, Dell Publishing, 1977.

and ideological roof it provides for much of the complexity of people, and therefore much of the complexity of disease and health, with corresponding diversity and complexity of treatment. It provides a form that accommodates information from most eras, most parts of the world, and most therapeutic approaches. Paradoxically, accounting for such complexities results in simplification, holism, unity, a broad but basically single approach to the problem of how to help people make themselves and keep themselves healthy. One or another of Shealy's individual approaches may turn out to be useless or harmful, as is true of all healing efforts; but his openness to the many possibilities of healing, if combined with evaluation of them, can only improve everyone's chances of being healed.

Chapter Eleven
Exploring the Personalities of Psychic Healers: A Psychological Test Study

RESEARCHERS ON PSYCHIC HEALING have largely focused on whether and how psychic healing works. They have paid little attention to the personalities of the healers. Yet, if psychic healers have personality characteristics in common, these may not only help explain why they act as healers but also shed light on the nature of healing.

Can one generalize about a person's personality on the basis of their profession or skill? In one sense, no; it would be impossible to say that all skydivers are the same, all computer technicians are the same, and all surgeons are the same. And yet, stereotypes and generalities have grown up around these and other occupations on the basis of unsystematic, informal observations that yield fairly accurate predictions. (Skydivers will likely be adventurous and more oriented toward action than toward reflection, computer technicians will tend to be more comfortable with things than with people, and surgeons will tend to be authoritarian.) By studying the personalities of healers I hoped to be able to find what they had in common.

How does one define a healer? How effective does one have to be in order to be called a healer, and how much healing must one do? Do healers who do one kind of healing have personalities as a group that are different from those who do another kind? Many people claim that healing skill is inherent in everyone. On that basis Delores Kreiger, and others, teach healing to people only grossly selected — for example, classes at the New York University School of Nursing. How, then, can there be a distinguishable healing personality? Lacking systematic answers to such questions as these, but having to start somewhere, I decided whom I would call a healer and study as such in this way: Eleven of the twenty-four healers that I studied are, in the world of healing, well-known as healers. Three of them were on a list of six people that I got from Dr. Norman Shealy (see Chapter 10). He offered his list in response to my request for people about whom there would be general agreement among partisans of unorthodox healing that they were authentic psychic healers. I learned about eight others of my subjects from reading scientific reports about them, by word-of-mouth, and through recommendations by Martin Ebon, a prolific author of books on paranormal phenomena who has also been active in the administrative and political affairs of organizations devoted to psychic work. Six other subjects are known as healers only in their local communities of Montreal, New York, and Kansas City. In regard to four people whom I studied, there is a pronounced question as to whether they are, in fact, healers. They are deeply involved in paranormal phenomena — one is Uri Geller — but their activities are substantially different from those who clearly identify themselves as healers. Three Philippine healers comprise another group, on two of whom the testing is incomplete because of their refusal to continue. While most healers consider their work to be at least generally spiritual, two of the subjects identified "religion" as their profession.

Other objections to my attempting to study the personalities of healers were offered by the healers themselves — for example, by a conventionally trained physician, Robert Leichtman, M.D. According to Leichtman, healing stems from a spiritual essence that is distinct from personality as conceived and measured by psychologists. He says that the personality is merely a vehicle for healing rather than its source. He likens the study of personality to the study of a television set when one is attempting to comprehend a symphony that appears on television, or to studying the fingers of the pianist in an attempt to understand their music. According to Leichtman, healing comes from a healer's "extraordinary compassion." This compassion is "laced with an orderly mind, which is necessary to focus healing power, and comes from a strong sense of identity and will so that the healer can remain sufficiently detached in order not to pick up the patient's disease" (Leichtman, personal communication).

Finally, it is difficult to know whether one's measurements and observations of healers refer to the healing personality or only to the personalities of those people who identify themselves as healers. Perhaps in electing to study people known as healers I would be less studying the healing personality than a particular kind of public personality. I quieted my scientific and methodological conscience with the recognition that the first order of business in science is to make observations.

I informally studied everyone with whom I came in contact in my healing travels, and those observations are included in what follows. But in addition, I gave psychological tests to twenty-four practitioners of psychic healing or related activities. Most of the time the test battery included the Early Memories and Thematic Appercention Test. (Early Memories is an inventory of memories from childhood that provides autobiographical information and an opportunity to learn how events in the subject's past were experienced and what meanings were attached to them. The Thematic Appercention Test is a series of ambiguous pictures to which the patient is asked to make up a story.) All of the subjects were given the Rorschach Test. This test is composed of ten ink blots; the subjects are merely asked to tell what they see in the blots. Some areas of the ink blots are sufficiently well defined as to be seen in the same way by a great number of people. By noticing the fit between what a subject sees and what most other subjects see, the tester can learn the degree to which the subject perceives reality in the same way as most others do, and is therefore a measure of what many people mean by the terms "sane" or "insane." For the most part the ink blots are highly ambiguous, so that what people see is more a function of what they impose, on the basis of their personalities, than of what is objectively, consensually there in the ink blot. Thus, one can learn from the Rorschach Test about a person's style or manner of thinking, wishes, fears, and other contents of the mind. Finally, how people react to what is, for most of them, an unusual task also provides information about their personalities.

Many people wonder about the mental stability of anyone who would claim to cure ills of the body just by touching or moving hands over it. That is the question most frequently put to me about the personalities of psychic healers. However phrased, people wonder whether psychic healers are mentally "normal." The healers themselves tend to be sensitive on this point; in one way or another they tried to find out, before agreeing to take the tests, whether I was mainly interested in their sanity. In this regard they differ only in degree from most others who consider taking psychological tests.

In fact, only three of the healers gave responses expectable from persons who are highly disturbed psychiatrically. Thus, the data do not support the contention that most psychic healers are just troubled people nourishing delusions. Almost half of the subjects were basically sound with regard to their testing of reality; they gave test records of about the same quality in that regard as would be had from your friends and mine.

The remaining subjects lie somewhere between the three disturbed people and the basically sound ones. Members of this middle group are somewhat inclined to reshape reality according to their wishes, sometimes more able to check such wishes against the facts, and sometimes less so. They are inclined to delude themselves, especially when their ideas have an external rationale and are supported by others. In the latter sense, they resemble many religious people or members of primitive cultures who believe in events that would be considered delusional in other contexts; their ideas escape psychiatric significance by being shared by others. The group decides to suspend disbelief on selected issues, leaving the way clear for the agreed-upon ideas: for instance, that the sea parted for Moses, that Jesus left his grave three days after dying, that Mohammed was taken into heaven on a white horse, that Joseph Smith found the Mormon scriptures on golden tablets, or that Quetzalcoatl left Mexico on a magical ship vowing to return.

The records of the three Filipinos should be considered apart from the rest, and are not included in my computations and conclusions. The responses of all three of them were highly deviant by Western standards — so deviant that I would have expected these healers to behave in overtly unusual ways during our interviews, and as I observed them interacting with others. The fact that they did not suggests that cultural and educational factors were responsible for their lack of attunement to the test requirements and for their test responses.

What I have been referring to so far is the machinery of the mind, the basic capacities to participate in consensually and culturally shared perceptions, thoughts, and reactions, if to do so is taken as a task. There are, however, other ways than through one or another kind of psychotic thinking to be deviant, to separate one's self from the usual run of people. Many personality characteristics result in being drawn to and supporting the less usual, and such characteristics were much in evidence in these subjects. Some of them showed a need to be different. For example, they would comment that a popularly given response was too obvious; they were interested in something more offbeat and original. Some were oppositional: they simply attempted to turn black to white, figure to ground, to say "no" in various ways when a simple "yes" would have been easier and better justified perceptually. Some said, in so many words, that they could see what was popularly seen, if they wanted, but chose otherwise. Many of them were fanciful. They would not only enliven their responses with embellishments, such as is often done by creative, imaginative people, but would build upon their embellishments, straying further and further from the test stimulus. They would redefine the task from a perceptual one, based on the instructions "Tell me what you see," to an imaginative one, sometimes independent of and to the detriment of what could have been their perceptual response.

Here we enter upon the psychology of creativity. Creativity is the capacity to produce something that is different, in important and substantive ways, from what is ordinarily produced. "Different" is a word that one also uses to describe disturbed persons, people who are different from the norm. There are different ways of being different. Some people, when shown a telephone as a stimulus, will say, for example, "that's a telephone," and when pressed to say more might say, "it is black" and "one can talk on it"; they will be hard put to say much else. Such people can be labeled as having constricted or banal minds. Others, after correctly identifying the telephone, will go on to describe how it brings geographically distant family members together; how, like other communication devices, it shrinks the world so that whatever happens anywhere can become known and influential almost instantly elsewhere; that Irving Berlin created what some have called the best first line of any popular song, "All alone by the telephone..."; and so on. Minds that deliver such associations might be called rich, elaborate, imaginative. And then there are those for whom, unfortunately, the phone will bring to mind a network of communication devices designed by aliens out to conquer us.

What is crucial in these differences? The unimaginative person recognizes the obvious and conventional dimensions of reality and leaves it at that. The imaginative person recognizes the conventional dimensions of reality, but chooses to embellish them; and if the person can capture the embellishment in a shareable and valued product, that person is an artist.

The delusional person embellishes reality, too, but seems not to have a choice, to be driven to impose idiosyncratic beliefs regardless of their ill fit with reality. And if such a person tries to put his ideas into a product, that product may repel rather than appeal to others.

Healers are not like artists in that they do not create a concrete, valued, shareable product. But they are like many artists in that they are disinclined to accept the world as it is; they are inclined to make something different of it. Upon asking artists about their work, not infrequently one gets an euphemistic or avoidant answer; they only do the work, they might say; it is up to others to explain it. Healers do the same, but in my experience to an even greater degree, and not only with respect to healing. Many of them have designed their way of thinking and the style of their lives according to the principle that they will not be pinned down. They show a kind of claustrophobia, as if some unnameable dread lies in wait should they, for example, respond to a direct question with a direct answer, should they name or categorize, should they trace out logical connections or attempt to specify cause and effect. Like mercury, they slither from one direction to another, making them difficult people to interview. My experience with this difficulty is evidently typical. Lawrence LeShan writes, "Indeed, it is well known among experienced psychical researchers that the best way *not* to get the answer to a specific question from a sensitive [psychic] is to ask it as a specific question. One can only introduce the general subject and, perhaps, leading a little to the general area, await results and hope that the answer will arrive *spontaneously*." Thus, the interviewer is forced into the same state of mind that the psychic uses in order to do his or her work, a patient, pervasive passivity. LeShan quotes famous psychic after famous psychic describing the state of mind conducive to their psychic work in Zen terms: they do without doing, they wait rather than strive. Rosalind Heywood: "To me quiet and a more or less inactive brain are important — and *no* expectation on the part of my conscious mind ... you don't do psi [psychic work] by trying to do psi. You do it by trying to do something else." Eileen Garrett: "The slightest effort to consciously produce evidence will inhibit this condition ... pressure for 'results' is probably the singly most destructive factor in mediumistic phenomena."

For such people, even answering a direct question is evidently felt by them as a threat to their receptivity, a receptivity that pervades their whole personality rather than just being restricted to the psychic task at hand. The most famous of the Philippine healers, Tony Agpoa, was described this way: "There is nothing Tony dislikes more than a rigid schedule ... he is especially attracted to improvising and he loves surprises above all. Perhaps his personal talents would suffer if he were forced to adapt to a 'normal' daily schedule and submit himself to rules we routinely accept" (Stelter, p. 160).

Such claustrophobic, mercurial characteristics offer the best way I could find to explain an unexpected test behavior. When handed the Rorschach Test cards, about half of the subjects turned the cards upside down or sideways. Almost always they turned the cards frequently; in other words, if they turned a card at all, they did so on practically every card, and a good many times on each card. I have been unable to find statistics as to the frequency with which this card turning occurs in the general population of testees. But on the basis of my experience giving or supervising some thousands of the tests, these healers did far more turning of the cards than I would expect.

What does turning the cards mean? None of the standard test explanations seem to me to explain adequately the card turning that I observed the healers do. I am more persuaded by the explanation, in keeping with the rest of the test material, interviews, and observations, that these are people who in a wide variety of situations simply refuse to accept the world as it is, to take the cards as handed to them. Rather, they reacted to the implicit constraint of taking the card as handed to them by looking at things from a different point of view, at odd angles, or upside down. They did with the cards what they did in response to my interview questions.

Since healers claim to do remarkable, seemingly miraculous things, it is no surprise that they offer many indications of expansiveness, grandiosity, belief in limitless possibilities. Here are some examples of what healers saw in ink blots: someone walking on water, regeneration of lost parts, "the unlimited possibilities of springtime overriding everything," super-rabbits and Phoenix birds arising from ashes, and an oracle. Elmer and Alyce Green, longtime observers, experimenters, and authors on the occult among other things, have noticed this characteristic also: "... grandiose behavior ... is a trait shared by many mediumlike persons" (1977, p. 285).

Expansiveness and grandiosity are often linked with being the center of attention. So it is not surprising that the subjects offered many evidences of an inclination toward display or exhibitionism, as in seeing in the ink blots Kabuki dancers and Las Vegas and Ziegfeld show girls. One of them suggested that the words "praise" and "punishment" were similar in that both were "attention-getters." They studded their test responses with references to such super-performers as Isaac Stern, Zubin Mehta, Paganini, and Einstein.

Such grandiose and exhibitionistic responses may well issue from the fact that these are people who need to exhibit themselves, and who have enough confidence in their abilities to identify themselves, and practice, as healers. Yet as a group, healers tend to characterize themselves as humble. Almost to a person they claim that they are merely vehicles for a healing Power. However, the idea that a healing Power should have chosen *them* in particular as vehicles suggests anything but humility. It could be that great confidence in one's capacities is at the core of healing. Indeed, many patients seek out and seemingly benefit from healers (whether psychic healers or physicians) who inspire confidence, who seem to say with their personalities that they can cure. Justa Smith, the biochemist whose research showing the effects of a recognized healer's laying on of hands on enzymes is reported in Chapter 6, also studied as "healers" college students who had no belief in themselves as healers. The students followed the same procedures as the recognized healer but failed to influence the enzyme. Dr. Smith notes with regard to her findings and informal observations of many healers she has met that the healers must have "... absolute confidence in what they are doing. I'm sure they never doubt." The college students presumably had no such confidence. It is unclear, of course, whether the confidence promotes healing or comes from being successful as a healer.

A healer, a healee, and I had a long night's discussion during which we tried to tease out the possible contributions of many plausible causes for the healee's success in overcoming his illness. The erstwhile patient said good night and left the room, only to return shortly saying, "just one more thing — love and caring." Until then we evidently had taken love and caring for granted. The healing process is frequently described as being an expression of love, often with love as the *sine qua non* for healing. "Only love can generate the healing fire," says Agnes Sanford. "We must care for others deeply and urgently, wholly and immediately; our minds, our spirits must reach out to them," say Ambrose and Olga Worrell. Between healer and healee, writes Lawrence LeShan, "... there must be intense caring ..."

A case can be made for healing being an expression of the kind of love that predominates early in life, a love that is based on the wish and expectation of mother and child that mother will "make it all right." Just as the mother-child relationship begins with a symbiotic or merging phase, so too, for example, does one type of healing. In discussing his experiences in training people to become psychic healers, Lawrence LeShan describes it as the healer becoming as one with the healee. Without that context, results tend to be transient, while *with* it, results tend to be permanent. In ingenious experiments, Dr. Lloyd Silverman has shown that behavior of people being treated for a variety of ills, from phobias to schizophrenia, improved after the message "Mommy and I are one" was tachistoscopically flashed into their consciousness though outside of their awareness. This condition of merging takes place during the so-called oral stage, a time when the infant's, and therefore to a large extent the mother's, experience is dominated and saturated by things to do with nurturing, food, digestion, the mouth, and when the main mode of interaction is cradling and other kinds of soothing touch. Healing could, therefore, be considered a latter-day expression, a useful and subculturally condoned expression, of orality. It could be considered a sublimation of the oral stage of life just as being a gourmet or gourmet chef may be.

It is likely that people who have sustained such oral commitments and put them to important use would show other oral characteristics. They might, for example, tend to be overweight and to use their mouth in much talking as well as much eating. Such did seem to be the case with many of the healers; they were over-talkative and overweight. While, as I have noted, they were adept at not answering questions directly, they often sidetracked my questions through substituting garrulous, tangential talk for a direct answer. Not only was talk, for them, a means of avoidance, but it seemed a means of pleasure, a joyful exercise of the mouth, the more the better. Just as children may avoid the later life demands for order, self-responsibility, and independence by staying as long as they can at the oral level of development and having others minister to them, so too did the healers attempt through the exercise of oral faculties to fend off my attempts with questions designed to impose order and structure.

To shamelessly generalize, then, the typical healer has basically sound reality testing though is open to self-delusion through being less interested in checking ideas with reality than having wishes supported by like-minded people. Made anxious by the hemming in of rules and structure the typical healer is committed to finding their own path and rejecting that of others.

The healer is aided in this by sublime self-confidence, however cloaked in humility, and is drawn, in fact or fantasy, to center stage. The healing behavior itself may stem from an infantile layer of the mind that includes such oral traits as eating and garrulousness and a merging givingness modeled on the mother-child relationship.

It could be that those who benefit most from healing have similar or complementary personalities. They too may be people who can suspend disbelief, submit easily to awe and admiration, who feel their needs exquisitely and expect help with them. Healing may indeed be a temporary, symbiotic return to a time when love between mother and child conquered all, when mother often did, through the laying on of her hands, "make it all right."

Such a possibility is likely distasteful to many people in Western cultures who prize individual initiative and swaggering independence, who insist that any external help should be in the form of the high technology of drugs and machines. In rejecting the healing properties inherent in human interactions, such people may undermine the very glittering healing technology on which they are willing to depend. All healing depends, ultimately, on the patient's willingness to take advantage of whatever healing measures are offered in order to heal himself. Differences in receptivity to the infantile core of the healing interaction may explain the notoriously variable way in which people respond to the same healing interventions and why some healers are more successful than others, whether they be psychic healers or medical practitioners of the bedside manner. If further study supports the personality contributions to healing that I suggest here, then healing of all kinds requires coming to terms with the basic needs and assumptions of the infantile years. It has implications for who should become healers, and how they should be trained. Such coming to terms, involving aspects of love and peace, also, places healing in the same context as a wide variety of social problems, all of which might best be settled by capacities to give help and be cared for. Much in life requires healing. The universal experience of the mother-child interaction if accepted and implemented may be the matrix that provides for the healing of the universe.

Chapter Twelve

Kinesiology: Bodily Truth and Consequences

THE SCENE IS THE LOBBY area of the American Holistic Nurses' Association annual convention. I have my arm extended at a right angle from my body, and a young woman is pulling down on it while urging me to resist her pressure. In the best macho tradition I hold my arm firm. She presses various points on my body, and I persevere, with increasing pride. Then she touches a point near my hip, and my arm collapses as if I have suddenly lost my strength. The points that she has been pressing allegedly correspond to various inner organs. The sudden weakening reflects a deficiency in the organ corresponding to the area touched. The area touched may be right above the organ in question, or it may be at some distance, usually along an acupuncture meridian point that corresponds to an organ elsewhere in the body. Or one may touch an area known to be injured — for example, she touched my tennis elbow, and again I was unable to hold my arm firm. With other areas I resumed my stiff upper lip and stiff outer arm.

The name of this dramatic diagnostic procedure is kinesiology. I had originally encountered it as a parlor stunt. It seems to be making the rounds of parties as a demonstration of how bad sugar is; one puts a bit of sugar on the tongue, and the arm, held rigid without the sugar, collapses.

The demonstration in the convention lobby, inadvertently, showed something besides the phenomenon of how arms apparently weaken as a result of various influences. The kinesiologist's explanation for the weakening of the arm provided an example of how disparate approaches may share fundamental similarities. Her explanation could serve just as well as the one that Dr. Pfeiffer gave for why legs change in length in response to touching parts of the body with magnets. It could serve, also, for the various "touch" therapies such as acupressure, polarity message, Shiatsu. In all of them stimulation of points on the body close or far from an organ being tested or treated influence that organ. When the stimulated organs are deficient, the brain, which kinesiologists call a "biocomputer," directs energy to that stimulated deficient part, incidentally depleting the rest of the body. Dr. Pfeiffer detects the depletion by way of spinal movements that show themselves in, among other things, the length of the legs; kinesiologists detect it by noting the weakening of the muscles controlling the arm. They agree that one can make such measurements elsewhere on the body, as well; arms and legs are chosen for convenience.

I remembered another bit of evidence supporting the kinesiologist's contention from a demonstration George Leonard gave at a human potential conference some years back. He showed that one could resist downward pressure from his arm, or be unable to do so, according to what the subject was thinking. For example, if the subject thought of extending the arm across the world, of anchoring oneself in the earth, and of experiencing the arm as firm and unbending, then that person would be able to resist the pressure better than if one had been thinking of, say, dinner.

So much for diagnostic procedures. Like Dr. Pfeiffer, the kinesiologists maintain that they can with kinesiology also test therapies for their likely effectiveness. Instead of dropping a pill on the chest, as Pfeiffer does, they put a pill under the tongue (a vascular region that absorbs quickly) and then do the arm test while touching near the organ or injury in question. If, with the pill, the arm that was weak before becomes strong, then the pill is the right one for that organ or injury. If the arm remains weak, then the pill is not doing its job.

Here, economics takes over with a vengeance. The Nature-all Formulas, the brand that the demonstrator was selling, includes, at this writing, some thirty mixtures designed for a wide variety of symptoms. These symptoms and illnesses include connective tissue conditions, problems with the cardiovascular system, the digestive system, and the building of red blood cells; impaired kidney function, and poor absorption of various nutrients. The mixtures are for the most part made up of vitamins, minerals, enzymes, amino acids, fatty acids, herbs, and cell salts. According to the Nature-all literature, the mixtures were formulated through consultation with "experts from every important field of nutrition ... herbalists, homeopaths, biochemists, chiropractors, and formulators of natural supplements." The formulas were then "tested and finely tuned for years in clinical practice internationally, where they demonstrated overwhelmingly great success in producing better health!!!" I could have done with less hyperbole, no exclamation marks, and the citation of some systematic evidence of fine tuning. But the muscle testing observation was there, and requires an alternate explanation if one does not want to credit the explanation that the kinesiologists offer. As it stands, kinesiology along with several other approaches, asserts the truth of a bodily system, independent of the familiar medical one, which, when measured and stimulated in various ways, makes possible diagnosis and healing. Such stimulations are simple, not invasive, with no side effects, and inexpensive.

John Diamond, M.D. is a psychiatrist who believes that he can help patients by attending to what he calls the energy level of the body better than he could by giving people understanding. He offers two explanations for the apparent weakening of muscles revealed by kinesiological testing of the arm. One stems from Western medicine's understanding of the thymus. The thymus is a gland that lies in the middle of the chest, just beneath the upper part of the breastbone. In calves, and on French restaurant menus, it is called sweetbreads. Its main function is to secrete lymphocytes or white blood cells, which are responsible for the action of the immune system. Lymphocytes begin in the bone marrow and mature under the influence of thymus hormones. They then leave the thymus and settle in the lymph nodes and spleen. There they create T (for thymus) cells. As a true endocrine gland, the thymus continues to influence the T cells by way of hormones excreted into the bloodstream. The thymus not only creates and maintains T cells, but "teaches" them to distinguish self from non-self, friend from enemy, so that T cells can destroy foreign cells while leaving the other cells intact. Thus, T cells are the body's major defense against infections and, according to some recent opinion, cancer. The incidence of cancer increases with age as the size of the thymus decreases. Aged mice, given thymus extract, develop less cancer than those not given thymus extract.

One can make the thymus more efficient, according to Diamond, not only by supplementing it with thymus extract, but merely by tapping the body ten to twelve times just over the thymus. He prescribes "thymus taps" for quick, though temporary, increases in energy. The remarkable thymus, according to Diamond, can also help make equal the separate functioning of parts of the brain. People who ordinarily are more left-brained can increase their employment of functions controlled by the right side of the brain, and vice versa, through increasing the energy of the thymus.

Clearly, a gland that helps fight disease (including cancer), strengthens muscles, and works against dominance of one side of the brain over the other is a sweetbread that is no small potatoes. One might think, therefore that the thymus would be the object of extensive and rigorous investigation. Not so. Should a physician want to conduct research in the United States on the effects of administering thymus material from animals to humans, he would be risking his medical license if not his liberty. In other countries he might be a hero. Thus, I had to meet in secret with a physician who did inject people with thymus taken from animals. His patients were thus saved an expensive trip to Switzerland, where "live cell therapy" is used routinely for prevention and cure of a variety of diseases. Furthermore, the resulting improved health has cosmetic benefits: devotees claim that with live cell therapy wrinkles are reduced, natural color returns to grey hair, and eyes regain their youthful sparkle. No wonder Switzerland is a movie star playground. Such results are no surprise to Dr. X, the California outlaw physician who has observed these salubrious effects from his treatment as well. And why not? he asked, as he reiterated Diamond's claims; the immune system is central to the contraction or prevention of diseases, including cancer, and the thymus promotes a vigorous immune system. I would have liked some research demonstrations backing up each step in this line of reasoning, as well as proof that injections of fresh thymus cells strengthen the thymus and in turn the muscles. A physician friend tells me an injection of milk would be as useful — any stimulation of the immune system is helpful; it need not be thymus extract or thymus tapping — but whatever is used, the results are only temporary. And so it goes in our land of claim and contradiction.

The process of getting live thymus into the human recipient is a lot harder on the calf who supplies the thymus than it is on the person who receives it. I, as a contributor to Save the Whales and who melts at the gaze of a dog, am troubled to report that the thymus is taken from a calf killed immediately after its birth. The thymus tissue and secretion are injected into the hip area of humans at the bodily cost of only a slightly painful prick and mild soreness for a day or two. Some people have a minor systemic reaction, usually in the form of general malaise. Dr. X claimed that a more than minor reaction, especially early in a series of injections, signifies considerable pathology.

If I would like to invest in prevention of future disease, rejuvenated appearance, and enhanced energy, he recommended some ten to twenty injections. The cost of this illegal procedure in the United States presumably varies widely; I was charged $100 for each injection, or $200 for a double dose if it turned out that I could tolerate that much all at once. Since I was in the area only on a brief visit, I was able to take only two injections, one per day. I did not notice any after-effects, though I almost wished that I had, since such a reaction would at least have reassured me that my money was spent on something other than caramel-colored water. As it happened, in the ensuing year I made several trips to the area for various reasons, and, with double doses here and there, was able to get ten injections. My hair continues to be silvery grey. My forehead still has toy train tracks across it. There are those who claim that my eyes are brighter, and that I look younger than I used to. But then I heard that even when I used to look older.

The seeming parlor stunt of testing by way of changes in muscle strength turns out to be ensconced in physiological theories, but with no way presented of ruling out suggestion as the sole or contributory cause of any effects. It provides an entry to ideas and practices that promise to be of great use in diagnosis and healing. It is promulgated outside the established medical system by a grab bag of either self-deluders, mountebanks, or creative, intrepid pioneers. The rest of us bumble along waiting for some definitive opinions.

Chapter Thirteen
Olga, Ambrose, and Robert: A Convention of the Unconventional

THE AMERICAN HOLISTIC NURSES' Association's Annual Conference included talks and workshops on biofeedback, healing through touch, preventive medicine, detoxifying the body, and holistic mental health. This year the conference was organized in cooperation with Holistic Institutes of Health, an umbrella term for several institutes sharing the common purpose of promoting education and research in health improvement, pain management and stress control. Holistic Institutes of Health is the creation of the ubiquitous Norman Shealy, one of its institutes being the Shealy Pain and Health Rehabilitation Institute described in Chapter 10. That is why the conference took place at Southwestern Missouri State University in Springfield, Missouri — the city where Shealy has his headquarters.

I find myself rapturously transported by any college campus. I am mesmerized by the recognition that on this battered and battering planet there are these few square miles whose purpose is devoted to learning instead of battering; a fitting place for explorations into improved health.

Tiny and modest SMSU looks like a movie set; but that was not the only connection the conference had with film and drama. Alan Newman, a television producer and a member of the Advisory Council of Holos who has made several remarkable films on healing, showed, during this conference, videotapes of Brazilian psychic surgery. "Dr. Fritz," who is said to have been the spiritual guide to the famous Arigo, "surgeon with a rusty knife," has now become the guide of an obstetrician and gynecologist in Recife, Brazil, who has put aside his shiny, hygienic instruments and collegial relationship with anesthetists. Now he too uses a rusty knife or his bare hands, *sans* anesthesia, as illustrated by Newman's pictures, and does his operations in such a way that the camera can practically poke its lens into exposed, gaping holes in the patient. There was more drama to come, in the form of assertions of reality which flatly contradict traditional conceptions of what is possible.

Also under the Holos umbrella is the American Institute for Holistic Ecology, devoted to the study of the ecological aspects of health such as the effects of chemical farming on produce; the Biogenics Institute of Health, which encourages research related to biofeedback, nutrition, acupuncture, and behavioral medicine; and the Self-Health Institute, whose purpose is to provide public health education. Finally, there is the Ambrose and Olga Worrall Institute of Spiritual Healing, whose establishment was celebrated at this conference. That Institute provides a permanent repository for material related to the work of Ambrose and Olga Worrall, and will support research projects related to spiritual healing. To commemorate the new institute, Olga Worrall was presented with a plaque in recognition of her many years as perhaps the nation's premier psychic healer.

Upon Norman Shealy's presentation of the plaque, this ordinarily loquacious woman was (for the first time, according to those assembled) at a loss for words; not, however, at a loss for tears. She wept not only because of what the presentation of the plaque and the establishment of the institute signified, she said, but because her late husband, Ambrose, had chosen to be present on this occasion. I learned of this, of the many times she had seen him since his death, and of his regular communications to her about life in the spirit world, from the Bennetts, longtime friends of the Worralls who happened to be seated next to me at the ceremony. The relationship between the Bennetts and the Worralls had begun with the healing of Mrs. Bennett; they were neighbors in Baltimore, and over their thirty-odd years of friendship the Bennetts had been privy to many of the Worralls' healing and psychic exploits and, in the last several years, to the relationship between Olga and Ambrose as it has continued after Ambrose's death.

While I, among others, was not privileged to see Ambrose, at least one person other than Olga has been so privileged. Dr. Adachi, a professor of law and doctor of political science in Japan, had never had a previous psychic experience, and did not know he was having one when, while attending a lecture by Mrs. Worrall, he saw the deceased Mr. Worrall sitting beside her. That is his verbal and published claim. Ambrose appeared to Adachi so clearly that Adachi invited Mr. and Mrs. Worrall to a dinner party prepared for them both; he was surprised when Mrs. Worrall appeared alone. The extra sukiyaki stood as mute proof of his vision. (Dr. Adachi had told his wife to prepare sukiyaki for *four* guests, Mr. and Mrs. Worrall and another couple.) He provided articulate proof in a detailed description of the event; even more curiously, although he had never seen Mr. Worrall in the flesh or in photographs, he described him in detail.

Olga Worrall was the doyenne of healers.* If healers were baseball players, she would have been Joe DiMaggio. If you saw her at a party, and you used to read the *New Yorker* cartoons, you would think that a Helen Hokinson lady had come to life. She is prim and trim in what always seems to be a print dress; she always wears a hat. But if you saw her at one of the many human potential meetings where she appears, you would see a queen. She is either always surrounded by an entourage, or looks as if she is. What has she done to deserve such adulation? Whether her healings are any more effective or durable than those of any other healer is hard to say. All healers carry in their wake a long train of testimonials that go like this: "Medical science had given up on me; [the healer] did her thing; the next day the doctor was amazed to find I was no longer ill. 'Spontaneous remission,' he said, muttering." Mrs. Worrall, then seventy-six, has been a healer for a long time, and if for no other reason had a larger collection of such testimonials than most. For the most part she gave up individual healings, which for her involved the laying on of hands, in favor of distant healings. The ill person was instructed to sit quietly, every night at 9:00 P.M. Eastern Standard Time, and think about his or her illness and about Olga while Olga sent forth healing to hundreds, maybe thousands, all over the country and the world. She continued to do laying on of hands on Thursday mornings at her New Life Clinic at the Mt. Vernon Place Methodist Church in Baltimore. Here she gave a healing service during which those who wished queued up for the touch of her hands. One more reason for her many testimonials, and alleged cures,

---

* Mrs. Worrall died during the preparation of this book.

was her charismatic reputation, which presumably encouraged maximum exploitation of suggestion and placebo. Healers beget healings that beget healing.

Olga writes and says, at many opportunities, that she considers it a sacred duty to advance the cause of spiritual understanding and healing by cooperating with scientific investigators. She has probably been the subject of more laboratory studies than any other healer or psychic. According to these researches, she can change the molecular makeup of water by holding a vial of it in her hands; concomitant with her prayer therapy at a distance, she brought about uterine contractions in guinea pigs; she has lowered blood pressure in hypertensive patients; she has stimulated plant growth by concentrating her thoughts upon the plants; she has by her presence caused turbulence in a cloud chamber, a device used to detect elementary particles and other ionizing radiation (as described in Chapter 5), and when absent from the cloud chamber she has caused the same turbulence by visualization and concentration of her mind; she has minimized the effects of poison on bacteria, changed the surface tension of water, repaired damaged enzymes, and effected measurable changes in subjects' EEG, EKG, pulse, GSR and respiration by sending healing from a distance.

I cannot attest to the scientific purity of any of these researches, but I daresay that they adhered more closely to the scientific method than I did with Olga. She and I had met at breakfast in a hotel. I tried to persuade her to take psychological tests as part of the studies I conducted on healers. Despite her cooperation with scientists through the years and her avowed intention to thereby contribute to the advancement of psychic healing, she drew the line at psychological tests. I was told that someone had once tried to spring a Rorschach Test on her at a dinner party, and she had never gotten over the shock of it. I failed to persuade her to consider the test as a means of understanding rather than as potential proof of pathology. As a sort of consolation, she put her hands around a glass of water on the breakfast table, concentrated for a while, and gave me the water to do with as I chose. It so happens that I was at that time the owner of a large India rubber plant that was clearly terminal. I watered the plant with the water Mrs. Worrall had treated, and the plant is blooming still. A friend of my daughter's appeared with a fresh gash in his leg, and I sprinkled the wound with the treated water. He too is still blooming, which is medically not surprising, but his wound did heal far more speedily than could have been expected.

Scientific investigations delighted Olga's husband, Ambrose. According to Olga, they continue to delight him. He was an engineer and a spiritualist, as well as a highly effective healer, and was always confident that spiritualism, healing, and science would eventually come together. While their psychic powers, in addition to healing, were always well known — Olga's started when she was three years old — after Ambrose's death there was, to put it mildly, increased opportunity for the Worralls to demonstrate their spiritualist capabilities. According to Olga, the two are in constant communication. She has a large notebook in which she records his comments. She hears him in what she calls her "inner ear" and writes down what he says in her usual handwriting. However, when Ambrose is finished, he "takes her hand" and signs his name in his own handwriting.

Ambrose claims to ache to comfort Olga with his physical presence, but he says that his faster rate of vibration makes it impossible for her to see him except at those few times when conditions are favorable. Such references to "vibrations," strange as they may seem to those unfamiliar with the language and concepts of spiritualists, are part of their ordinary discourse. The reference stems from the belief that people, and indeed all "objects," have unique rates of vibration. These rates of vibration determine whether, and under what conditions in the viewer, the person or object is available to perception. Thus, a person may be there, in a certain sense, but invisible to any particular viewer if that viewer's requirements for a level of vibration are not met by the subject's vibrations. Strong emotions, particularly grief, are among the favorable conditions that make Ambrose visually available to Olga. She and Ambrose do get together, in a manner of speaking, when Olga sleeps, there perchance to slip out of her body on an astral trip with her husband. Olga recalls little of what she sees or experiences on such trips, though Ambrose refers to them often. He tells Olga of his life on the other side of death. I was delighted to learn from Ambrose by way of Olga that there is a Spirit World Library where one can "receive" the essence of a book (for more details of the other world, see Cerutti, 1975). In addition, Ambrose offers a theory of spiritual healing, central to which is what he calls para-electricity. The healer projects the electricity into the mind of the patient from which it moves to the cellular level in the area of the body that requires healing.

The last event at the Holistic Nurses convention, appropriately enough on a Sunday morning, was a healing service conducted by Mrs. Worrall. She declared the several hundred participants as attendees at a church service, and in so doing made it legally possible for her to heal the sick through the laying on of hands. (Ministers can perform such feats as part of a putative religious practice without being accused of practicing medicine without a license.)

According to Olga, even when one is free of disease, one can benefit from her touch for purposes of prevention of illness and for a sense of vibrant good health. Consonant with my usual procedure, I would have found a way to have those famous hands on my head. This time, however, I realized that a number of people had come there with serious illnesses in the desperate hope that she would heal them. Indeed, before the service, I saw in the audience Mr. and Mrs. D, whom I had seen and talked to from time to time at various healing meetings. They were taking every opportunity of which they could avail themselves, within conventional medicine and alternative medicine, to halt the potentially fatal inroads on Mrs. D of amyotrophic lateral sclerosis — Lou Gehrig's disease. Smiling, indomitable, yet with creases of anxiety around their eyes, they were here, as I have always seen them, with modest expectations from hard-edged reality, yet hoping for a miracle. They had driven several hundred miles for the healing service. Although they knew that Mrs. Worrall no longer does individual healings, they still hoped that somehow or other Mrs. D could have her chance to be healed by Olga. I learned that people in the audience would have hands laid upon them if they took their places in a queue. I told the D's of these plans and suggested that they try to station themselves near the podium where Olga was to be seated. They were delighted at the prospect of receiving Mrs. Worrall's attention; yet worried that because of Mrs. D's difficulty walking and maneuvering her steel walking aid, they might not be able to take advantage of this opportunity. In the milling about before the service, I apprised Mrs. Worrall of the situation. "Honey," she said to me (she calls everybody honey), "you know I don't do any individual healing anymore." A wink passed between us as I mumbled something about any opportunity to be helpful that might present itself.

We were to be treated to a facsimile of the weekly healing services that Olga has conducted these many years in Baltimore. Because of the large number of people, she had three other healers with her. She assured the audience that those who came up to be healed would receive equal benefit no matter whose hands were on them, and asked those who wanted to be healed to come forward as each row in the audience was called. I found her nomination of a healing quartet unsettling. I wondered glumly whether she meant by "equal benefit," *no* benefit, that all would receive equally. The arrangement seemed to imply that the others had the same healing skills that she had, though she was supposed to be the premier healer.

However, now with clear conscience, I was able to take my place in line and was eventually able to feel on my head the storied hands of Olga Worrall. Just after I left those cradling hands, I turned to point my camera, only to find that Olga was no longer there. She had walked to the audience and found Mrs. D, whose head she was now holding. Was it my imagination or was the whole assemblage frozen into a tableau of hushed reverence? Perhaps it was my imagination, also, that Olga looked like an angel and that Mr. D was crying, and that everyone around them seemed to be praying.

I saw Mr. and Mrs. D about a week later. She said that she felt better. She was breathing easier and could climb some stairs that had previously been too much for her. No miracle cure, but maybe a small miracle; or maybe just the small yield of anecdotal evidence.

WHEN OLGA INTRODUCED HER longtime friend and associate, Dr. Robert Leichtman, to the Sunday morning healing service, she referred to him as "Buttercup." Duke Ellington referred to *his* longtime associate, Billy Strayhorn, as "Sweetpea." The comparison is apt: Both Buttercup and Sweetpea were people of enormous talent in and of themselves — Strayhorn was Ellington's arranger, and a composer and pianist; Leichtman is a medical doctor, writer, psychic, healer, medium, and ordained minister who served Olga as her assistant at her weekly healing services, and as confidant on her professional activities. Both Strayhorn and Leichtman bask in the light of the highly publicized leaders with whom they are associated, and they are both partially obscured by those leaders' shadows.

Olga's choice of "Buttercup" for Leichtman was presumably based on his smooth-shaven, sunnily rotund appearance. Many people would, no doubt, consider his mind on the flabbily accepting side also. He not only practices psychic diagnoses and healing, but he claims to converse with people who are technically dead (see below). Such beliefs and practices could easily be explicable in terms of the personality of healers described in Chapter 11: a refusal to accept the world as it is in favor of a creative restructuring of it, with thinking dominated by wish-fulfillment relatively unchecked by logic, to say nothing of the scientific method. As will be seen, some of the things that he claims to do, to put it mildly, strain credulity. And yet, apart from some of his beliefs and activities, he is in many ways impressively sharp. He is articulate and lightly humorous; he thinks subtly about personality and the human condition; he draws from his background as an internist and upon a wide knowledge of contemporary culture. I particularly enjoyed and respected his initial reaction to my proposal to test healers. He suggested in a letter to me that one's capacity to heal was separate and superordinate to one's personality as measured by psychological tests. Examining healers' personalities is "... as unimportant as knowing which oil well was the source of the gasoline in the tank of your car." He warned me that "ordinary psychological testing would not only miss the mark, it might throw undue emphasis on unimportant points in the healing phenomena."

As a medical student Leichtman made medical diagnoses intuitively rather than deducing them from conventional medical examinations. The accuracy of his diagnostic inferences made that way are such that physicians use him as a diagnostic consultant. Unlike Edgar Cayce, who made such diagnoses while in a trance, Leichtman makes them in his usual consciousness, with the patient present or absent. Under either condition he claims to analyze a person's personality and physical situation from various bits of information that he gets psychically from their present and their past lives. He is reputedly as effective in the laying on of hands as Olga is. He gives lectures and courses in how to develop one's self spiritually and psychologically. He has codified his teachings in a series of thirty published essays entitled *The Art of Living*.[3]

Leichtman's capacity to overcome skepticism with wit and erudition is put to its most severe test in his series of books entitled *From Heaven to Earth*, which purport to be records of conversations with the spirits of William Shakespeare, Carl Jung, Sigmund Freud, Thomas Jefferson, and psychics such as Arthur Ford, Eileen Garrett, and Edgar Cayce. The *modus operandi*: Leichtman's associate, medium David Kendrick Johnson, goes into a trance which supposedly enables him to contact the spirit in question. The spirit uses Johnson's voice to answer questions put to him (them) by Leichtman.

I have before me a scribbled note from my then-sixteen-year-old son who was with me in an audience to which Leichtman presented this project, and during which Leichtman recited snatches of conversations with his esteemed communicators. (Leichtman refers affectionately to the communicators as "spooks.") My son wrote, "How can you find out whether or not one is capable of talking to spooks and about other psychic tricks — how do you know you are right? Is it really Will Shakespeare and not *you* out of your gourd?" I assume that the *you* in my son's question was somewhere in between the impersonal "you" and a specific questioning of my own gourd. He went on to ask if there was any evidence that dead people continued to learn and develop psychologically, whether persons who died in their youth remain as they are or become wiser as time goes on in the spirit world, and if they do become wiser, how? How do the dead keep up with events in the living world without the aid of a living medium? Do all spirits do so, or only those who were psychic in their earthly lives? Was Shakespeare "psychic"? My son wondered whether the dead transcend the language barrier — did Jung and Freud speak English? (Jung was articulate in English; Freud was less so and did not write professionally in English as Jung did.) Leichtman tries to explain the language issue by saying that Johnson receives the ideas and translates them into his own words, using his own language and vocal rhythms. That does not quite come to grips with the question of whether the spook has to speak to Johnson in English, or whether he can communicate thoughts in ways that transcend language. The issue is important, particularly for those who would cherish the idea of learning Shakespeare's thoughts, for as my son pointed out, Shakespeare's Elizabethan idiom could not be readily understood by most speakers of contemporary English.

My son's questions serve as openers to the question of validity: is Leichtman really transmitting the thoughts of dead people? According to him, in his Preface to Volume I of the series, the reader can measure the validity of the interviews — and the continued existence of the communicators — by the value of what is said. In Leichtman's view, the communicators all had "the spark of genius," which presumably Johnson does not have, and so if this spark of genius is manifest in interviews, it must come from the communicator. Leichtman believes that the spark of genius is abundantly manifest throughout the series of interviews. I failed to find it. When I am told that I am to be privy to the words of William Shakespeare or Sigmund Freud, I expect repartee of more than average intellectual substance, and evocative style. Maybe that's not fair, either to Leichtman or, considering the special circumstances of the interview, to Shakespeare and Freud. While the remarks of the communicators are not without wit, charm, and knowledge specific to their fields, they are not so witty, charming, and knowledgeable as to be outside the repertoire of less gifted living persons. The key to the question is Johnson. Either he is a person who in his usual consciousness can speak as the "communicators" did, or only in his mediumistic life does he have the requisite knowledge and style of speech and thought attributed to the communicators, or specialized knowledge is made available to him in the trance state by the alleged communicators.

Leichtman tells me that he has himself served as a medium for communications with illustrious dead persons. He describes the experience much as Olga describes her communication with Ambrose. Neither he nor Olga need a trance for such communication, they just listen to "an inner voice." From what I know of Leichtman, he, as a living, breathing mortal, might be sufficiently knowledgeable as to supply the information that comes out in these communications from notables on the other side.

At one point during his interview with Leichtman, Edgar Cayce "pointed" to the medium's cigarettes and asked for one, even specifying which of two brands on the table next to the medium he preferred. The cigarette evidently did not disappear. Thus, if discarnate entities are going to enjoy cigarettes, then the cigarette has got to become discarnate also, or else some mechanism would have to be specified to get the cigarette enjoyment to them psychically. The cigarette issue is but one detail in a mosaic of questions that any scientist, detective, or ordinary citizen who is devoted to logic, would level at the spook project. I halfway expected that the urbane, intellectual part of Leichtman would disavow the whole thing when I questioned him about it. But unflappable as always, he had some kind of answer for everything that I asked. What these interrogations boiled down to was whether I wanted to believe or not. As always, I tried to keep an open mind, even tried to tilt toward only mildly critical acceptance, but the spook project remains a bit too much for me.

There are serious problems connected, too, with the evaluation of Leichtman's psychic readings, as there are with those of others. Leichtman did a series of readings of some of my professional acquaintances, my cancer patients, and myself, sometimes with the subject corporeally there, and at other times when the subject was not there. When one considers the difficulty of the task, it is of course amazing that he or any psychic could get anything right. Leichtman offered many instances of apparently correct information along with many instances of apparently incorrect information, as well as information the accuracy of which could not be determined at the moment; especially predictions. I use the words "correct" and "incorrect" glibly; such judgments are difficult to make. The chief difficulty in judging the accuracy of the inferences offered — not only by psychics, but often by psychologists and psychiatrists — lies in the generality of their comments. People are sufficiently complex and their bodies have so many aches and pains that one could consider almost anything said about personality or bodily functioning to be true in some sense. I inadvertently demonstrated this difficulty when I was going over the transcriptions made from tapes of Leichtman's psychic readings. As a result of a secretarial error I read material about one subject while I was thinking it was about another subject, and I scored a number of comments as correct. They *were* correct, in a sense: the sense supplied by me. I could have judged them as correct had they been appended to the names of dozens of other people as well. Leichtman's saying that such and such part of a body was unhealthy would result in correct diagnostic statements a certain number of times even without psychic skills.

With all that, he did make some diagnostic statements that were difficult to explain away. In giving names of subjects for Leichtman to "read" psychically, I gave him a pseudonym once used by one of the subjects. I also gave him that subject's real name as if it belonged to another subject. Since the two names referred to the same person, their readings could have been expected to be the same. Leichtman's first comment about the pseudonymous person was, "I first get the image of two very different people." He had not made that comment with regard to any other subject, and so that comment was impressive. Yet he described the person as different from the same person with a different name. Enter here two major methodological problems: (1) Since one "person" was reacted to on the basis of his name only and the second "person" was present during the reading, these different conditions could have influenced Leichtman's differential readings. (2) If one reads the unconscious of any person, one is likely to come up with comments about them that seem different from the way they appear on the surface. In a sense everybody is two or more persons and has various sides to his character. Some of Leichtman's comments were subtly descriptive of the subject and too specific to dismiss them as lucky guesses or as applicable to anyone.

My experience evaluating Leichtman's work was an extreme example of my frequent experience with psychics: his audacious claims stimulated a quick rush of skepticism, and yet his demeanor, reputation, and quasi-persuasive demonstrations at least keep the door open to definitive study.

For what it is worth, Leichtman was the third psychic to place one of my past lives in France at the time of the Revolution. How he arrived at his arcane information may or may not have had something to do with his whistling, in-between his psychic revelations, "Thanks for the Memories."

Chapter Fourteen

Tripping the Light Fantastic: The Possibilities of LSD

I WAS INVITED TO PARTICIPATE in an annual convention of the American Academy of Psychoanalysis because of my published remarks about possible applications to psychoanalysis of insights and practices from the new therapies.[1] As the representative of therapies outside of and challenging to psychoanalysis, I assumed that I was to be the heavy. I prepared myself for sharp questioning, and the sometimes indignant dramatics characteristic of many such confrontations.

None of that took place, however, because of a sharp dialectical shift to the left which left me in a relative rightist position. This shift was supplied by another member of the panel, Stanislav Grof. Though trained in Czechoslovakia as a psychoanalyst and medical doctor, he offered ideas not only outside and antithetical to some aspects of psychoanalysis, but which challenged basic assumptions of the reality of practically every person in the room. Not only that, but he had been a leading researcher in LSD. Had *LSD* been a stimulus word on a word association test given to people in that room, myself included, likely responses would have been "acid," "kids," "sixties," and "craziness." The attitudes implied in such associations were largely responsible for LSD's being declared illegal, including even use for research purposes (with the exception of limited use with cancer patients). The data for the revolutionary ideas that Grof asserted were drawn from his decades of research with about four thousand LSD experiences. For that, if for no other reason, he was a hard man to argue with. Nobody else there had observed patients and normal subjects during LSD experiences under controlled conditions as Grof had; he was the only one with data.

As a person Grof may seem contradictory. Somewhat overweight and burly, he nonetheless gives the impression of hard-muscled litheness. Though a member of the counterculture and dressed accordingly, there is something of the three-button suit about him. As I subsequently learned, he is generous and warm. Yet he has a slightly forbidding, no-nonsense surface. At first he may give the impression that he is not listening, while in fact he is listening carefully and, moreover, is patient and accepting of whatever is being said. As with many people for whom English is a foreign language, he is highly precise and articulate in its use. (English is one of eight languages he knows, including Sanskrit.) In his presentation and in response to questions he was low-key, well-organized, and had clearly given his subject much thought. As a result of his demeanor, his ideas, which under other circumstances might have been met with derision and dismissal, were met with thoughtfulness — although consternation certainly did show around the edges.

His two main assertions were (1) that life in the womb and birth are, like post-birth experiences, recorded in the brain and influence the development of personality and later-life symptoms, and (2) that people are capable of experience that is *transpersonal*, above and beyond the personal, and that what we are ordinarily aware of by way of our five senses is merely a sliver of the reality that we could be aware of — a reality which has vastly different characteristics from the five senses one. According to Grof, the transpersonal experience provides a basis for understanding paranormal phenomena and psychic healing. And if my patients were being influenced by prenatal life and birth experience, then I was missing one way of helping them master influences from their past on the present. So I eagerly absorbed the following, condensed from Grof's remarks at that conference, from later opportunities that I had to talk with him, and from his books. But first some introductory remarks about regression, which is one way of conceptualizing the process by which knowledge of the transpersonal and prenatal states is achieved.

"Regression" is one of those psychiatric-psychoanalytic-psychological words which means different things to different people, and sometimes different things to the same person, depending upon the context. Regression may be used to refer to a back ward hospital patient's regressing to the point of smearing feces on the walls, or to the joyful regression of being silly on Saturday night. Whatever the degree and circumstances, it occupies a point on a line between daytime objective problem solving using a highly focused turn of mind; and the night time — as reflected in dreams — of diffuseness, imaginativeness, rules or grammar of thought that violate conventions of time, space, and cause and effect.

It is less a matter of how "deep" the regression is than of who is doing the regressing, the capacity to control and use such oscillations. For example, when Jung declared James Joyce's daughter to be schizophrenic on the basis of her disordered thinking, Joyce remonstrated by saying that her thinking was like his writings. Jung is said to have gently replied, "But Mr. Joyce, you are able to turn it on or off." So from time to time one may choose to loosen the bonds of ordinary, focused reality in favor of reverie, daydreams, producing and enjoying works of art, experiencing sexuality, or taking a vacation, especially to places where the culture and way of life are greatly different from one's usual ones.

One is aided in regressing when the environmental stimuli are minimal or unclear. Thus, people become "regressed" under conditions of stimulus deprivation, as when in a dark enclosure or floating in a tank of water. In highly structured situations, where the task is clear and the choices are few, people fasten themselves to a limited reality, to the detriment of regressive possibilities. As the situations become less structured and the task ambiguous, they regress, in the sense of drawing upon deeper levels of their personality and imagination to fill in the blank screen. In talking to patients in psychotherapy, face to face, one provides a degree of structure which limits regression. When the patient lies on the couch with the seemingly clear but fundamentally ambiguous task of saying whatever comes to mind, it is often found that ideas ordinarily held outside of awareness come more easily into awareness.

According to Grof, the psychoanalytic method of inducing regression is sound and useful, but only to a point. Its regression-producing circumstances are insufficiently powerful to allow revelations from the deepest levels of consciousness. While Grof acknowledges that some symptoms and symptomatic behaviors do change in the course of psychoanalysis, these are ones that have had their inception or greatest impetus in later states of infantile life, and which can then be summoned by way of verbal connections, with ordinary language. Psychoanalysts themselves have been responding to the challenge to go back to earlier periods in patients' lives. While Freud emphasized the so-called phallic or oedipal stages of the years four through six, many psychoanalysts since then have emphasized the so-called preoedipal factors from birth through four years of age, and some claim that in the first year of existence there is a well differentiated mental life which includes developmental challenges thought by most other psychologists to occur much later.

The body, which after all is there before language, is a mediator of a deeper level of experience than the mind. Some view it as a kind of tape recorder in which physical trauma, disease, operations, and even psychological events translated into physical terms are laid down, there later to be discovered and amplified. This may be done through direct physical intervention such as the deep massage and manipulation of such body therapies as Rolfing, bioenergetics, or the Alexander Technique, or through psychological regression.

The next, deeper level is perinatal, which refers to life around the time of birth, available to awareness if one can find the means of promoting deep enough regression. Grof emphasizes the seemingly obvious — that birth is intimately connected to death. Ordinarily, no one is closer to death than at birth, when the child's life hangs in the balance. Freud said that we could not know death because we have not experienced it; our knowledge exists only in our fantasies about it. According to Grof, we do experience it, or at least its proximity, during birth. That experience is indelibly imprinted on the mind. But, one might understandably ask, what of the conventional medical opinion that the neonate's brain is too little myelinized, its nervous system insufficiently covered with that organic sheath to record memories, or even to transmit pain? Grof argues that the standard medical opinion is wrong. He has observed hundreds of LSD experiences in which people relive perinatal and birth events which are highly differentiated and of great emotional significance. He cites an obstetrician, David Cheek,[2] who took notes on the birth circumstances of his patients, and twenty years later with hypnosis had those same patients recall their birth. He found a high degree of correlation between his notes and their memories. There is an accumulating literature of investigation using a variety of means which promote prenatal and birth regressions. These investigations report the appearance of bodily manifestations which according to records occurred at that time but had since vanished, birthmarks, for example. Memory can be demonstrated in fish, which have no cortex, to say nothing of inadequate myelinization of the cortex. One can condition even unicellular organisms. Surely, then, an infant is equipped to evaluate the many hours and powerful events of the birth process. The most impressive and obviously useful aspect of these studies is the fact that symptoms often disappear when a person re-experiences such early life events — symptoms that have proved intractable to explorations at less deep levels of experience.

At this point in his discussion, Grof remains within the tradition of psychoanalysis and other environmental approaches conveyed through the five senses which posit that life events lost to awareness nonetheless continue to influence behavior. His novel contribution to this model is to include within it earlier life events, earlier environmental stimuli, than most disciplines have allowed for. His next step, however, marks a radical departure. By contrast with influences conveyed sensorially from the environment, he claims that there is a *transpersonal mind*, a cosmic consciousness which is standard just by way of being alive.

In ordinary consciousness, modeled on the philosophical beliefs of Descartes and the physical beliefs of Newton, one's identity is coexistent with one's body. Mind is a function of brain. Bodies have fixed and clear boundaries that separate themselves from the environment. Experience is limited to the present as mediated by the senses. One calls up the past into the present, and the future is knowable only through fantasy taking place in the present.

By contrast, the transpersonal hypothesis includes a conception of mind as primary rather than as a function of brain; the body is merely a temporary mediator of mind, which continues when the body is gone. Mind or spirit may continue in the cosmic sphere or, according to Grof, may invest itself in a new bodily mediator, as is the case in reincarnation. Separateness is an illusion promoted by limitations of the senses. For a dog who can hear it, very high-pitched sound is part of reality, while to a human who cannot hear such a high pitch, that sound does not exist in their reality. A drop of water is one thing to the naked eye, and quite another under a microscope. The reality that ordinarily seems so palpable has, in fact, to be learned. When congenitally blind people are given sight, they cannot at first make out what the sightless consider to be reality; they have to learn about it. Some of them resist that learning, preferring the previous familiar reality conveyed by their other senses. In transpersonal reality, Newtonian conceptions are replaced by Einsteinian ones: quantum physics, the recognition of relativity, flux, permeability, and oneness. While an object may appear solid, when scientists probe deeply into the nature of matter, supposedly solid matter is revealed as being made up of swirling energies, particles, some of whose existence are calculated mathematically rather than observed — reality is less discrete *things* than it is *relationships*. Time and space are seen as inventions of the mind superimposed upon a reality which has no such inherent dimensions. Past, present, and future occur at the same time and so are knowable at any given instant, as countless psychics have implicitly claimed in their readings of past and future. Since boundaries are illusory, psychics can learn about a person by way of temporarily becoming that person, or animal, or leaf, since all of nature is organized by one consciousness. For example, people may discover in themselves an identification with an animal and perform the mating dance done by that animal, even though in their usual consciousness they do not know those movements. Healing can take place across thousands of miles, as healers who practice distance healing claim, since space is only a construction of limited consciousness, irrelevant to the communication possible between parts of an all-embracing whole. Seeing what is or is not occurring out of the viewer's eyeshot — so-called remote viewing — becomes understandable if we accept the idea that if the idea of space does not intervene, then one simply views what is there.

The contents of consciousness, since it is unitary, can be found in all cultures and in all times. Grof has some five hours' worth of slides of drawings done during and after LSD experiences — and of cave paintings and paintings through time from various cultures; their themes and images are strikingly similar. The subjects who drew while under the influence of LSD were almost without exception unfamiliar in their non-LSD consciousness with these paintings and drawings. Jung captured the idea of a unitary consciousness in his concept of a collective unconscious which included archetypes — images that influence all people, regardless of their environmental training. Herein lies the means of understanding how it is that a fetus can be influenced by, and make sense of, intrauterine environmental events. The fetus has not yet learned postnatal consciousness. It is unimpededly tied to the transpersonal, cosmic consciousness, and it is the contents of that consciousness which are activated by the environmental events of the birth process.

While Freud criticized Jung for deserting the dynamic unconscious and the recognition of the influence of environmental, and especially psychosexual events, Freud himself was neither insensitive to nor above using speculative, sometimes quasi-mystical ideas. In attempting to account for the occurrence of the Oedipus Complex, he took recourse to a wildly speculative phylogenetic hypothesis, as propounded in his *Totem and Taboo*.[3] With little biological justification, he posited a death instinct, an entropic force returning people to their basic organic state after the hiatus called life. He suggested that anxiety had its beginning in the birth trauma, an idea that most of organized psychoanalysis has chosen to ignore (along with his ideas about the death instinct and his views on non-medical analysis). Freud as a grand speculator and perhaps a closet mystic can be seen especially in his last books. There he considered, albeit ambivalently, the possibility of psychic phenomena. Were it not for sociopsychological influences, including the need of his time and place to be acceptable to materialistic science, he might have implemented and embroidered his speculation with transpersonal and mystical awareness. His follower, Rank, did exploit Freud's ideas on the importance of birth trauma to later personality. Another of Freud's followers, Sandor Ferenczi, claimed that the wish to return to the womb reflected a wish to return to the ocean, suggesting that humans are something like dolphins and whales, who had a try at the earth and heeded the call of a return to the sea. These expansionistic tendencies lost out, however, to an uncompromising reductionism in the battle in Freud's mind and consequently in the history of psychoanalysis. Every psychological event, according to Freud's reductionistic view, is potentially understandable solely in terms of a sensorially-mediated reality and according to the tenets of the psychoanalytic theory of personality.

LIKE SO MUCH MEDICAL vocabulary, "intractable symptom" has an authoritative ring, and often stimulates a knowing, sad shrug of the shoulders. But such a judgment may be less authoritative than relative. Who has decided that a symptom is intractable, and on what basis? Is its intractability a function of any individual practitioner's lack of skill, of knowledge available in a particular discipline but which might be available in another discipline; in fact, has everything been tried, or only those measures that are geographically or financially available?

Grof suggests that all possible sources of symptoms have *not* in fact been dealt with. In addition to those stemming from environmental events after birth, there are also those stemming from environmental events before birth, and from the collective unconscious and past lives as they function by way of cosmic consciousness. In his view the post-birth environmental influences, useful as they may be for some purposes, may not be sufficient for other purposes, and they reveal their bankruptcy when symptoms persist. He creates the image of well-meaning, often highly proficient, psychological practitioners lengthening the time of treatment to Woody Allen dimensions, in the hope that more of the same will finally turn the tide. Yet such practitioners are doomed to failure for want of an approach that accounts for all the major forces influencing the symptoms.

Anxiety is the engine that runs the psychopathological machine (as it does in normal and sometimes superior functioning). Anxiety is the expected and necessary response to danger. While a conventional point of view might indict the danger as being to one's masculinity (especially as embodied in sexual functioning) or of loss of love, abandonment, or loss of control, the fundamental basis for anxiety may be *birth* anxiety, stemming from the time when life itself is threatened, when basic survival is at issue. A claustrophobia, for example, may be maintained less out of a fear of being overcontrolled by a powerful parent than by the memory of an actual situation in the womb when circumstances produced the danger of never being born or of intolerable, seemingly trapped conditions.

Aggression, which might otherwise be traced to one or another kind of post-birth deprivation or threat, might in addition be understood as a response to the fear of life-threatening events at or before birth. The depression often linked to deprivation of oral supplies — food, warmth, protection of the early years — might additionally be linked to the loss of the maternal organism and its umbilical cord connection. Post-birth deprivations of basic supplies may reactivate and reinforce still earlier losses. In and of themselves, post-birth deprivations might never have led to a particular symptom — obesity, for example; that symptom may resist change until the earlier sources of loss are dealt with. Those suicides whose purpose seems to be an escape into peace and reunion with a lost love object, may be an attempt to return to the oceanic condition of birth, before the activities of the later birth process. Such suicides distinguish themselves by their passive nature: overdosing with drugs or submitting to escaping gas in a closed area. One explanation for the not infrequent cutting of wrists while in a water-filled bathtub might be a wish to reproduce the fluid sac of the womb. That one kind of suicide, at least, may not be a wish to kill or be killed, but rather an attempt to find transcendence, a mystical union — experiences felt to be irreparably missing in life. Other suicides are traceable to the no-exit situation that obtains at the onset of the birth process: an inexplicable powerful pressing on the neonate begins before the cervix is open and thus before there is apparent hope for escape.

The inclination of severely regressed people to eat excrement or drink urine, as occasionally some children do, may reflect that period in the womb when the child is in fact surrounded by such biological substances. *Vagina dentata*, the fantasy that the vagina has teeth which can destroy parts or all of the person, may have its source in the painful, frightening, life-threatening moments when the child enters and moves through the vagina, sometimes with great difficulty, on the way to being born. The common fear of being cut may be traceable not only to the castration complex but to cutting involved in the birth process, episiotomy, umbilical cord, or Caesarean section. Migraine and other headaches and asthma may be traceable to the crucial moments during birth when the head is impinged upon, and the infant may have to gasp, sometimes unsuccessfully in the case of a twisted cord, for air. Tremors and tics may have their inception in motor inclinations in the womb that have no place to go, whose expression is restricted to brief, abortive actions. Perhaps the myth of the Garden of Eden has its beginning in the expulsion of the infant from its oceanic condition in the womb.

If, as has been observed to many people's discomfort, infants have a sexual life (for example, they masturbate), then they may have a sexual life in the womb as well. Thus, sexuality becomes associated with events of the womb: excretion, pain, and forces over which one feels one has no control. Such conditions are reproduced in such perversions as requiring excretory acts or products for personal pleasure, in masochism, and in the common fear, resulting in various impairments of the sexual response, of being swept away by sexuality — a diffuse and pervasive fear of surrender to orgiastic experiences.

What could be expected in the way of effects on personality of having been born by elective Caesarean section? People born that way would be subject to influences from time in the womb, but not from labor and birth itself. (Those Caesareans undertaken because of unsuccessful labor would provide still different experiences.) It seems that people born through elective Caesarean section miss not having experienced the later stages of the birth process: for them there is always something undone, a sense of wrongness leading to the consequent need to get into situations that require breaking out, challenges. If not kept in the birth canal too long, they are likely to be optimistic and have the expectation of easy success. If kept in the womb too long, they have feelings of inferiority, as if somehow they failed to do what they were supposed to do. They tend in later life to have easier access to transpersonal experiences, which implies that in non-Caesarean births the agony of birth forces a shift away from the prenatal transpersonal to the postnatal environment. Grof states that people born by way of Caesarean section have difficulty defining their position in the world, are unsure how much they can ask of it, and do not know where they belong. Also, they have an affinity for knives, presumably reflecting the scalpel that released them to independent existence.

This topic was a matter of more than pedestrian interest to me since my own children were born by way of elective Caesarean section, without experiencing labor. I thought about having brought my son a collection of knives as souvenirs from countries that I had visited. Was I responding to something in me or in him? Then I saw among the slides in Grof's collection a painting by modern popular artist Frank Frisetta — a painting whose prominent feature was of a man in armor with upraised sword. Knives are prominent in a number of pictures drawn by Frisetta, who for a long time was one of my son's favorite artists. My son had the painting represented in Grof's slide on his wall for years. Coincidence, of course, or was it? I later noticed on the wall of his college dormitory, incongruously surrounded by examples of the fine arts, a knife I had given him fifteen years earlier. He had no clear explanation as to why that odd item was ensconced on his wall, though he offers clear and forceful opinions about most things. Like a person behaving according to post-hypnotic suggestion, he seemed blankly puzzled about his action. (A psychoanalyst's explanation having to do with the vicissitudes of father–son relationships is, of course, plausibly available.)

Grof offers a cartography of the stages of birth which he calls "basic perinatal matrices." Each of these is recreated during LSD sessions, has its analogue in Freudian erogenous zones, results in specific symptoms, and finds its way into interests, activities and personality traits in postnatal life.

Matrix I is the primal union with the mother, encompassing intrauterine experiences before the onset of delivery. Without noxious stimuli interfering, this matrix includes the symbiotic, oceanic condition of optimal security, protection, and satisfaction of needs. Noxious stimuli range from occasional, brief interruptions of this ideal state — such as mild disease, occasional dietary indiscretions including the use of cigarettes and alcohol, excessive noise, gynecological examinations, sexual intercourse in later months of pregnancy — to severe and extended interferences with the ideal state, such as serious diseases in the mother, unremitting tension and emotional stress, excessive noise and vibrations, chronic drug and alcohol addictions, cruel and violent treatment of the mother, and crude attempts at abortion. The ideal oceanic aspects of this matrix appear in LSD sessions in the experience of the world as friendly and secure; subjects display a resulting confidence that needs will be met, often with little effort on their part. Such a background gives rise to peak and transcendental experiences. When noxious interruptions are relived, the person may report ecstatic episodes which are suddenly interrupted by visual or somatic symptoms. While tranquil intrauterine experiences are closely related to religious and mystical enlightenment, disturbances of the intrauterine life also appear to be the source of schizophrenia and paranoid conditions, perhaps explaining the sometimes precarious boundary found between schizophrenia and spiritual enlightenment.

In Matrix II the mother and child are in conflict with one another as the ideal comes to an end, first through chemical influences, then by uterine contractions. There is extreme emergency and a sense of vital threat, along with intense physical discomfort. With the cervix closed, and as yet no progressive movement, the fetus has no evidence that things could ever be different. It experiences terror and discomfort as timeless and forever, therefore leading to a sense of hopelessness. It is a world of "no exit," "hell," claustrophobia. In later life a person excessively influenced by Matrix II is selectively aware only of the ugly, evil, and hopeless aspects of existence. The person shows empathy and identification with the victimized, downtrodden, and oppressed, and exists in a dehumanized, grotesque, meaningless, and absurd world. Coinciding with the deadly clarity about the meaninglessness of existence, is a desperate need to find meaning, perhaps issuing from any attempts of the fetus to escape from the closed uterine system.

In Matrix III, mother and child work together to bring about passage through the birth canal. While there is a great struggle for survival, with crushing mechanical pressures and often a degree of suffocation, with the cervix open hope is in sight, and the interests of mother and child coincide as they strive to end the painful condition. There is light at the end of the tunnel. In the titanic struggle of Matrix III there is a mixture of inflicting and receiving pain, considerable sexual excitement, and scatological preoccupations.

In Matrix IV there is the separation from the mother (termination of the symbiotic union and formation of a new type of relationship). The agonizing experiences connected with propulsion through the birth canal come to a climactic end; tension and suffering are followed by sudden relief and relaxation. Psychologically, the fetus experiences the death of all that has gone before, and rebirth in a new context. This provides the basis for all later life change which by definition involves ending or giving up what one knows in favor of the danger, and hope, of what one cannot as yet know.

While all the matrices leave their marks on the personality, one or more may be of heightened significance, and thus disproportionately influence later personality, symptoms, or behaviors. Any such special emphasis shows itself in its centrality and emphasis in the LSD sessions. If the stirred-up thoughts and feelings derived from any matrix are not adequately worked through during or after the LSD session, they may continue for weeks or months to influence mood, thought, and behavior.

Grof was confident about what could be accomplished therapeutically through confrontation with one's birth process and extended consciousness. According to him, such confrontations, induced by psychedelics or precipitated by other mind-expanding means including emotional or spiritual crises, can eliminate the fear of death, lead to a life transformation, overcome psychosomatic and other symptoms, and produce beneficial change even in instances of severe mental disturbance such as schizophrenia. Indeed, according to Grof, many people labeled currently as psychotic might be merely stuck in a process of expanding awareness. If such people successfully move through the labyrinth of altered consciousness, they can turn what otherwise might be called pathology into one of restructuring, opening, and elevating existence. Was this, I thought, the myth of the happy lunatic surfacing again? How was I now to think about the view of the mind that I had observed for years?

I would soon have a chance to try to answer such questions, and to formulate new ones. It just so happened, Grof told me, that a few weeks hence, he and his wife and colleague, Christina, would be giving a five-day workshop at Esalen — a New Age center in Big Sur, California — using "holonomic integration," their method of exploring transpersonal consciousness. I went through the usual inner debate and outer juggling of the calendar, but the conclusion was foregone. There was too much promising material here for the study of psychic phenomena and healing to cavil about details.

A FEW WEEKS LATER, I found myself, once again, in Esalen. How would it be the same, I wondered, and how different from the way I had found it some seven years before? It is still, as I wrote in *Out In Inner Space*, "a choice spot on one of the world's most beautiful seacoasts, an Eden cliff above the Pacific Ocean and below the Big Sur mountains." I found it, however, even more breathtakingly beautiful than I had remembered it. The air seemed more crystalline, the waves to leap higher, their crash against the rocks more resonant. I roved deeper into the Nature of the place, went further along the roads and paths. I felt (or thought I felt) an "energy," a sense of new possibilities. As it happened, I learned that when people with particularly strong psychic abilities came to Esalen, they too noted such an energy, and even localized it in one spot where, it is said, the Esalen Indian medicine men had performed their rites.

Since the geography hadn't changed, what, I wondered, had changed in me? Among other things, on the previous trip I had been more introspective about myself, a state of mind allowed if not goaded by a steady diet there of Gestalt practices and encounters. I had been softened by body work such as Rolfing, and been blown open by culture shock, since the human potential represented at Esalen was at that time new to me. I was too absorbed in what it meant to me, on making my first trip to nude bathing in Esalen's sulphur tubs, for example, to make such quizzical observations as the following which I made on this trip: not wanting to bother to get undressed and dressed in the Spartan conditions around the tubs, and taking advantage of a balmy night, I simply wore my towel down the long path that led from the central activities to the baths which are nestled on the side of a cliff. As I walked the path, from *de rigueur* clothing to *de rigueur* nudity, I found myself trying to decide at what point on the path I could remove the towel, when a social sin and legal offense would become acceptable.

The Esalen format was as before. The days were full of ways of experiencing and studying body, mind, and spirit. Some people were there for two-day weekends, others for a week or a month, and others were long-term scholars. The people, however, seemed to me to be less spacey, more down to earth, a bit more organized than they had seven years ago. I also detected a bit more shortness and irritation than I had remembered as the more usual open, welcoming, and gentle human potential ways. The change that I sensed was illustrated in an evening presentation of thoughts about mind-body interaction. The audience sat on chairs rather than lolling on the floor. The presenters were seated on a makeshift stage, and the whole was bathed in lights for videotaping. Though the participants were barefoot and dressed informally, there was a spot of lipstick here, a new or just-cleaned garment there. Instead of an immediate free-for-all discussion, the program began with prepared remarks. These were augmented by a dean of the medical school at the University of California who suggested that a challenge of our time was to integrate experience with knowledge. Some years back, such intellectual presentations might well have been met with derision, as alien intrusions from the technological, bourgeois outside world. One lonely audience voice from the past was still there. He interrupted the speakers by complaining that they were just *talking* about the body; they were not experiencing it, or offering experience, or esteeming experience, or doing something about experience. Words, words, words, he complained. Just how one was to have a discussion *without* words was not clear to anybody. The voice was now an embarrassment, an interruption to people wrestling with issues — not intellectualizing them away, but attempting to guarantee their survival and flowering without doing violence either to experience or thought. I heard someone mutter that the dissident must be on drugs. That used not to be so disapproved of either.

Approximately thirty people — housewives, priests, psychiatrists, businessmen — were enrolled in the workshop co-led by Stanislav Grof and his wife Christina. Composed and warm, Christina stands as a glowing testimonial to the curative power of confronting one's transpersonal consciousness. She described her first experience of such confrontation as occurring when she gave birth. Worriedly puzzled as to how to think about her unaccustomed awarenesses, she was faced with the choice between keeping them quiet, concluding that they were symptomatic of mental disturbance and turning herself over to psychiatric treatment, or pursuing with herself the hypothesis of transpersonal awareness. She chose the latter, and the rest is history.

But how did she, and how were we, to achieve such awareness since LSD, the fastest and easiest means of achieving deep awareness, was now illegal? The method to be used was simplicity itself, and indeed when I first was apprised of it I could hardly believe that it would have much effect. That method was to lie down on a mattress, relax all the muscles of the body, and hyperventilate. During this process, powerful classical music was blared into the room. Four such exercises were included over the period of five days of the workshop, which alternated with didactic lectures by the Grofs, the showing of their slides of paintings and drawings, and people telling of their experiences during the exercises. During two of the four exercises, one served as "sitter" to a partner. The sitter was to be available to physically protect the person doing the exercise and, if necessary, to remind the person to continue to hyperventilate. At the first meeting, following brief self-introductions by the members, Grof suggested that we find partners of our choosing. He suggested, however, that those of us who were there with spouses or close friends might not want one another as partners. The reason was that it might be difficult to see someone near and dear go through the apparent agony of the experience. I thought, "He really means it, he really does think that people are going to have LSD-like experiences without LSD." And I noticed the huge pillows and mattresses, with renewed respect for the understanding that they were there so that people would not injure themselves in the course of thrashing about. I mused, also, about Grof's comment that people might try to avoid the experience out of their fear, and that one way to do that was to stop the deep breathing. He instructed the sitters to gently, with a slight touch or whispered word, remind the person to continue.

I would be just the one, I thought, to blow this opportunity to have the experience, remembering a major attempt I had made to be hypnotized. I had sought out the hypnotist who had made it possible for Elizabeth Kübler-Ross purportedly to go back to a past life in which she was a Spanish priest, and to recite, into a cassette which I heard, the sunrise service in Latin, a language that she claims barely to know at all. Her hypnotist, however, proved no more successful in hypnotizing me than others who had tried, though he and I worked at it off and on for two days.

My fears were realized at the workshop. Once again I stayed on the periphery of the regressive experience I was putatively trying to achieve. And the way I apparently did it was to do the deep breathing minimally, and sometimes not at all, despite the reminders by my sitter. If this failure resulted from my fear of the unknown in myself which might be revealed, what was I to make of my years of being psychoanalyzed? Even without being idealistic about the goals of analysis, shouldn't it at least have dispelled enough fear for me to enter into this experience in the way so many others did? That question illustrates Grof's contentions: analysis does not go deep enough to gain mastery over fears stemming from the birth process and transpersonal or past life events. Analyzed or not, in Grof's experience certain types of people find it difficult to avail themselves of this breathing technique or even of LSD itself. Perhaps the explanation was merely that, for them and for me, the difficulty was the same as is shown by a percentage of people who seem not to be hypnotizable. That difficulty could be biological or psychological, or both.

Approximately half of the other participants had no such difficulties. The music crashing into the darkened room was soon punctuated by groans, cries, and shouts. Occasionally someone would utter a scream that seemed to come from the depths of his being. Such screams seemed to me to be primal expressions of long-pent-up anguish, like the screams produced by Primal Therapy. A woman near me threw her legs up and down repeatedly with such force as to take her off the mattress and across the floor. Her sitter and others gathered around with pillows as shields, stepping backwards so as not to interfere with her movement, but ready to prevent her coming into violent contact with a wall or another person. According to Grof, these people were discharging tension associated with the content of their experiences, and it was important that the tension be fully discharged. Thus, we had to put aside concern, worry, or anything more than minimal protection, in order to allow the person fully to discharge the energy — to express in whatever way, through body or voice, what needed to be expressed. I was, frankly, terrified. My healing self wanted to reassure the participants, to interrupt their frenzy. I checked Stan and Christina's faces for any indication of worry on their part, but they seemed to be entirely at ease with what was happening. Toward the end of that procedure Stan went around the room and asked each person whether there was pain in their body, which implied a blocked discharge of energy, and he urged the person to "let it out, let it all out," as he pressed selected areas of the person's body.

As the driving music, flailing bodies, and piercing screams roiled into a *Götterdämmerung*, I wondered whether the people would emerge from their trances, their altered states, their alleged confrontations with birth and cosmic consciousness, in any kind of reasonable condition. Between one and two hours later, things began to simmer down, and candles were brought out. By the light of these candles, people drew mandalas, filling in circles using supplied crayons, with whatever came to mind — drawings which, presumably, reflected their experience during the exercise. Where a moment ago someone was in convulsions, that person was now sitting peaceably drawing like a child at school. Shortly after, as people wandered off toward dinner, they seemed just as they had been before their experiences.

Yet here is a sample of what they claimed, in the discussions afterwards, to have gone through: "I was upside down, there was pain in my legs, and I just surrendered. There was a red sky, black earth, hands like claws came at me and I panicked in a world of war, horror, a sub-world, I had no strength, I became a red giant with three eyes, snakes were coming out of my mouth, a river of snakes, and I was guided to another world. In that world there was a balloonist, air and water; I had a wonderful, loving feeling, and I did not need to breathe anymore ... hands were choking me ... I had sexual feelings, I felt like throwing up, a somersault, I felt that I was floating, felt that I was a rock, it was sweet and calm, there were Indians by the fire, I was one of them and I was also a rock."

At the next session, I was the sitter for my partner. He worked hard at the breathing, and there was little that I had to do in the way of reminding him to keep at that task. Since he kept his occasional writhings on the mattress, I did not have to protect him either. I did have to dodge the flying feet of others, and was pressed into the service of holding protective pillows for other sitters and subjects. As before, about half of the people had obviously intense experiences, as could be seen from their bodily movements, cries and shouts, drawings, and verbal reports to the group. The week was structured so as to make it possible for each person to have two breathing experiences, and I approached my second and last chance determinedly. I did somewhat better in the sense that many images crossed my mind, but I was unconvinced that I had any more striking or revealing images than I could have gotten from a moderately deep meditation. I was bitterly disappointed. Excited by the potential importance of Grof's hypotheses, and needing to convince myself one way or the other about them, I had hoped such conviction could be had through personal immersion in a regressive experience. There, I could, ideally, learn firsthand the kind of data that Grof claimed to have amassed. I resolved not to let the matter rest here on the dusty floor and dank mattresses of Esalen.

I visited the *Spiritual Emergency Network* (S.E.N.), a nonprofit research and study center a couple of miles from Esalen, developed by Stan and Christina Grof as an expression of their belief that a substantial number of people are erroneously and harmfully labelled as mentally ill. Instead, they believe that such people are having "spiritual emergencies" or "transpersonal crises," which are opportunities to transform and heal themselves. Such moments may come about through meditation, self-exploration, or life stresses, or occur spontaneously. The typical psychiatric approach, according to the Grofs, is to suppress such experiences through tranquilizing drugs, and to isolate the experiencer physically as in hospitals, or emotionally through psychiatric labeling. By contrast, many ancient and non-Western cultures have welcomed and institutionalized such experiences in rites of passage, shamanistic procedures, and healing ceremonies. The Spiritual Emergency Network makes itself available to people in such circumstances as an alternative to conventional psychiatry. At the time some 4500 people from 27 countries had contacted the Network center. Many of them are counseled over the telephone. The center also maintains a roster of people, including many professionals, who are sympathetic to the opportunities offered by such altered states of consciousness, and callers are referred to them throughout the country and world. Also, these practitioners are helped to overcome any geographical or emotional isolation through using the center as a clearinghouse and point of contact.

The Grofs recognize that not all individuals suffering from mental or emotional disorders are necessarily involved in a spiritual emergency. In their words, as criteria for a spiritual emergency, "There must be significant spiritual emphasis in the person's unusual states of consciousness, e.g., experiences of Kundalini, or energetic awakening, death and (re)birth, past incarnation sequences, archetypal phenomena, extrasensory perceptions, animal or plant consciousness." Moreover, "The person must be willing to approach their experience as an 'inner process' without projecting it into the world of persons around them." Among other criteria are "absence of severe persecutory hallucinations and delusions." The problem with that, of course, is to know whether a person's preoccupation with spiritual themes and claims of such experiences are delusional or not. That ticklish point seems to me to require skilled conventional diagnostic understanding.

There are, indeed, many practitioners, as well as cultural forces, devoted toward suppressing what seem to be symptoms of emotional disorder through drugs and other practices. Yet many — perhaps the majority of — traditional psychotherapists eschew suppressive means, believing that it is therapeutic for people to express their thoughts and feelings, preferably in words. The jargon for such an approach is *expressive psychotherapy*. Many of Grof's basic understandings of people are identical to those of traditional, or psychoanalytic, psychotherapists: he believes that (1) events in the past influence the present; (2) symptoms are an expression of inadequate repression, i.e., something is too close to the surface for comfort; (3) a person repeats the past, at least in part, in order to solve it, which in a psychoanalytic context might be called repetition compulsion; (4) responses in the past which may have been appropriate at the time, no longer are; and (5) there is great healing power in intense expressiveness. The one or few sessions of intense expressiveness during LSD sessions, often held to be useful in and of themselves, hearken back to the early days of psychoanalysis when Freud attempted to produce cures through the abreaction of traumatic events. That is the Hollywood version of psychoanalysis — the present is the result of a past awful happening. The usefulness of recovering such early memories in psychoanalysis is still accepted, though it is less central now than it used to be, and its limitations are better known.

Grof differs from conventional psychotherapists through extending the realm of data backwards from birth to conception, and upwards and outwards into universal consciousness. In so doing he makes crucial assumptions which many people do not accept. In my opinion, he should address himself more to what connection there may be between the Freudian primary process — the way people think in dreams — and how patients think, perceive, and feel during LSD experiences. It may be that LSD simply activates the primary process in a more basic and primitive form than is available in most dreams, which would make the transpersonal hypothesis a less parsimonious and perhaps unnecessary explanation.

Be that as it may, most traditional psychotherapists have never addressed themselves to data such as his, and so can hardly expect to have informed opinions about his assumptions. I do hope that he focuses more on the continuity, similarities, and bridges between his approach and that of conventional psychotherapists and less on the differences in order better to encourage conventional psychotherapists to experiment with the data that he suggests are relevant to healing.

To a limited extent I did some such experimentations when I returned to my patients. With many of them I asked what they knew, or could find out, about their gestation and birth events. Most people seemed unsurprised at the question, and easily understood the possible usefulness of such information. I am aware that any new procedure is inclined to "work" at first, whether that procedure be a new line of inquiry or a new drug. The history of healing is replete with instances in which new healing procedures lose their effectiveness as time goes by. So one might assume that the effectiveness was due to the novelty of the procedure, a break in the routine, an extension of hope, or enthusiasm on the part of the treater. I tried, therefore, to make allowances for the dramatic and useful material that emerged with my patients. As far as I can tell, even with such allowances, I was able to draw plausible inferences confirming a fit between hypothesized prenatal and birth experiences and later personality development and symptoms. To a lesser degree and more speculatively, some patients even began to offer evidence supporting both transpersonal ideas and the opportunities for transformation inherent in what, from another point of view, could be seen as emotional disturbances.

One highly intelligent patient nonetheless had great difficulties in finishing college. As we began to discuss the circumstances of his birth, he acknowledged for the first time a repetitive fantasy consisting of a long passageway at the end of which was himself — tiny and vulnerable, as yet ill-equipped for what lay ahead. It turned out that his mother's labor had been induced, and so he perhaps was born before he was ready for birth and subsequent challenges. One way that he now viewed his circuitous path was as a way of staving off the usual progression of developmental challenges, not only through school but through the dislocations of life brought about through his emotional turmoil. All along he had been what he called a "night person," whenever possible sleeping late into the day and working in the night. He disliked the day, recoiled from light upon awakening, and was soothed at dusk. Could it be, we wondered, that night reminded him of the safety *in utero* before his abrupt and untimely delivery toward the blinding light of the typical delivery room? Throughout his life he had been chronically late, for any and all events. He now said that his lateness was less an attack on others than it was done with a sense of rightness, and so he was never ashamed of it. Could it be, we wondered, that he was feeling the rightness of being born in the natural rhythm of things, and resisting having to be somewhere prematurely at a time determined by others?

Another patient, in connection with our discussion of birth issues, told me, for the first time, that she often had the image of a column with a light at the end. Her mother's labor with her had been extremely difficult. She offered the opinion that perhaps she had resisted birth; indeed, she organized her whole life according to the theme that she must always be in charge, active, and could not afford to let things happen to her. She wondered whether her mother's seeming lifelong antipathy toward her may have stemmed from this labor in conjunction with the mother's disinclination to have a child, as perhaps could be seen in her having to withdraw her breast after only two weeks and developing gallbladder disease during pregnancy with consequent refusal to eat. The battle between mother and child that had apparently begun at that time continued through life to the point that the two rarely visited or communicated, to the apparent disappointment of neither of them. At this point during the discussion the patient contributed the idea that her longtime love and daily practice of swimming was encouraged by the joy she felt at hearing her breathing during the swimming, a possible reference to the halcyon days in Matrix I, before the hard labor of birth began. While she had previously believed that her mother's resentment centered around jealousy at the good relationship between the patient and her father, she now saw it more as mother's rejection of her just because she was a person, *any* person, as reinforced, intensified, and illustrated by the hard labor. Following several hours of this discussion, the patient embarked on a spurt of emotional growth. She claimed that the anxiety that she had felt for years had now diminished and that she was no longer troubled by persistent suicidal fantasies. She understood the latter as issuing from a feeling of having no control, being passive and at the mercy of (presumably) the birth process — the state of affairs she worked so hard throughout her life to overcome with activity and dominance. She visited her mother in a distant state and reported having, for the first time, a good visit with her. She was critical of the same things about her mother that she had been critical of previously, but she felt in their relationship a new warmth and willingness to be mother and daughter. When she came back from that trip she found herself better in tune emotionally with her own daughter and able to deal creatively with previously troublesome issues between them. She was determined, now, to change her employment, which she had for a long time wanted to do.

In addition to my work with patients around some of Grof's ideas about perinatal phenomena, I did some reading in the standard scientific literature; much of this literature is summarized in *The Secret Life of the Unborn Child* by Thomas Verney, M.D.[2] Among many other observations, Verney states that a fetus can discriminate between sounds, that prolonged emotional stress during pregnancy results in infants who weigh less than average and have high levels of activity, and that a positive relationship has been found between the mother's level of anxiety during pregnancy and the amount of neonatal crying. Research has demonstrated that babies who move the most *in utero* grow into the most anxious children, and that the children of schizophrenic and psychotic women have more physical and emotional problems at birth than the babies of non-schizophrenic and non-psychotic women. Verney assumes that such mothers are able to give less emotionally to their unborn children than are the other mothers. The child suffers, also, when the father abuses or neglects his pregnant wife; indeed, the father's commitment to the marriage affects the well-being of the child as measured in the uterus and at birth. That the child hears and responds emotionally to the father was demonstrated by instructing fathers to speak to their unborn children *in utero* using short, soothing words. At birth, children who had been so spoken to were able to pick out their father's voice even in the first hour or two of life, and would stop crying upon hearing the father's voice. It is as if that soothing voice is familiar and tells the child it is safe, according to Verney. In other words, we are back with grandmothers who for generations told us that what happened during a mother's pregnancy would influence the child. Along with the grandmothers, there is evidence from the Chinese of a thousand years ago, from primitive cultures which had strictures against pregnant women exposing themselves to fearful situations, from Hippocrates' journal, and from the Bible. Leonardo da Vinci wrote in his *Quaderni* about the effect on the unborn child of the mother's thoughts and feelings. Music lovers will, depending on their preferences, be pleased or irritated to learn that fetuses respond differentially to composers. Vivaldi and Mozart are among their favorites, Brahms and Beethoven are disliked, and all forms of rock music "drove most fetuses to distraction." The criterion was the amount of kicking in response to the playing of such music. Shining a light on the mother's stomach results in the fetus turning away. Contrary to the conventional medical opinion about inadequate myelination of the brain before birth, Dr. Dominic Purpura, head of the study section on the brain of the National Institutes of Health, notes that the fetus's neurocircuits toward the end of pregnancy are just as advanced as a newborn's.

While investigators differ as to just when a child begins to remember, there is some evidence that a child does remember events that take place *in utero*, probably between the sixth and eighth month. Grof, of course, would put the time much earlier. And so it goes through Verney's volume, a long series of observations and formal studies, all adding support to the hypothesis that the unborn child can and does learn, remembers what it learns, and is affected emotionally and physically by what it learns. It follows, then, that learning about and working through such prenatal experiences may result in healing to the same or greater extent than discovering and working through learnings that take place after birth.

Finally, I read carefully Grof's detailed reports of his researches, as included in his published books (Grof, 1976, 1980) and the manuscript of his then-unpublished *The Nature of Reality: Dawning of a New Paradigm*. In that manuscript he extends and elaborates his earlier assertions that the transpersonal phenomena discovered in LSD sessions and through other means of altering consciousness are an expression of a reality alternative to the conventional one. In short, he says things are not what they seem to be: we had learned a view of reality limited by our senses and canonized by Newtonian and Cartesian physics and philosophy. Now the post-Newtonian Einsteinian physics supports alternative and extended views of reality which are consonant with ancient and Eastern views of reality.

The twin hypotheses set forth by Grof — the effects on later personality of pre-birth experiences and the existence of a transpersonal, cosmic reality — aroused in me corresponding excitements: my therapeutic self was aflame with the possibility that patients could be helped even more than they are now through a psychotherapy which would include pre-birth data. My philosophical, social and questioning self was excited at the prospect of being able to secure data about such questions as the fundamental nature of persons, the universe, and God. I had to find a way to alter my consciousness sufficiently so that I might gain a firsthand appreciation of the data that gave rise to these hypotheses; LSD, as far as I could tell, was the best way to do that.

DR. GROF HAD DONE MUCH of his LSD research at units especially equipped for it at Spring Grove Hospital in Maryland. One of his colleagues there was Francis Di Leo, a fellow psychiatrist, who continued the research to the extent that the law allowed. At the present writing, that allowance is only for the purpose of working with cancer patients. According to Di Leo and others, cancer patients who are given LSD have less pain, accept their illness and the idea of death better, and perhaps make gains against their illness. Di Leo has been trying to get permission from the Food and Drug Administration to expand his research, in particular by adding other populations including professionals who want the experience for academic study. Grof suggested that if I wanted to have an LSD experience, I might be able to get one, should that pending request for permission be accepted.

Di Leo works under abysmal conditions. He supports himself financially with a partial private practice while devoting what time he can spare to the LSD research. The research is poorly funded; he has only limited access to research consultants, statisticians, even secretaries, and so he writes or types his own letters. One has to include, as an additional burden, the subliminal drain on him of pursuing a research in a hostile cultural environment as epitomized through governmental regulations and outright prohibition.

There are dangers in the indiscriminate use of LSD, as there are dangers in the indiscriminate use of any number of drugs. The way the problem is ordinarily handled is to control the availability of drugs through restricting them to licensed professional workers. With LSD, however, Di Leo, and anybody else who wants to use LSD legally, must submit a formal experimental design to a designated governmental committee, the Human Volunteers Research Committee of the Food and Drug Administration. The government's hard-nosed attitude toward the experimental and clinical use of LSD stems no doubt in part from the lurid and notorious associations with the drug in many people's minds. LSD achieved that notoriety by becoming one of the playthings of the counterculture, anti-Vietnam rebelliousness of the '60s — and a dangerous plaything it was. In examining people with psychological tests in the '60s at the Menninger Foundation's psychiatric hospital, I saw sufficient numbers of post-LSD "psychoses" to be able to develop criteria to discriminate between disorganization which was a consequence of drugs, whether LSD or the cornucopia of other illegal drugs popular at the time, and disorganization that was independent of drugs.

Not only did some of the users of LSD harm themselves through its unsupervised and indiscriminate use, but they elaborated their experiences into a pompous, self-serving philosophy: They had seen the truth of existence, and the rest of us were self-deluded. One wonders what the gurus of the time expected to happen when the Establishment heard that their children were being told to kill their parents, and that there was somehow a greater nobility in dropping out than catching on.

I am rubbed the wrong way by such puerile narcissism. One ought to be able to discriminate between using LSD for kicks or rebellion, and exploring its possible use for psychological and philosophical investigation and for healing. As to protecting citizens against the risks of LSD, from what I can gather from Grof and others, the dangers stem from the context in which it is given. As an unlawful and unregulated substance, it may be of poor quality, and is taken in uncontrolled dosages by a self-selected group of people with widely varying reasons and capacities to manage it. Rarely do these people have trained or even concerned people available for help or support; psychological preparation for reentry is even more rare.

By contrast, Grof's criteria for safe and effective use of LSD for healing purposes include having sitters, preferably male and female, available full-time to the subject. Such sitters are trained generally in psychotherapy and specifically in how to deal with events created by LSD. The procedure is preceded by interviews in which the subject is prepared for what is to happen. Ground rules are laid, and objectives clarified. The experience takes place in a protected and preferably aesthetically appealing environment. It is followed by a process of reentry which includes discussion of the experience and its wider implications for the person. The person continues to be protected for the day or so that it might take to dissipate the intense effects of the experience. According to Grof, I would not see patients who take LSD under those salubrious circumstances in a psychiatric hospital, as I had in the '60s. In his experience with thousands of patients, hardly anyone sustained severe or long-term harm. Assertions have been made from time to time that LSD adversely affects chromosomes and causes genetic mutation and malignancy. Citing study after study in what appears to me to be a fair and thoughtful systematic evaluation, Grof amasses evidence that suggests that none of these dangers is backed by convincing experimental or clinical data when the drug is administered under controlled conditions.

However, there are a few specific contraindications. Pregnancy is one, possibly because of the danger of disturbing the biochemical balance between the fetus and the mother, and because of intense uterine contractions that may occur as memories of the mother's own birth process are evoked during the session. Although some people with epilepsy have responded favorably to LSD treatment, there is the possibility of LSD's triggering epileptic attacks. Those for whom excessive muscular activity poses a danger would also be at risk: for example, those with pathological fragility of the bones, insufficiently healed fractures, or disposition to dislocation of the joints. Those with severe liver damage may take more time in detoxifying LSD and excreting it and so might have prolonged reactions.

The psychological consequences of LSD are more severe, but of a different order. One thinks about them in the same sense that one thinks about the pain and distress attendant upon any powerful psychotherapeutic intervention. The more powerful the intervention, the more likelihood of pain and distress at certain points during the process. As in psychotherapy, such pain and distress signals what is important and what needs to be overcome through therapeutic work. LSD patients may show their temporary disorganization with such symptoms as suffocation, physical pain, blacking out, or violent seizure-like activity. They may face what is likely to be the humiliation of vomiting, losing control of bladder and bowels, sexually unacceptable behavior, confusion and disorientation, and the making of inhuman sounds.

Added to these temporary expressions of vicissitudes of the therapeutic process is the danger that thoughts and feelings troublesome to the patients will be activated in the sessions and not adequately dealt with. These can then influence behavior in dangerous and potentially destructive ways. Grof and other LSD therapists assert that practically all such consequences can be eliminated through optimal therapeutic conditions. Instead of staying stuck in an arousal mood and perception, the subject works through it to liberation, not only from its LSD activation, but from the hold it has had on the whole of life.

Much of this information, these distinctions and niceties of work with LSD, is unappreciated or unknown by most people still caught up in the horror of its irresponsible use. It is just such ignorance and fear that could be dispelled through adequate opportunity to research its use. Instead, we have the ludicrous situation of LSD being freely available on the streets, to be used dangerously, while unavailable to responsible practitioners who could use it safely and for the potential benefit of knowledge and healing.

This is the context in which Di Leo conducts his lonely investigations and repeated pleas to the government for support. This is the context in which the document on the desk before me was created: the verbatim transcript of the hearing held by the Psychopharmacological Drugs Advisory Committee, Department of Health and Human Services, Public Health Service, Food and Drug Administration, on February 24, 1983. Its 133 pages add up to the following: (1) Yes, LSD is probably safe if used as specified in the research protocol. (2) The research will not be funded because it will be unable "to generate reliable scientific data." The main reason for rejecting the research was that "There are no objective methods of assessment that are suggested here ... they are all highly suggestive, inferential judgments ...."

At that I had for myself a silent, hollow laugh. Psychotherapy journals are filled with studies in which objective methods have been used, and most of them are of little use because they were designed to answer questions whose answers were of little use. These questions were, however, amenable to study according to the ideal rule book of science. The real challenge is to ask questions of sufficient depth and gravity as to be potentially useful and still conform to the rule book of science. Or one can recognize that the rule book of science needs to accommodate itself to the question, not the other way around: The experimenter formulates a question whose answer may make a difference, and then sees what can be accomplished in the way of finding an answer. I wrote a book some years back reporting on a psychotherapy research project that took some twenty years to complete and cost over a million dollars, much of it from the government, in the days when a million dollars was a lot of money even to the government. The major source of data for that research was subjective clinical judgments, just the kind that the LSD committee objected to. The judgments were treated with some sophistication in order to make them reliable, but basically the research team recognized that they were studying clinical activities in a field which is as much art as science, whose intricacies do not easily lend themselves to simplistic methods — and anyway the clinician's subjective experiences, judgments, and inferences were an integral part of what was being studied. It is an old debate in psychotherapy research. The FDA committee came down solidly on one side of it. The record of their deliberations suggest that they tried to be fair. At times they implicitly acknowledged that they were just administering the law, not making it, implying that they were sorry about doing what they had to do. Their deliberations seemed sober, conscientious, and no more influenced by the dynamics of groups than practically all committees are. The committee members were not entirely innocent of the key differences between LSD and the usual run of drugs, yet none seemed too conversant with that difference either. Their deliberations lacked the overall sense of excitement, the possibilities of discovery, the great gains that might accrue from the freedom to do the research. From reading that transcript I failed to get the sense of possibility with which I was imbued, either from the committee members or to some extent from the researchers. The latter seemed to have been beaten down by the suspicious, hostile atmosphere in which LSD is embedded.

What all this meant to me at the moment was that I had reached an apparent dead end to my hopes of learning about LSD firsthand as a research subject. I opened my desk and mused over a tiny square of paper permeated with LSD which originally came from a college community. Perhaps I would have to take my chances with its quality, see whether I could find some trustworthy, responsible person with at least some background and interest in the procedure to be on hand if needed — or maybe just do it alone, come what may.

I realize as I write this that thousands of people are in a position to read it and laugh at me. LSD is easily available and frequently taken by any number of people; what was I waiting for? I was beginning to wonder the same. But instead of plunging ahead at the moment, I thought I would take a bit more time to see whether I could find a context in which to take it that would be safe and more likely to yield the information that I wanted. Grof and Di Leo were the obvious sources, but just because they were so obvious, they were in no position to help me; they would, after all, be breaking the law in so doing. Give or take an occasional parking ticket, breaking the law is not my thing either. It is at once trite and profoundly true that at times one has to decide between the law and a higher law. In psychotherapy as in life, salvation lies in having the freedom to learn and come to one's own conclusions.

Exploring LSD was for me a step toward possible intellectual, and for that matter perhaps personal, salvation. In addition I could, perhaps, benefit others if I found out anything of general social or scientific usefulness. So with reasonably clear conscience I researched the highways and byways of the professional and quasi-professional ranks until I found what turned out to be pretty close to the ideal situation for the experimental self-study of LSD psychotherapy.

My sitters, whom I shall call Reggie and Joan, would work with me in a — should I call it, a safe house? — in Oregon. The external environment met the criteria of pleasantness, and the internal one did also, since it included many stimulating books, paintings, and sculptures. I flew there the night before the session, after having dreams full of anxiety. I spent the first night and morning having a psychiatric interview and a preparation for what was to come. I was told that I would lie down on a mat and wear eye shades and stereophonic headphones. The purpose of the eye shades was to cut down external stimuli, thus driving me deeper into the regressive process. The headphones were to enable me to receive a constant flow of music. Music, too, has a regressive effect and cuts down any extraneous material that might interrupt an internal voyage. I was assured that either Reggie or Joan would be there the whole time, usually both of them. The mat was covered with a rubber sheet, and a bucket was placed nearby. I thought to myself that they take seriously what was written in the books, that patients may lose control of their bladder or bowel functioning, may vomit, may thrash around violently. I was informed that the effects of the drug would last six to eight hours. There was then some discussion about the size of the dose. Some people get an intense experience even out of a small dose, others require a large dose, and for some it seems not to matter what size dose they get. Ever acting brave as a way of dealing with terror, I suggested the highest of the dosages discussed. I had not come this distance to have a pallid experience or to be disappointed.

At 12:30 P.M. I chewed on a square of paper about the size of a single block in a newspaper's crossword puzzle. Amid nervous banter, while waiting for the drug to take effect, I uttered a silent prayer that I would, after all of this, go through all of the expected stages of LSD regression, as described by Grof, in order to get the answers I was seeking.. Those stages include: (1) a sensory level characterized by seeing brilliant colors and usually artistic shapes, many of which are observable in the paintings of other cultures and other times; (2) the biographical level which includes influential scenes from one's life, particularly one's childhood; (3) the perinatal material, experiences from the four stages of uterine life and birth experience; and (4) the transpersonal.

Twenty minutes after ingestion I lay down on the mat, put on the ear phones and eye shades, and received a pat on the shoulder and the words, "Have a good trip." The music began (Resphigi). The music was selected for its evocative power, sometimes crashing and frantic, sometimes pastoral and soothing, conventional Western music and occasional Eastern or Oriental selections or animal sounds, but always having the capacity to evoke strong emotion. Some other selections were by Schumann, Mahler, Brahms, Rachmaninoff, and Peruvian flute music.

I was warned that getting into the experience and sometimes during the experience, I could be subject to panic, often at the no-exit claustrophobic experience of Matrix II or at facing the self or ego death of birth. That ending or death of the prenatal period can seem terrifyingly equal to final death, or at least to people's fantasies about mortal death. I had gotten a chill signal of Matrix II from Reggie's remark that there was no turning back once the LSD was taken, no antidote for it. It would have its way with the mind, brain, or self until it wore off, and that was all there was to that. The only way to try to minimize the experience that I knew of at the time would be to open myself to external stimuli, such as taking off the eye shades and earphones, getting up from the mat, trying to move around or do unrelated things. But I had entered into a pact with Reggie and Joan that no matter what I would stay with it.

A few minutes into the experience, I jumped bolt upright. I had to stop, I had to get away! Instead, in honor of either the pact I had made with them or the inner pact I had made with myself, I stayed with it. I struggled against the full impact of my terror by attending to the music, drumming up topics to preoccupy my mind with, chattering and intellectualizing, and occasionally finding relief in waves of tranquility which accompanied brilliant visions of stars and other seemingly celestial forms.

What follows is substantially taken from a running verbatim account written by Joan, including the time, musical selection, any activities of mine, and what I said. When I try to recall the many hours of the LSD session, I am amazed at how little I remember of seven hours of an almost exclusively mental experience. Did I employ a massive repression of what I otherwise would remember, as with those people who claim that they do not dream or cannot remember dreams? Or maybe nothing much did happen beyond the repetitive designs and brilliant colors characteristic of the first level of LSD experience. Remarkably, once past the initial burst of terror, I moved around and spoke very little, at least by comparison with the many other subjects that Reggie and Joan had observed. Toward the beginning I saw a series of shapes and brilliant colors such as I had seen in slides, books, and movies depicting drug experiences. Many of the shapes were classical, ones that could be seen in paintings from past centuries and in other cultures, and the colors were indescribably brilliant. Perhaps I saw the shapes by way of suggestion and association to slides and paintings, but the sheer brilliance of the colors could only have come from some alteration in my perceptual capacities.

"I'm seeing jewelry."

"I'm solving the problems of the universe, facing existential problems ..."

At several junctures Reggie or Joan would ask how I was, did I feel like saying something. Usually I did not. I was absorbed in what I was seeing, and when not having fits of anxiety, I relaxed into an absorption with what would happen next — with a disinclination to be interrupted by the workaday world.

"I'm drugged. Right now it's an empty battlefield, echoes."

4:30 P.M.: "Tell me it's over, all hell's breaking loose, overwhelming, I'm so hot. Do I want to get over it, that's the question?"

"Are we talking about coming out of it or going into it?" Here, perhaps I was facing a death-rebirth decision, undecided.

The "trip" image seemed right, as I decided to go around again, to embark on another voyage rather than come out of the experience.

"Back for centuries ... defiled by vomit and stench, blood, entrails and nausea."

"No matter what key the orchestra is playing in, they're playing our song." (I rather like the feel of that comment, though I do not have the faintest idea why I said it.)

"I'm tired, it's black and awful, and I am getting a pain, or is it a pleasure?"

"I can't tell my waking life from the crazy life."

"Now I'm feeling nausea, over and over again, blockage."

"Molten lava, fireworks, cannons, a big curving arc, I can feel it all up and down my legs."

"It gets dark and awful and quiet. The silence is deafening."

I offered a series of comments about bodily sensations, and then an actual memory from college days. The existence of such a memory suggests that in the midst of the regressive experience and altered consciousness and perceptions, there is still access to ordinary thought, ordinary memories, material that is, for example, commonplace in traditional psychoanalysis.

Joan asked if I saw anything of the birth process, to which I responded, "Caverns, I feel like an egg attached to a wall." I do remember having a vision of an egg which looked like a pea attached to a wall, but I have no way of knowing whether that vision and my comments would have occurred spontaneously, or were pressed into the service of responding to Joan.

"I am cradling a child in my right arm. It's mine and it's me."

6:30 P.M.: I was beginning to emerge from wherever I was, back from a trip to I know not where. In this half-and-half existence, Reggie and Joan would hold, manipulate, push against various parts of my body, all the while encouraging me to scream and to make animal sounds. They would sense bodily areas where I was holding tension, and my screaming and growling were ways of reducing that tension. The sounds were unearthly, rumbling out of my inside, streaking down from my brain, catching hold of my vocal cords and exploding.

7:00 P.M.: "I hate to think I will come back to daily life without solving anything."

"I see a battlefield — red, guts."

"All those fountains of lights."

"The only way out is out." (A birth experience?)

When I got up, everything seemed dark, and momentarily I could not tell whether it was an inner darkness fastened over my eyes or that the day had gone into darkness by then. I felt a band around my head. Perhaps that was an evocation of the head at birth encircled by the cervical opening.

The sitters brought out some light food; I remember thin slices of oranges. I assumed that I would be hungry since I had not eaten all day, but I couldn't eat a thing. I would take a bite or two, then literally spit it out. Somehow it seemed the thing to do, and I was reluctant to resume the polite, labored encumbrances of removal and deposit. I remember launching into a long piece of autobiography. Reggie and Joan were as unfailingly attentive to that as they had been to my needs throughout the day.

That night I had extreme difficulty going to sleep. To lie down and close my eyes was to recreate the sense of sinking into the initial terror of the LSD experience. I was to have that trouble at least intermittently for the next couple of weeks. The following week when I was on another, this time geographical, trip gathering material for this book, I was able to get only a few hours' sleep over three days. I resisted taking any sleeping medication for the same reason that I resisted sleep, fearful once again of losing control and drifting back into the world of elsewhere. What to do in such a situation? (1) I could take tranquilizers or barbiturates or other depressants. Those, I thought, would merely suppress the experience, leaving it unaltered and in a position to send its reverberations into symptoms, behaviors, and other life experiences. I was tempted by that but refused to give in. (2) I could work through — intellectually, emotionally, in consciousness, ideally with the help of further LSD sessions — the loosened, but unintegrated, thoughts and feelings. At the moment I felt as if I wanted no more of LSD, though if it was available I would have continued working with it. Instead, I used introspection on the double. (3) I could let the passage of time seal over the loosened, unintegrated material. It's not really "time," of course, but the reparative processes of the person, and I cheered them on. (4) I could take Tryptophane, a soporific amino acid nutritional supplement, which at the time was available in health food stores (though it has since been removed from the market). A welcome find. Perhaps it was in response to my occasional penchant for hyperbole that the person who suggested Tryptophane thought I should take sixteen per day, when less than half that would probably have been sufficient. The result was a fatigue hangover added to the fatigue hangover of several days' sleeplessness. That, too, however, passed. Tryptophane did finally make sleep possible.

Upon awakening that first morning after the LSD ingestion, among my first thoughts was that the yogis, esoteric wisemen, and self-denying ascetics were right in their pursuit of Truth, while the rest of us were squandering ourselves in the pursuit of irrelevancies. Philosophical speculations are expectable sequelae of LSD. I spent the rest of the day as a walking, or rather shuffling, exemplification of the list of characteristics described in Grof's book of people who have had a bad trip: lack of appetite, extreme fatigue, lack of interest in sex, suicidal thoughts.

It was a bad trip in another sense also: as far as I could tell, I had mainly experienced during the LSD the first or sensory level of experience. I did not unearth convincing memories of intrauterine or birth experiences, and certainly not transpersonal ones. Some would say that it was unrealistic to think that I could have done so in one session anyway. Grof, however, reports that sometimes one session is sufficient, not only to enter those realms convincingly, but to therapeutically integrate material stemming from those realms.

In the days following the LSD experience I felt relief that I had finally found both a way logistically to get it and the courage to do it. Indeed, I felt slightly heroic — which must come as a joke to the thousands of adolescents who have tripped the light fantastic presumably without my internal fanfare. I also felt disappointed, mostly in myself. I wondered and worried at the extent of my inhibitions such that even a hefty dose of LSD could not sufficiently dispel them. Was I that afraid of my feelings, I asked myself, I who cry at movies, parades, photographs in musty albums, and whose saxophone playing has often been called passionate? Was my immersion in feelings all sham, synthetic display, compromise expressions of a soul still encased in Matrix II, or whatever the dungeon? Were all those psychics who placed me in a dungeon in France in a past life correctly reading my past life or instead correctly sensing the person before them?

I felt also the cold hand of the suspicion that there might not be anything more to learn. Perhaps I had only taken a psychedelic trip like any modish psychedelic trip, full of sound and fury signifying only that weird things happen in the head under the influence of chemicals. Perhaps Grof, whom I intellectually and instinctively trusted and admired, was no less a muddleheaded zealot than many of the others I had encountered in my explorations. And if that was so, was I not also muddleheaded?

Finally, I felt disappointed and frustrated at the loss of opportunity to learn matters of potentially great importance, and I was enraged at the bureaucratic mentality which made further exploration so problematic.

As time went on, the bad trip effects and keenness of the disappointment wore off, but my interest in the possibilities raised by Grof's work did not. I continued to wonder what "early life" referred to in the statement of belief that events from early life influence later life.

Before Freud, early life was taken to refer to any time in childhood. After Freud's elucidation of the determining importance of the first five years, early in life was taken to refer to the first five years. In the last decade, consistent with the psychotherapeutic treatment of an increasingly wide variety of people, and generally more troubled ones, the importance of the first year of life has been emphasized. Thus, in principal there was good precedent for pushing early in life back still further, to include birth and pregnancy. I listened to the thoughts and dreams of my patients with that in mind, and I asked many of them about any such memories or family stories that they could learn from relatives or from hospital records. With a few patients I did the LSD-like breathing procedure. What I saw and experienced in these ways supported Grof's hypotheses. But as scientific, confirming evidence, it is pitifully weak. I could have been hopelessly biased, even eliciting confirmatory material spuriously. The putative recreation of pre-birth and birth experiences and hypothesized influence on later life could be nothing more than a shared collusion between me and the patient. It could have "worked" as so many things do when first introduced, when enthusiasm, interest, and hopes are high.

I am only partly dismayed by these considerations. A part of me shares with our culture the incredulity, if not indignation, at the complexity of adult personhood being definitively influenced by infantile experiences. On the one hand we have perinatal events determining not only later health and illness, but also personality traits, choice of mate, school grades, interests, occupations, and hobbies. On the other hand we have the conventional medical belief that the infant's insufficiently myelinized brain prevents registration and memory. In an ideal rational system, ways would be found to convincingly evaluate medicine's evidence for its belief against the evidence provided by Grof's thousands of cases and the researches reported in *The Secret Life of the Unborn Child*. But there the matter stands. And stand there it must until the government legalizes the use of LSD at least for research, as a necessary beginning on the way to wholehearted support.

Down the street kids are ingesting black-market LSD of unregulated and questionable quality, and doing so as criminals. The policies that create such circumstances, and the vendetta against knowledge which they represent, deserve our resentment. If the truth shall set us free, and that is the way we deal with the possibilities of truth, then we shall never truly be free.

Chapter Fifteen
Beating the Bushes: Folk Medicine in Belize and Beyond

For those who have not kept up with the decline of the British Empire, Belize — to the east of Guatemala, south of Mexico, north of Honduras — before gaining its independence in 1981 was called British Honduras. With a population of less than 200,000, it is rich in many things (for example, over 90 percent literacy) but is poor in other things such as an organized Western-influenced health care system. (Whether that really qualifies as poorness, at least with regard to many ailments, is another matter.) Instead of either the black-satcheled caller at your house of the past or the high-tech wizards of the present, many Belizeans rely upon folk medicine.

Thus, I found myself seventy miles into the interior in the private community of Gallon Jug, a cattle, coffee, banana, corn, cacao, etc., farm hard by a vacation resort called Chan Chich (Mayan for "little bird"). "Resort" arouses tacky images which are quite unsuited to its exquisite setting on a small plaza surrounded by six Mayan burial and ceremonial mounds, its thatched-roof buildings, lovely plantings and visited as much by ornithologists, zoologists, and other naturalists as by casual tourists. How many resorts exist where one is awakened by sounds of wild parrots, toucans, and monkeys, and with the knowledge that jaguars, ocelots, and tapirs may be not far away? Both Gallon Jug and Chan Chich were hacked from the jungle by Barry Bowen, the 46-year-old descendant of the Bowens of England who came to Belize around 1750. When not leading his country into the 21st century as one of its premier citizens, Bowen slakes the sub-tropical throats of Belize by making and distributing Coca-Cola, beer, and other assorted thirst quenchers. He can also be seen in reruns of *60 Minutes*, which temporarily gave up muckraking to do a laudatory piece on Belize, and in *National Geographic*, evidently dazzled by Belize's rainforest, barrier reef, and Mayan ruins.

"What does one do in case of sickness?" I asked members of the Bowen family and others. Those with major illnesses and means are likely to get on the next plane to Mexico, the U.S., or Costa Rica. Those with access to the few medical doctors get a screening and maybe limited treatment for limited problems. But many of the citizens draw upon the wisdom of thousands of years, wisdom that probably began with the Maya, who owned the place from around 600 B.C., and was maintained by a steady succession of grandmothers and purveyed by natural healers scattered through the towns and rural areas.

My first stop in pursuit of local folk healing was a rural village built by Bowen near his Gallon Jug farm primarily to house his workers. No indoor plumbing, but running water, electricity, cleanliness, a school built and maintained by Bowen for all the children of the area — all in all, for this part of the world, a nice suburb.

The local health care system is named Rosalita and is short and round, flashes a brilliant white smile, and wears the traditional white Mayan garment, a seemingly all-purpose housedress-nightgown called a *huipil*. Like a petitioner to Western medicine's Latinate gobbledygook, I struggled with halting Spanish and an interpreter to bridge the linguistic and cultural differences. It turned out that Rosalita conceived of her job as primarily being a pharmacist. Eschewing such common folk options as rituals, laying on of hands, manipulation and massage, she relied upon plants which were easily available from the scrubby land, often right around her house. She glowed as she picked the plants and held them up for me to admire. Several of the plants, she said, were specific for the treatment of premenstrual distress if made into a hot tea to which cinnamon is added. Headaches were said to yield readily to tobacco leaves saturated with olive oil, put on the head as hot as one can stand. Lower back pain, that bane of civilized citizenry everywhere, was no problem to Rosalita's pharmacopeia. She and other local healers get rid of back pain with a plant called *dormadioi*, or "12 o'clock," spoken of in this region as the poor man's Vicks Vap-O-Rub. But not only poor men use it. Barry Bowen, smitten with lower back pain, chose not to fly off to the U.S. in favor of using "12 o'clock," with, he reports, excellent results.

Humberto, my guide through the rain forest surrounding Chan Chich, pointed out the Mayan mounds with their tunnels made by robbers of its antiquities, the cave paintings by which anthropologists had been able to date the civilizations of the epoch, and the species of trees, plants, tracks and specimens of wild life. (I was sorry not to see the monkeys, and especially the rarely-seen tapirs, but not sorry to have missed seeing a jaguar on the path, despite Humberto's reassurance as to their tractableness.)

Humberto became most animated, however, when he pointed out, picked, smelled, and pulled apart plants and barks. These had various uses, but most prominent among them were their medicinal properties. It turned out that Humberto was another local health care system. In his fifties, he likely had forty or so more years to live, for his father was going strong in his nineties, and his mother, albeit younger, was past the biblical allotment too. Of his thirteen children, the father had found Humberto to be the most interested and adept in learning healing, and had passed on to him his knowledge of the forest as medicine cabinet. Here is a sampler:

- *obel* — used as an anesthetic and for mosquito bites. Humberto demonstrated its anesthetic properties by breaking into it and sucking on the juice, which he said produced a tingling then deadening feeling similar to Novocaine. He broke open a stalk for me, and there was opium for the masses. I can't say I would have been sanguine about having a molar pulled under its influence, but it did tingle and deaden as advertised.
- allspice — the leaf is boiled, cinnamon added, and then used for stomach distress, which distress Humberto assured me would yield to its healing properties within five minutes.
- *copal* — a nut resembling a coffee bean which, when added to alcohol and rubbed on the offending part, dispels pain, particularly arthritis and rheumatism pain. As Humberto acknowledged in his best scientific variable-separating manner, one could not tell whether the relief came from the copal or the alcohol. Or, one might add, from the suggestive effect of Humberto's understated but unmistakable confidence in copal, and from its reputation as a painkiller.

- "give and take" — a bark which when split reveals a substance the color and consistency of cotton. It is used to stop bleeding from wounds, as anecdotally attested to by Humberto, who claimed to have stopped serious bleeding from an accidentally self-inflicted machete gash.
- *pichoja*—a root which when boiled, again combined with cinnamon, is a cure for diarrhea.
- *kapok* — a tree which yields a substitute for those afflicted by allergies to down and other bedding materials.
- cedar bark — scraped, boiled, and served cold, it is good for the kidneys.
- *tukis Mayan* — for those afflicted with asthma help is on the way, so long as one's stomach and sensibilities can deal with the remedy. After peeling the shell from a small young turtle, the animal is toasted, then eaten.

Additionally, I have forgotten, or never was told, the name of a vine which when opened afforded water. Such water can be considered medicine for the terminally dehydrated, and for those afflicted with pinkeye and other eye ailments for which in the United States Visine would be recommended.

What a contrast these remedies are with expensive prescriptions, prescribed by medical authorities, backed up by million of dollars of research and testing, and certified as safe and effective by a U.S. government agency. It's enough to make one laugh and sympathize with poor, innocent Rosalita and Humberto.

But maybe Rosalita and Humberto should have the last laugh, for some 40 percent of Western medicine's high-tech drugs are made from plants and herbs: digitalis from foxglove, aspirin and quinine from tree bark, coumarol from sweet clover, reserpine from snakeroot. Anti-cancer drugs made from plants are a virtual industry used within as well as outside of orthodox medicine. Lilly Co. researchers found that the Madagascar periwinkle provided anti-cancer activity, and from it have been derived two modern anti-cancer drugs, vincristine and vinblastine. Bristol Myers derived etoposide (or vepeside) from a favorite folk anti-cancer source, the mayapple. Folk healers have been said to have used over 3,000 plant species to treat cancer. "Somewhere in the tropics, there are probably compounds that will alleviate or correct every ailment known to mankind," says James Duke, botanist with the U.S. Department of Agriculture. Packaged, distributed, and high-priced, the drugs made from plants are said to be purified of extraneous matter in favor of their active ingredient. Maybe so. Or maybe the reason for the notorious side-effects of drugs is the isolation of the active ingredient from its natural form — a form that just might include elements designed by that other drug company, Nature, to neutralize toxicity.

Botanist turned Harvard-trained physician and author Andrew Weil would doubtless support at least the approach of Rosalita and Humberto. In his book *Natural Health, Natural Medicine*, he reports that for every pharmaceutical drug that he prescribes, he prescribes forty or more plants and herbs. He recommends a basic medicine chest of fourteen herbs for a variety of common ailments. The Chinese, having beaten the Mayans by 2.5 times in longevity, to say nothing of survival, are unsurprisingly the world's greatest resource for plant and herb healing. Weil recommends the *shiitake* mushroom for lowering cholesterol, and the *enokitake* mushroom as a preventive for cancer. Now, if we were walking in a forest in Canton province, with Weil as our native guide, and he picked up a mushroom which he said could prevent cancer, we might laugh indulgently. Some American drug companies wouldn't laugh. They have signed contracts with the Chinese government to develop drugs from mushrooms. The Germans and Japanese would laugh at our laughing. The German FDA has approved the over-the-counter sale of botanicals for explicit use as treatments and preventatives. The Japanese sell through vending machines foods developed from Oriental medicinal plants.

The great barrier reef running alongside of Ambergris Cay, a small, thin island just off the coast of Belize, is second in size only to the more famous reef off Australia. Surely, I thought, it was worth a look from a glass-bottomed boat. So I set off in such a boat under the captainship of Ramon Badillo, a leathern old man of the sea — and the area's best-known folk healer. Or at least he used to be. Like any disillusioned veteran of the go-go '80s, Ramon decries the passing of values and lack of appreciation of the old. He associates newness and technology with emotional coldness and lack of appreciation. He used to get appreciation as value received for his healings, but now complains that the more educated and prosperous that people became, the less respectful and grateful they became as well. "The sharks," he said, gazing at the sea, "are more on the land."

Too bad; my guess is that he was a hell of a healer. For one thing, his garrulousness and hint of grandiosity peeking through humility and givingness conformed to the psychological profile of healers delineated in Chapter 11. For another, many a citizen of San Pedro, the main town on Ambergris Cay, has a personal testimonial to his healing prowess. I ran into one such when I met, on the beach, a Harvard Ph.D. in education who was spending his sabbatical helping out the local school system. His young daughter had dislocated her arm; they had it treated by the local physician with less than desirable results, and took her to Ramon, who took care of the problem with dispatch.

That sort of thing was Ramon's specialty. Somehow he had learned, in effect, chiropractic, and that along with massage were his favorite treatment modalities. Not that he eschewed other remedies. He described a process of burning a candle in a glass which sounded like the Oriental practice of moxibustion. He used local botanicals as medicine to the point that he worried about their becoming unavailable as the result of development of the land. (Lemon grass boiled in a tea is specific for gaseous distress; garlic and honey are specific for coughing, and so on.)

How did Ramon learn his healing trade? Through necessity — or at least, necessity forced attention to the healing wiles that descended orally and by example through the ages. "I can't teach anybody," Ramon said, "because I never learned it." In other words, healing lore was inherent in his growing-up reality, no more "learned" self-consciously than was speaking.

Once past the xenophobia of the Western world view, one finds it easier to recognize that far more of the world's population is treated with folk medicine than by modern medicine. Belize is a tiny piece of the globe, and it is also a teacher: Less developed in terms of the practices of the present, it can more easily maintain connections with its past. The main side-effect of its medicine is to instill a respect for the past and a recognition of its sequestered wisdom.

Chapter Sixteen

Endings and Beginnings: Conclusions

THIS TRAVELOGUE BEGAN WITH the observation that diverse healings produce cures, and so they may have elements in common. The first category of such common elements can be labelled suggestion-placebo. Having said that, I must acknowledge that I have not said much beyond what we usually say in reference to the fact that something not understood has influenced a change. Such terms as *hope, expectancy, positive attitude*, as applied to the patient, and *bedside manner* or *charisma* when applied to the healer, represent attempts to specify suggestion and placebo. All such terms can be subsumed under the idea that a particular reality inhibits or facilitates healing.

We live in different realities all the time, from the dream reality where anything is possible, to the sharply focused reality of, for example, adding up a column of figures where only one answer is permissible. Day and night we drift in and out of different realities. At any given moment we are only relatively awake, more or less conscious. Each kind of consciousness constitutes a different reality, encouraging or discouraging different events. The psychological reality that facilitates performing brain surgery is usually inimical to the writing of poetry; the psychological reality that facilitates composing music likely inhibits the selling of farm machinery.

Studies in academic psychology have demonstrated that people tend to perform according to what they and others expect of them. Such "level of aspiration" studies provide realities that define what is possible or impossible. For decades conventional reality decreed that it was impossible to run a mile in less than four minutes. Then Roger Bannister ran a mile in less than four minutes, thereby creating the new reality of the under-four-minute mile. In swift succession other runners broke the four-minute-mile barrier. Runners had not suddenly become more efficient physically; rather, they responded to a new reality.

In a well-known study it was shown that people put on a clinic's waiting list for psychotherapy turned down the therapist when their turn came to get one because their symptoms had gone away. Healing was probably generated simply by the act of deciding to get help with one's life, or by the feeling that help was on its way, or of the fear that they would soon have the responsibility of telling about their inner, heretofore guarded, selves to an intimidating stranger. The almost-patients had removed themselves from the usual workaday realities and inserted themselves into a new, putatively healing reality. They had come to a healing building, they were acknowledged as patients in a healing organization, they were thought of in healing terms. That put into action their reparative capacities, their healing response; or in the case of a "flight into health" to avoid self-exploration, their protective capacities were stimulated, which is also a variety of healing.

A healing reality is created and sustained by social agreement as to what healing methods are effective. Whether such methods are technologically effective may be less important than the fact that people believe them to be so. Rituals, setting, and paraphernalia enhance that belief. In pre-industrial society these included incantations, dancing, demonstrations of special and presumably supernatural skill (imperviousness to fire, surgery with bare hands). In post-industrial society these include hospitals, machinery, degrees on the wall, and language that is unintelligible to most patients — all of which creates the impression of arcane and esoteric knowledge and skill. In these realities one expects healing to take place. At the least the normal curve, or something like it, takes over as it does in so many human affairs; some people have remarkable cures, some are therapeutic failures, and most people fall somewhere in-between. The healing reality exerts an effect by its very nature; a good many people are going to be healed pretty much no matter what.

Jerome Frank offers Lourdes as an example of how the psychology of a healing reality is concretely tied to a geographical reality. He notes wryly that people who live in the vicinity of Lourdes fail to benefit from the supposed healing powers of the spring waters there. Instead, those who make the trip there join with others who also believe such a trip to be worthwhile, participate in processionals and other rituals, see piles of crutches discarded by those who supposedly have been healed, and respond because they have entered a reality in which they expect to be healed.

A famous experiment with rats, who depend on their whiskers for sensory cues, provides an excellent opportunity to see how a changed reality can change behavior. The rats drowned quickly when their whiskers were trimmed, while with whiskers left intact they could swim for hours. The experimenters concluded that trimming the whiskers gave the rats a feeling of hopelessness and so they gave up; they were put into a reality which permitted no other alternatives. When the rats were briefly released from the water tank, and then put back, they did not give up; evidently they now experienced themselves in a reality in which there was hope for the "healing" of their predicament — if it happened once, it could happen again.

"Voodoo death" in humans occurs in the reality where hexes produce death, as noted in Chapter 9. When freed from that reality, people recover from illnesses supposedly caused by hexes, and voodoo is no longer capable of influencing their health.

Five thousand years ago, yogis declared that the mind creates its own reality. They have certainly demonstrated it dramatically through the centuries by enduring heat without pain and blisters, sticking needles through their flesh without pain or scarring, or going without much air, food, and water for long stretches of time. Through training their minds with meditation they created a reality in which such things were possible. When they created mental images of the reality they wanted, their bodies responded as if that reality was there, and indeed for them it was. Biofeedback, currently so popular as a means of healing a wide variety of ailments, is based on these yoga ideas. Basically, biofeedback can be thought of as meditation with machines, dials to cue and monitor the mind's efforts to bring about the desired reality. Like mini yoga masters, biofeedback patients assert control over aspects of the body conventionally thought to be uncontrollable. When the medical textbook authors declared aspects of the nervous system to be "involuntary," they were right — in one reality. They failed to realize that in another reality, what was supposedly involuntary could be voluntary — heart rate, blood pressure, basal metabolism, and much more.

Positive thinking — Christian Science being the epitome — is also founded on the idea that the body responds to the reality created by the mind. If one thinks one is healthy, then one is healthy, so professional healers are unnecessary. The latter live and work in a reality in which there is disease, a different reality from that of the positive thinker.

The effect of any reality is enhanced by the evocative effects of drama, which makes healing reality an especially potent force, for illness is dramatic. Anyone can get an audience to hear about one's operation (if one doesn't go on too long about it). The newspapers say that we fight illness, we wage valiant battles against it. It is as if anyone who gets cancer, takes a long time to die from it, and follows doctors' orders without making a fuss is a hero. There is the rising action of symptom and diagnosis, the climax of cure, the falling action of going off into the healthful sunset; or, if it is a tragedy, a significant mournful death takes center stage. Doctors in hospitals are probably second only to lawyers in courtrooms at providing fodder for dramatic productions. The ill person is the center of an audience's attention; all that goes on is stimulated by and designed for that person. For many people, caught up in what they may experience as the humdrum of life, illness is high adventure. By developing and keeping (or imagining) illness, some people try not to leave center stage.

The Filipino psychic surgeons openly acknowledge exploiting the dramatics of their role. Whether or not they actually do what they appear to do, they are happy to fake it in order to dramatize the healing power of God. Group contagion can heighten dramatic effects just as viewing a play or movie in a group can. Being a member of a horde bathing in the Ganges, or of a healing processional in Lourdes, probably leads to healing better than a solitary trip to either would. It is doubtful that if one went through Shealy's Pain Clinic singly one would derive as much benefit as accrues from joining with others in that program.

The success or failure of healing depends upon the ratio between the *context* of healing — those elements in the environment that promote or inhibit healing — and the *technology* of healing: designated healing interventions such as surgery and medicines. The more powerful the healing reality, the less powerful the technology of healing needs to be to produce cure, and vice versa.

All the healings reported in this book, indeed all healings everywhere, take place in some sort of healing reality which exists in the mind. We are thus confronted with the perennial question of how one's mind can affect one's body. A part of most of us is aghast at the possibility that the mind can have any effect at all. We automatically separate mind from body, even derisively characterizing an illness for which no organic basis can be found as "all in your mind." We do so even as popular culture has adopted the notion that "stress" causes illness and that certain personalities dispose one to certain illnesses, as with Type A personalities and heart disease. We do so even in the face of evidence from our own bodies: an embarrassing thought causes our bodies to blush; a sexual thought causes our bodies to respond with swelling and secretions.

Freud called the connection between mind and body "the mysterious leap." True to his training as a physiologist and neurologist, he hoped to find a physical substrate for personality. He tried to at least supply such a substrate hypothetically in his concept of libido. Here he joined many traditions through the ages and across the world which included a concept of energy to supply the driving force of life — *orgone, prana, bioplasm, chi* were some of the names given to it. In recent years discoveries of substances secreted by the brain, endorphins and enkephalins, may finally provide a physical analogue to hypothetical energy. These morphine-like secretions appear to be addictive, as in runner's high and the craving of those Chinese regularly treated with acupuncture for continued treatment with the needles. In other words, physical secretions of the brain supply motive force for experiences and behavior.

Freud's "mysterious leap" occurs in clinical medicine by way of the infamous placebo effect. Most of us fail to grasp fully the awesome implications of therapeutically inert substances, offered as medicine, sometimes having as great or greater beneficial effects than active medicine. Placebos may even produce side-effects such as rashes and nausea. By the same token, many of us fail fully to grasp the awesome implications of hypnosis. Even as we know that hypnosis is the best cure for warts, that dentists can slow with hypnosis the flow of blood to a tooth, and that some surgeries are conducted with hypnosis as the anesthesia, we relegate hypnosis to a sideshow curiosity. As long as healing can occur through placebo and hypnosis, then anything that enters the mind in the context of a healing reality can provide healing impetus. That fact troubles those who would like to isolate, work with, and credit only their particular modality or belief. The rest of us bless placebo and suggestion as constituents of a healing reality. Instead of controlling for them, we should find ways of maximizing them.

The second category of common elements in healing has to do with love. That may come as a shock to those who are imbued with a reliance on machinery and physical sciences, and who are squeamish about love. Love is, to many people, unmasculine; it belongs in the province of art, about which we stereotypically are ambivalent, rather than science which we stereotypically worship. We are not trained for love; it is to be distrusted if not over-controlled, like so many other natural tendencies. In describing his medical training, a physician writes in *The Townsend Letter for Doctors and Patients* "... love was never taken seriously as a real entity or was dismissed as some sort of infantile holdover." Dean Ornish writes in his book *Love and Survival: The Scientific Basis for the Healing Power of Intimacy* that we don't learn about love in medical training despite its powerful impact on health and disease. Yet, note what happened when David McClelland in a research at Harvard showed students there a film of Mother Teresa taking care of dying patients. He measured immunoglobulin A in their saliva before and after their exposure to the film's portrayal of selfless love. Half the students objected to Mother Teresa's religiousness and considered her a fake, yet as a group the students' immunoglobulin level increased significantly. Since, among other things, immunoglobulin A is a defense against colds, it seems that exposure to the portrayal of love, which presumably stimulated some variety of loving reaction in the viewer, has an immunosupportive effect, even when the person consciously rejects the experience. (In recognizing love as a variable in healing, one has to discriminate between the love as stimulated in McClelland's experiment and love in greeting-card, instant friendliness, unbridled eroticism, or hypocritically intellectualized forms.)

Healing encounters involve great and existential need, which leads to heightened suggestibility, a turning to others for help in a wish-driven reality where anything is possible. That description characterizes the early relationship between mother and child. Thus, a good mother-child relationship can be considered a healing, a healing of the question of survival — illness.

Many traditions have grasped and embodied the connection between healing and certain kinds of need-fulfilling love relationships. Those who are said to have achieved the highest spiritual attainment, to have truly understood the dimensions of love, were also healers — not only Jesus, but Christian, Sufi, Hasidic, and other saints, Tibetan lamas, and Hindu gurus. On a more mundane level, George Meek, an explorer of unconventional healing, writes, "healers are almost invariably warm, loving people with great concern for their patients, and they are almost as invariably spiritual." I found such traits, also, by way of observation, interview, and psychological tests, as reported in Chapter 11. Among the elements that healers had in common was am affinity for the "oral" stage of development, the time in early life when mother and child are united in the task of survival and growth. The guarantor of that survival is love.

Lawrence LeShan trained himself and large numbers of others to heal through learning to achieve a feeling of oneness with the patient, an experience saturated with compassion and love. In that reality he not only healed by way of laying on hands but, eschewing physical touch, healed simply by "being with" the patient in that special consciousness, that healing reality.

Perhaps Jesus, in his role as healer, knew that healing comes about through relationships: "Where two or more are gathered in my name, I am in the midst of them." He may have been acting upon the same intuition when he adjured his disciples "to go two by two." The rapture and transcendence of religious conversion experiences, when the seemingly impossible comes true and when one seems at one with the One, can be seen as a recreation of the magic of the mother-child relationship. Religion began, and continues, as something to turn to when frightened, whether of mysterious thunder and lightning or while waiting for the results of a surgical operation.

If it is true that the capacity to heal oneself, and health in general, has as its matrix early healing relationship experiences, then it follows that destructive early relationships would produce anti-healing and illness. (If love produces healing, then lovelessness can produce illness.) By "destructive early relationships" I do not necessarily mean obvious abuse and destructiveness. Rather, I am referring to the wide range of behaviors that are inimical to health. These may be sufficiently pervasive as to handicap almost any expression of healthful living, or be restricted to narrowly specific inhibitions and patterns. These patterns are legion. Two examples: A child with self-absorbed parents may get the idea that only through illness will he or she be able to gain a parent's attention. A mother unsure of herself as being a desirable woman, and fearful that her daughter may supplant her, may unconsciously persuade her daughter to be weak and unattractive through poor health among other ways. The gritty reality is that parental attitudes vary from open hatred and destructiveness, as in overt child abuse, to parents who *consciously* accept, esteem, and love their children even as the parents' unconscious difficulties encourage illness. Since ambivalence is a fact of human existence, there is something of both good and bad relationships in all people. And not by coincidence, no one remains in perfect health or heals expeditiously all the time. Which relationship predominates, or can be summoned, is therefore crucial to health, illness and cure as it interacts with organic or hereditary factors.

There is much precedent for believing that early relationships influence the nature of healing which takes place years later. The whole edifice of dynamic psychotherapy rests on the idea that the past influences the present. "Repetition compulsion" is Freud's term for the recognition that people inexorably and regularly repeat the past. We less create our lives than we re-create them. One knows only the reality that one has learned. If mothering, and by extension other relationships, are healing ones, then that is what one expects and duplicates. The influence of this line of reasoning on healing is both esteemed and disregarded. Like some other facts of life we register them, but draw back from their implications. Part of us would like to think that we start with a clean slate, can create our destiny, are free of the past, and that the healing relationship will be successful no matter how unsuccessful other relationships may have been. And yet we accept as unremarkable the fact that a puppy should not be taken from the mother before it is six to eight weeks old, for without these early weeks, corresponding to about a year in humans, the dog's behavior later in life will be impaired. A famous research series showed that monkeys deprived of maternal touch, or its equivalent, at the beginning of life were, among other things, unable to copulate in later life. *Marasmus* is the name given to a condition of human babies who die in infancy, well cared-for physically but deprived of mothering in other respects such as touch.

That those who have good beginnings tend to have good later healing experiences, and vice versa, was supported by a research project conducted over many years at the Menninger Foundation. In assessing results of psychological tests given before, just after, and two years after psychotherapy I noticed that the greatest gains were found among those who were best established psychologically to begin with. In the course of psychotherapy, the rich got richer, while the poor stayed the same or only slightly improved their lot.

We may call the way people respond to healing opportunities "the healing response." Recognizing such a response shifts the emphasis from the technology of healing to the context of healing, from the skill of the healer and the inventiveness of modern medicine to the nature of the patient. The healing interaction now must include, along with what one person *does to* another person, what the patient brings to the encounter.

If there is a heal*ing* response, then for the same reasons there should be a heal*er* response. The healer, too, reacts to the healing situation on the basis of the healer's early healing relationships. Those healers who have received healing love in their most formative years, in whose reality people can heal one another, are likely to be able to give healing love. In a grand synergy, the healer, through offering a healing stimulus, summons the patient's healing response. That is the essence of the "bedside manner," the otherwise mysterious capacity for healing that some people have, and others have less of. A long series of researches have shown that psychotherapy patients do better with therapists judged by others to be warm and accepting, and whom their patients like. Understanding the differences among healers in this regard helps us understand the otherwise mystifying fact that people respond so differently to healings that are ostensibly similar.

One may wonder how the loving healer transmits healing love. Obvious ways include dedication to and respect for the healee, kindness, concern, and compassion, a proper balance between the needs of the patient and the needs of the healer, the ability to convey that the patient is valuable and so should be healed.

At the same time, however, interpersonal love often is not enough. It needs vehicles of expression, concrete actions such as proper food, felicitous touch, and physical protection, indeed a kind of technology. One frequently needs to express love by, of all things, technology — what one specifically does for the healee. After all, mother gave not only of her nature, but milk, touch, and physical protection. Interpersonal love is aided by such concrete actions as concrete action is aided by interpersonal love.

The synchronous balance between the interpersonal and the technical is in constant danger of being lost. Take psychotherapy, for example. In this age of often chaotic and unsystematized training there are psychotherapeutic healers who try to substitute a healing personality and the suggestion-placebo effects of the healing reality for a thorough grounding in the craft, for the technology of concrete action, usually in the form of therapeutic intervention. That extreme of mindlessness is unfortunately matched by the opposite extreme: the image of the cold, intellectualizing, interpersonally heedless or hypocritical healer who overlooks — or at bottom may disbelieve — that anything is curative other than medicine, surgery or psychological interpretation.

One bridge between these two polar extremes is the concept "energy," whether called *orgone, libido, prana, bioplasm,* or *chi*. Especially among unorthodox healers it has been considered to be an actual substance with quantity, direction, and direct healing capability. Others think of it merely as a metaphor or a hypothetical construct.

The dispute may be at least partially resolved by recent discoveries of substances secreted by the brain, as noted earlier. These can be seen as the physiological substrate for energy and thus underlie a limitless number of psychological and physical events that are held to be influenced by energy. Freud's hope and expectation that his psychological discoveries would one day be seen as the function of physiological events would be realized. The Cartesian separation of mind and body would collapse into a researchable, conceptually powerful holism. The boundaries between body and mind, feelings and thoughts, interpersonal influence and concrete actions would become more plausible, be rearranged or even dispensed with.

How does one bring to awareness, and work verbally with, influences stemming from pre-verbal times? The usual psychoanalytic answer to that problem is that words, if used creatively and evocatively, can recreate non-verbal experiences, as can dreams which involve visual images antedating words. Indeed, much can be accomplished in such conventional ways of working. Some patients, particularly when they are granted the opportunity for long-term and frequent meetings, do recreate what look to be very early experiences.

But perhaps there are more direct ways of doing that. Hypnosis is an obvious opportunity, and a few hypnotherapists take advantage of it. But for the most part, psychoanalysts and other psychotherapists follow Freud's path of eschewing hypnosis. Not much in the way of convincing formal research is available to substantiate the decision to eschew it, or for that matter to use it. A still bolder approach would be systematic use of either LSD or the breathing procedure as described in Chapter 14. A variety of other mind-altering or mind-expanding agents offer possibilities. Their misuse by questionably trained therapists as well as irresponsible street use have given these approaches a deserved bad name. What has not yet been done is to use such agents in the context of ongoing, sophisticated psychoanalytic explorations. The situation is identical to the opportunity to employ body therapies, such as Rolfing, bioenergetics, or the Alexander Technique as I have suggested elsewhere.[34] In principle, these various approaches to the sensory, feeling, pre-verbal states by way of the body may enhance psychotherapy and shorten the time that it takes.

To summarize, the degree to which people heal and are healed stems from their early experiences, especially the mother-child interaction. Since people differ in their early experience, with consequent differences in their healing response, it is no surprise that the "same medicine" administered and taken by different people will have different effects. The plot is thick indeed when one tries to solve the mystery of healing.

These ideas have important implications for the selection and training of healers. Where does one find, and how does one train, people with healing characteristics? One source is, perhaps strangely enough, fellow sufferers. Those who select candidates to become psychotherapists know that one unlikely source for healers is overly conventional, bland people. Such people find it difficult to empathize with the misery presented by patients. Modern Western neon-and-chrome culture is in general unconducive to healers; our present culture puts a premium on action more than reflection, progression more than regression, defining boundaries more than relaxing them, goal-directed thought more than intuitive feeling, self-reliance more than mutuality, and stereotyped masculinity more than stereotyped femininity such as in the giving of compassion, nurturance, primitive caretaking and being comfortable with touching.

Those who qualify for advanced degrees in general, and medical degrees and psychological degrees emphasizing academics and research in particular, are questionable sources. The premium put on intellectual skills necessary to win the competition for such advanced degrees predisposes such people toward intellectualization more than feeling. Much of the course work necessary to earn such degrees, for example, in chemistry and physics, draws upon skills often different from those that facilitate the healing response. The raw material for healers in the sense described here is more likely to be found among those who become artists, historians, literary scholars, those who have emotional sensitivity and curiosity about what makes people tick. Women may be better suited to be healers than men since, whether through biology or culture, they tend to be more nurturing than men. As a society we have not systematically selected people to become healers with due regard for who will make a healer in the sense described here. Rather, we have blithely assumed that the general requirements for membership in the officially designated healing professions would suffice for the specific requirements of healers.

By the same token, we have failed to devote ourselves fully to the training of healing characteristics. To maximize his healing potential, Lawrence LeShan[2] spent over a year improving his skill at meditating. I, too, have found that my capacity apparently to perform psychic healing is facilitated by an altered state of consciousness brought about by brief meditation. A complete psychoanalysis as the cornerstone of training to become a psychoanalyst is probably on the right track, though the quality of such analyses vary with the participants and situation and may or may not provide all that could be done to facilitate the healing response as described here. Rollo May cried out for educating psychotherapists in the literary classics, and assigned his students Sophocles, Dante, Ibsen, Melville, Dostoyevsky, Kafka, and Mann along with standard psychological texts. Whatever the details, if one takes the healing response seriously one will think through and probably renovate the means of selection and training of healers. Healing is too precious to be left to the vagaries of history and chance as it largely has been and is.

Here are some practical conclusions and recommendations to people in need of healing. Such people are often in a difficult position with regard to what to do about their illness. The welter of claims and counterclaims, differences of opinion, the latest scientific journal article or *Time* magazine, a friend's personal experience or advice from one's brother-in-law contribute to confusion and indecision. Part of the seduction of modern medicine is its air of precision and clarity about what should be done. Unorthodox healing, on the other hand, presents the patient with myriad possibilities offered by a grab bag of diverse healings whose independent validating support ranges from none to only a little. Many people feel embarrassed, sheepish, at turning themselves over to such healing, and are often afraid of displeasing orthodox healers as they were once afraid of displeasing their parents. Some orthodox practitioners drive the point home by implying, or declaring outright, that they will not be available to the patient unless the patient evinces faith in them exclusively. A person who chooses to pursue unorthodox healing in the face of these discouragements is probably thereby offering a good prognostic sign. That person is able to convert the traditional passive patient role to an active role marked by self-responsibility and independent action. All other things being equal, that stance would likely make for better healing.

Of course there are unscrupulous charlatans who bilk the unwary; money and precious time might be wasted by misguided, fruitless efforts. Unorthodox healings have to be investigated, assessed, and compared with what orthodox medicine can offer, and with clear-eyed recognition of the balance between side-effects and expense, and likelihood of gain. But especially in those instances when orthodox healing extends little or no hope, it seems only logical to explore other possibilities.

The mysterious leap between mind and body, the contribution of each to sickness and healing, is by now well substantiated. Those in search of healing should take advantage of that. They should use the powers of the conscious mind, as through meditation, biofeedback, imagery, and hypnosis. They should exploit the possibilities for healing through improved nutrition and exercise. And they should explore the deeper, usually unconscious, contribution of the mind to illness and healing. We can no longer simply register idly the repeated suggestions that specific illnesses meet specific unconscious needs — such as that some cancers are suicide equivalents, ways of dealing with life situations experienced as otherwise hopeless, or that autoimmune diseases may reflect difficulty establishing and demarcating psychologically the self from the non-self as the immune system fails to do in lupus erythematosus.

Unorthodox healings offer society, and its agent science, a free laboratory which has yielded many hypotheses. If the body really does emit electrical energy, we need to know of its healing possibilities. If LSD or other mind-altering drugs can increase the efficiency of psychiatric treatment, we should know about the parameters of that path — administered by whom, to whom, with what illnesses, to yield what results as compared to results from other healing modalities. And if LSD can teach us more about the existential nature of life, as its proponents claim, then let us take advantage of it.

The fact that unorthodox methods *do* sometimes produce healing should imbue orthodox practitioners with some often unwonted humility. The effects of one's pet technology have to be assessed alongside the contribution of contextual healing reality such as suggestion and placebo and other factors inherent in the patient. These constituents of the healing reality should be recognized and used as befits a therapeutic ally, rather than treated as confounding one's preferred beliefs with pesky uncontrolled interference.

With regard to love as a curative agent, the healer is in a position similar to that of the patient. Healers need to attend to the conscious exploitation of their healing selves — compassion, respect, and appropriate selflessness. Healers should become imbued with the clinical position toward the healee of non-judgmental acceptance, of a benevolent neutrality that contradicts any healee fantasies about harmful, non-healing relationships. In order best to do this, the healer must come to grips with the unconscious sources of healing and anti-healing trends that the healer has learned in early relationships.

The healer is in a position similar to the healee, also, with regard to unorthodox healing possibilities. The healer, too, can honor limiting fears of departing from orthodoxy, imagine or knuckle under to disapproval, straitjacket imagination and courage. Or the healer can proceed from the objective appraisal of what orthodox healing might offer, and assess the costs and benefits of trying alternatives.

Now, as to the search for a white crow — I was being less than candid with myself and everyone else when I included that as a reason for this odyssey. I am reminded of the physicist Peter Phillips's comments with regard to my study of the Philippine psychic surgeons, that many formal and elaborate investigations had already resulted in equivocal findings and divided opinions. In short, he thought that I would not be able to prove a thing. In conducting any research one traverses a mine field of potential error. When research takes a white crow as its object, the mines are strewn all the more densely. To find a white crow would require that one could rule out any other possible explanations for the event in question. That is hard enough for a team working full-time at it; it is unlikely for a solitary and part-time investigator. And that, too, is something to be learned, by would-be investigators, but also by the rest of us. If society wants to improve healing — and the discontent one hears expressed about all healers suggests it certainly does — then society has to provide the necessary resources. I count as resources not only financial ones, but also the support provided by tolerance and encouragement, and the imagination necessary to suspend disbelief. The guiding credo should be that all sincere attempts at healing are judged innocent until proven guilty.

Instead of "proving" anything, I did examine the habitats where such crows might be found, and I spotted such possibilities as the photographs of Uri Geller's presumed psychic energy and his projecting an image for me to draw, some of Donald Galloway's messages and the time that he could not get any, people who gave up symptoms under my touch, Jean Pease's visualizations of a true-life situation, the psychic surgeon anecdotes and the psychic tooth pulling in the Philippines, and the viability of folk health systems.

I am inclined to believe that some people have an effect on other people without recourse to any third factor such as medicine or psychological interpretation; in short, that there is a possibility of psychic healing. I am inclined to believe that information can be transmitted from one person or animal to another apart from the five senses as they are ordinarily understood. I am inclined to believe that the mind can bring about varied effects customarily thought to come about only through physical means, whether this be bending keys, growing enzymes, or what used to be called "psychosomatic medicine," now more likely to be called "psychoneuroimmunology."

It makes good evolutionary and physiological sense to look at paranormal phenomena this way: the primitive old brain still exists underneath the later-developed folds of the cerebral cortex just as raw passions exist under the veneer of civilized behavior. The old brain's powers have diminished, a notable example being the sense of smell. It is logical to assume that before the development of language people used other means of communication such as sign language, grunts and groans — and extrasensory perception. The atrophy of such skills as extrasensory perception would be greater in some than in others. People with psychic powers could be those who have retained those primitive capacities more than the rest of us. The same line of reasoning could be applied to the capacity to transmit healing energy; it survives still in the primitivity of mother-child interaction where touching makes it better, as well as in those who evidently heal through the transmission of healing energy.

I had plenty of self-appointed guides in the habitat of alleged white crows. Hawkers of healings are everywhere, their claims resting more upon vociferousness than evidence. While this is patently true of unorthodox healings, it is true to a lesser but significant extent of orthodox healings as well. A systematically collected series of follow-up cases, judged alongside controls, did not determine the zooming popularity of open-heart surgery. Instead, a culture created the charismatic Cooleys and DeBakeys, encouraging them to behave in ways Americans like best: going in and doing something, preferably dramatic. Never mind that subsequent studies seem to be demonstrating that longevity is not increased by such operations any more than intensive care units increase longevity for heart patients beyond ordinary home care.

Hawkers of single-cause explanations are ubiquitous — it is all the fault of the body, of the mind, of zinc deficiency, of karma. Despite the seductions of simplicity of such claims, I am more than ever convinced that events are the results of many causes. Hardly anything is the sole result of the mind, or of suggestion, or of bacteria, or of surgery. Cause is composed of a multiplicity of factors arranged in a hierarchy of importance. Instead of "either-or," we should think in terms of "the contribution that such-and-such makes." Complexity reigns.

The search for a white crow could be doomed from the beginning for all of us who continue to encase ourselves in Western science and philosophy, for what we observe is already influenced by our capacity to observe. I had looked for a white crow through the lenses of Twentieth-Century Western Science, albeit ones tinted with liberalism. That approach subsumes the ideas that reality is mechanistic, composed of cause and effect sequences whose causes are physical and can be learned through physical means; that consciousness is nothing more than a secretion of the brain; that all information is available only through the usually agreed-upon senses; that observable boundaries rigidly surround all objects; that life begins at birth and ends at death. But the crow, the phenomena, the reality of psychic healing, may be quite different. To psychic healers, or believers in the paranormal, some events cannot be circumscribed and limited to tidy, predictable cause and effect sequences; the universe was designed for a Purpose; consciousness transcends the brain and connects all objects, which are only separated by fluid and permeable boundaries; and the period between birth and death is merely an episode in the existence of indestructible spirit. To the believer in psychic phenomena, the universe is a veritable aviary of what to believers in conventional reality are white crows.

According to the reality of believers in psychic phenomena I should throw away my lenses in order to see fresh and anew with other ones. But to do that I would already have embraced their world view. I would merely swap one set of prejudiced lenses for another.

I cannot take the metaphor of the lens any further for the same reason that so many of us seem to be stuck when it comes to evaluating psychic phenomena and psychic healing. What is missing is a way of seeing things that is not circumscribed and limited by prejudice, that is marked by the suspension of disbelief and a readiness to set up and follow rules of belief appropriate to and respectful of the subject. (How something is studied should be determined by the nature of what is being studied.)

Explorations conducted in that way may yet come to naught. The observations on which they are based may prove to be faulty, and conventional explanations may be found for these observations. Or, perhaps, we are in for a big surprise. It may be that those white crows were black all along; we just did not look at them in the right light.

References

Chapter 2
1. Galloway, D. *Inevitable Journey*. London: Frederick Muller Ltd., 1974.

Chapter 4
1. Nolen, W.A. *Healing: A Doctor in Search of a Miracle*. Greenwich, CT: Fawcett, 1975.
2. Stelter, A. *Psi Healing*. New York: Bantam, 1976.
3. Seutemann, S. In Meek, G. *Healers and the Healing Process*. Wheaton, IL: Quest, 1977.
4. Sandweiss, S. *Sai Baba: The Holy Man*. San Diego: Birth Day, 1975.
5. Kammann, R. *The Psychology of the Psychic*. Buffalo, NY: Prometheus Books, 1980.
6. Krippner, S., & Villoldo, A. *The Realms of Healing*. Millbrae, CA: 1976.
7. Valentine, T. *Psychic Surgery*. Chicago: Henry Regency Co., 1973.
8. Watson, L. In Meek, G., *Healers and the Healing Process*. Wheaton, IL: Quest, 1977.
9. Meek, G. *Healers and the Healing Process*. Wheaton, IL: Quest, 1977.
10. Fernandez, C. *Tooth Pulling Among Filipino Folk Healers*. Unpublished Ph.D. dissertation, University of the Philippines, 1981.

Chapter 5
1. Krippner, S. *Human Possibilities*. New York: Anchor/Doubleday, 1980.
2. Grad, B. Some biological effects of the laying on of hands. In Approaches to Healing: Laying On of Hands. *Human Dimensions*, 5, 1&2, 1976, 27-38.
3. Grad, B. The "laying on of hands": Implications for psychotherapy, gentling and the placebo effect. In Approaches to Healing: Laying on of Hands. *Human Dimensions*, 5, 1&2, 1976, 39-45.
4. Smith, J. Can Human Hands Heal? *Human Dimenions*. Buffalo, NY: Human Dimensions Institute, 1972.
5. Smith, J. Enzymes As Activated by the Laying on of Hands. *Human Dimensions*, 5, 1&2, 1976, 46-48.
6. Smith J. Further research into a chromatographic analysis. *Human Dimensions*. Buffalo, NY: Human Dimensions Institute, 1973.
7. Becker, R. Stimulation of partial limb regeneration in rats. *Nature*, 1972, 235, 109-111.
8. Becker, R. *The Body Electric: Electromagnetism and the Foundation of Life*. New York: Morrow, 1985.
9. Miller, R.N. In Hammond, S., *We Are All Healers*. New York: Harper & Row,

1974,
10. Miller, R.N. *Science of Mind.* 1974, 47, 112-116.
11. Miller, R.N. Paraelectricity, a primary energy. *Human Dimensions,* 5, 1&2, 1976, 22-26.
12. Appelbaum, S.A. *Out in Inner Space: A Psychoanalyst Explores the New Therapies* New York: Anchor/Doubleday, 1980.
13. Smith, J. Enzymes As Activated by the Laying On of Hands. *Human Dimensions,* 5, 1&2, 1976, 46-48.
14. Smith, J. Paranormal effects on enzyme activity. *Human Dimensions,* 5, 1&2, 1976.
15. Grad, B. The laying on of hands: implications for psychotherapy, gentling, and the placebo effect. In Approach to Healing: Laying On of Hands. *Human Dimensions,* 5, 1&2, 1976, 39-45.
16. Hunt, V. *A study of structural integration from neuro-muscular energy-fields and emotional approaches.* Unpublished manuscript, 1977.

Chapter 6
1. Frank, J. *Persuasion and Healing.* New York: Schocken Books, 1963.
2. Branch, R. *Harry Edwards.* Great Britain: The Awake Press Ltd., 1982.
3. DiOrio, R., & Gropman, D. *The Man Beneath the Gift.* New York: Quill, 1980.
4. Randi, J. *The Faith Healers.* Buffalo, NY: Prometheus, 1987.

Chapter 7
1. Gordon, R. *Your Healing Hands.* Santa Cruz, CA: Unity Press, 1978.
2. Krieger, D. *The Therapeutic Touch.* Englewood Cliffs, NJ: Prentice-Hall, 1979.

Chapter 8
1. To locate an approved practitioner of chelation, contact Association for Cardiovascular Therapies, Inc., 120 Mountain Ave., Bloomfield, CT 06002.
2. See Walker, M., & Gordon, G. *The Chelation Answer: How to Prevent or Reverse Hardening of the Arteries and Rejuvenate Your Cardiovascular System.* New York: M. Evans, 1982.

Chapter 9
1. Davis, W. *The Serpent and the Rainbow.* New York: Simon & Schuster, 1985.

Chapter 10
1. Shealy, C.N., with Freese, A.B. *Occult Medicine Can Save Your Life.* New York: Dial Press, 1975.
2. Banjaree, H.N. *Americans Who Have Been Reincarnated.* New York: Macmillan, 1980.
3. Shealy, C.N. *The Pain Game.* Berkeley, CA: Celestial Arts, 1976.
4. *Ninety Days to Self-Health.* New York: Dial Press, 1977.
5. Shealy, C.N. *Biogenics Health Maintenance.* C. Norman Shealy Health Maintenance Systems. Available from Shealy Pain and Health Rehabilitation Institute, 1919 South Fremont, Springfield, MO 65804.
6. Assagioli, R. *Psychosynthesis: A Manual of Principles and Techniques.* New York: Viking, 1971.

Chapter 11
1. Krieger, D. *The Therapeutic Touch.* Englewood Cliffs, NJ: Prentice-Hall, 1979.
2. LeShan, L. *The Medium, the Mystic, and the Physicist.* New York: Viking, 1966.
3. LeShan, L. *Toward a General Theory of the Paranormal* (Parapsychological Monograph, No. 9.) New York: Parapsychology Foundation Inc., 1969.
4. Stelter, A. *Psi Healing.* New York: Bantam Books, 1976.
5. Green, A., & Green, E. *Beyond Biofeed-*

back. New York: Delacorte, 1977.
6. Smith, J. Enzymes as activated by the laying on of hands. In Approaches to Healing: Laying On of hands. *Human Dimensions, 5*, 1-2. Buffalo, NY: Human Dimensions Institute, 1976.
7. Sanford, A. *The Healing Light* (8th ed.). St. Paul: Macalester Park, 1949.
8. Worrall, A., & Worrall, O. *The Miracle Healers*. New York: New American Library, 1968.
9. LeShan, L. *The Medium, the Mystic, and the Physicist*. New York: Viking, 1966.
10. Ibid.
11. Silverman.L., Lachmam, D., & Milich, R. *The Search For Oneness*. New York: International University Press, 1982.

Chapter 12
1. Diamond, J. *Your Body Doesn't Lie*. New York: Warner Books, 1979.

Chapter 13
1. Cerutti, E. *Olga Worrall: Mystic with the Healing Hands*. New York: Harper & Row, 1975.
2. Miller, R.N. Paraelectricity, a primary energy. *Human Dimensions, 5*, 1&2, 1976, 22-26.
3. Leichtman, R.R. *From Heaven to Earth*. Columbus, OH: Ariel Press, 1977.

Chapter 14
1. Appelbaum, S.A. Challenges to traditional psychotherapy from the new therapies. *American Psychologist* (September 1982), 37, 1002-1008.
1. Appelbaum, S.A. Out *in Inner Space: A Psychoanalyst Explores the New Therapies*. New York: Anchor/Doubleday, 1979.

2. Cheek, D. In Verny, T., & Kelly, J., *The Secret Life of the Unborn Child*. New York: Dell, 1981.
3. Freud, S. *Totem and Taboo*. In *Standard Edition, 13*, 1-162.
4. Grof, S. *Realms of the Human Unconscious*. New York: Dutton, 1976.
5. Grof, S. *LSD Psychotherapy*. Pomona, CA: Hunter House, 1980.
6. Grof, S. *Beyond the Brain: Birth, Death, and Transcendence in Psychotherapy*. Albany, NY: State University of New York Press, 1985.
7. Grof, S. *The Adventure of Self-Discovery: Dimensions of Consciousness and a New Perspective in Psychotherapy*. Albany, NY: State University of New York Press, 1987.
8. Appelbaum, S.A. The *Anatomy of Change*. New York: Plenum, 1975.

Chapter 15
1. Walters, R. "Herbs and Plants Against Cancer." *Townsend Letter for Doctors*, April 1991.
2. Weil, A. Boston: Houghton Mifflin, 1990.

Chapter 16
1. Meek, G. *Healers and the Healing Process*. Wheaton, IL: Quest, 1977.
2. LeShan, L. *The Medium, the Mystic, and the Physicist*. New York: Viking, 1966.
3. Appelbaum, S.A. *Out in Inner Space: A Psychoanalyst Explores the New Therapies*. New York: Anchor/Doubleday, 1979.
4. Appelbaum, S.A. Challenges to traditional psychotherapy from the new therapies. *American Psychologist* (September 1982), 37, 1002-1008.

Index

A

absent healing. *See* distant healing
abuse, effects of on the unborn, 237
Academy of Parapsychology and Medicine, 174
acupressure, 129–130, 200
acupuncture
　application, 185–186
　meridians, 102, 130
　restoration of energy through, 141
　used at the Pain and Rehabilitation Institute, 174, 176
Advisory Council of Holos, 204
affirmations, 92, 94–96, 179. *See also* positive thinking
African religions, similarities to Catholicism, 160
aggression, roots of, 223
Agpoa, Tony, 44, 195
Akashic Records, 19–20
alcohol and blood pressure, 154
Alexander, Grete, 114–115
alfalfa, 115
allergies, 254
allspice, 253
alpha waves, 72
Ambrose and Olga Worrall Institute of Spiritual Healing, 205
American Academy of Medical Preventics, 156
American Academy of Psychoanalysis, 216
American Holistic Nurses' Association, 204
American Institute for Holistic Ecology, 205
American International Ethics and Review Board, 136
American International Hospital, 128, 135–137
American Medical Association (AMA), 156
Americans Who Have Been Reincarnated (Banerjee), 175
anemia, diagnosis of, 138–139
anesthesia. *See* pain control
animals
　healing abilities of, 67
　sacrifice of, 169–171
　use of in treatments, 202
anxiety, birth trauma as source of, 222
apportment of objects, 44
apricots. *See* seed pits
Aquinas, St. Thomas, 51
Archbishop of Canterbury, 101
Arigo, 205
arthritis, 78, 253
Assagioli, Robert, 180
asthma, 224, 254
astrological readings, 9. *See also* psychic readings
atheism, effect of on healing, 181
atherosclerosis, treatment of, 156–157
auras, 73, 83–84
autogenic training, 179

B

back pain
　psychic surgery for, 31
　remedy for, 252
Badillo, Ramon, 255
Banerjee, H. N., 175
bath, in voodoo healing, 170–171
Beauvoir, Max, 166–172
Becker, Robert, 71
bedside manner, 150–152, 265
behavioral change through affirmations, 96
Belize, folk medicine in, 251–256
Bible, used in psychic surgery, 38, 41, 47, 52
biofeedback, 64–65, 177, 186, 259
Biogenics, 177, 178–179
bioplasm, 73, 266
birth process and regression, 219, 222–228
Blanché, Juan, 33–43
bleeding, 254
blockages, 142
blood lipids, 154
blood pressure, 64–65, 154–155
body, connection with mind, 220, 260–261
Body Electric: Electromagnetism and the Foundation of Life (Becker), 71
Bowen, Barry, 251–252
brain, chemistry of, 266
"brain equalizer" machine, 186

brain waves, 72, 93
Branch, Ray (Ramus), 100–103
breathing exercises, 102
British Medical Association, 101
Brown, William C., 19–29
Bruyere, Rosalind, 77–84
Buddhism, 62
Burn Center at Sherman Oaks Hospital, 79–80
Burrows Lea, 102

C

Caesarean sections and post-birth effects, 224–225
Caminong, Rodolfo Laganzod, 58–60
cancer
   diagnosis of, 110–111, 113, 120–123
   diet to combat, 123, 125, 128
   LSD used in treatment of, 239
   meditation in treatment of, 127
   pain control of, 63
   pre-cancerous state, 150
   psychological approach to combating, 127–129
   psychological cause of, 81
   treating with psychic surgery, 36, 45–46
Cancer Control Society, 135
candling, 133–134
carcinoma, 110–111
carrot juice, to combat cancer, 125
catalepsy, 24
catharsis, in Unity method, 95
Catholicism
   in Philippine healing, 56
   similarities to African religions, 160
cedar bark, 254
chakras, 73, 81, 83
channeling. See mediums
Charismatic Renewal Movement, 103
Charles II, 3
checkup, 111
chelation therapy, 155–157
chemical reactions, healers ability to affect, 72
chemotherapy, low dose, 135
chi, 73, 266
chicanery. See validity
Chinese Medical Journal, 61
chiropractic medicine, 25–26, 111–113, 116–121
cholesterol, 154, 255
Christian Scientists, 98, 109
Christian Travel Center, 44
circulatory disturbances, diabetic, 141
City of Faith medical complex, 88

clairvoyance. See psychic readings
clouds, disbursement of by psychic means, 70–71
Coca-Cola, in voodoo healing, 165
Colcol, 57–58
colitis, 147
collective unconscious, 221
colon cancer, 125
colonics, 25, 123
Committee for Scientific Investigation of Claims of the Paranormal, 36, 43
communication, pain as, 2
compassion, role of in healing, 190
confession, role of in healing, 161
confidence, as a personality trait in healers, 196–198
consciousness, 5, 221
context, as a factor of healing, 4, 260
conventional medicine. See orthodox medicine
copal, 253
corrective emotional experiences, 95
cortisone, 166
cost of healing
   in kinesiology, 200–201, 203
   Oral Roberts University, 88
   for psychic surgery, 50–51
   refusal of payment, 66
   for voodoo ceremony, 165, 168
Coue, Emil, 179
counseling, 181–182, 181n
courses in healing, 78
creativity of healers, 193–194
cultural considerations in personalities of healers, 192
culture and perspective in healing, 55
curses, healing with psychic surgery, 48
Cushing, Harvey, 22–23
cystometrogram, 146
cystoscopy, 146

D

dead, communicating with, 210
DeAngelis, Pat, 128
death, 63–64
   as experienced in the birth process, 227
   healing after, 90, 107
   in infancy, 264
   voodoo, 259
death instinct, 222
delusional personality traits in healers, 192–194
denials, 92
dentistry. See psychic tooth pulling

Department of Health and Human Services, 242
depression, rooted in birth trauma, 223
detoxification, 176–177
deviancy in personalities of healers, 193
Di Leo, Francis, 239–242
diabetes, 35, 69
diagnosis, 109–152
    chiropractic, 111–113, 116–121
    kinesiology in, 200–201
    legal issues of, 147
    magnets used in, 116–120, 129
    psychic, 114–115, 184
    traditional *versus* alternative, 146
    use of seed pits in, 119–120
    variations in, 153, 157–158
    of vascular system, 157
    visual, 124
    x-ray eyes, 52, 80, 129
Diamond, John, 201–202
diarrhea, remedy for, 254
DiOrio, Father Ralph, 103–108
Disciples of Christ, 140
diseases and disorders
    as attempts to gain understanding, 81
    causes of, 81, 272
    Kirlian photography of, 74
    not treatable by etheric surgery, 25
    questions of psychogenic source, 103
    treated by Bruyere, 80
distant healing
    in response to mailed requests, 100
    at a standard time, 71, 206
    through prayer, 16
    using a photograph, 184
Divine Healing, as opposed to faith healing, 107–108
divine intervention, 160
Doctor in Search of a Miracle, A (Nolen), 43
doctor/patient relationship, 150–152, 172
doctors as healers, 267
Dominican Republic, 160
Doppler Study, 157
dormadioi, 252
dorsal column stimulator, 174
drama, role of in healing, 57–58, 260
drugs. *See also* LSD
    natural sources of, 254
    in voodoo, 166, 171
Duke, James, 254–255
dwende (dwarfs), 56

E
ear wax removal (candling), 133–134
Early Memory Test, 191
Ebon, Martin, 190
Eccles, Sir John, 173
Edward the Confessor, 3
Edwards, Harry, 99–103
élan vital, 73
electrical equipment, effect of, 71
electro-sleep therapy, 177
electrodes in pain control, 174
electromagnetic energy, 82–83
    charges in humans, 71, 117–118, 142
    charges to release serotonin, 186
    in diagnosis, 116–120
    in healing, 72, 208
Elliotson, John, 175–176
emotional health, healers', 75–76
endometriosis, 1–2
enemas, 123
energy, healing, 72–73, 120–121, 129, 266
enokitake mushroom, 255
environment, significance of in healing, 182
enzyme activity, 69, 81
Esalen workshop, 228–233
Esperitista, 54
Estebany, Oskar, 68–70, 75–76
ether, nausea from after surgery, 27
etheric body, 73
etheric surgery, 19–29
ethylene diamine tetracetic acid (EDTA), 156. *See also* chelation
exercise, relation to blood pressure, 154–155
exhibitionism traits in healers, 195–196
exorcism, 56–57
expressive psychotherapy, 234
extrasensory perception (ESP), 271

F
facet rhizotomy, 176
faith, role of in healing, 53, 98–99, 107–108
Faith Healers, The (Randi), 105
faith healing, as opposed to Divine healing, 107
Faith of God Foundation, 15–16
falling, frequency of in healing ceremonies, 106
familiarity, importance of, 172
fasting, 113–114
Federal Trade Commission, 43
Fernandez, Constanza, 58
Filipino psychic surgeons, 260
Fillmore, Charles and Myrtle, 92
Flores, Juan, 53–54

folk medicine, in Belize, 251–256
Food and Drug Administration, 155
fractures, setting without casts, 166
Frank, Armong, 56–57
Frank, Jerome, 258–259
fraud. See validity
Freudianism, 81, 180–182, 261
Fritz, Dr. ("surgeon with a rusty knife"), 205
From Heaven to Earth (Leichtman), 211

G

Galloway, Donald, 7–15
ganglionic cysts, psychic surgery on, 37–38
garlic pills, 115
Garrett, Eileen, 194
Geller, Uri, 74–75, 190
gender, role of in healing, 267
General Medical Council, 101
genetic mutations from LSD, 240–241
Ghede, 163
"give and take," 254
God
    concepts of, 85, 181
    healers as conduits of God's power, 7, 21, 61
    healing as demonstration of power of, 107
    as the source of all healing, 85, 99
Golden Rule, as applied in healing, 181
grace, healing as evidence of, 67
Grad, Bernard, 68–69
Grand Oloffson Hotel, 165
grandiosity in behavior of healers, 195–196
Grof, Stanislav
    background and theories of, 216–221, 223–228
    reports on research, 238–241
    views on spirituality and mental illness, 233–234
groups, effect of in healing, 260
Guardian Angels, 16
Gutierrez, Virgilio, 45

H

hair analysis, 112–113
Haiti, 160–162
hands of healers, energy associated with, 72
handwriting samples, used in psychic readings, 16
Hanscom, Daniel H., 43
headaches
    related to birth trauma, 224
    treatment of, 64, 141, 252
healers, 3, 102, 183
    as conduits of God's power, 21, 61

healers *(Continued)*
    education of, 22, 78, 256, 267–268
    personality traits of, 46, 189–198, 267
    physiological changes in, 64–65, 105
    psychological testing of, 80, 190–192, 207
    qualifications for, 267–268
    seeking intervention from, 21
    spiritual, 99
    as subjects of research, 68
healing groups, 124–125
Healing Light Center, 77
healing reality, 260–261
healing services, 90–91, 208–209
Health Maintenance (Shealy), 186
heart attack, chelation as preventative measure, 156
heat, felt during healing, 105
hemocrit, 138
hemoglobin, 138
herbs, wormwood for colonic irrigation, 25
Heywood, Rosalind, 194
hiatal hernia, 147
high density lipids (HDL), 154
Hispaniola, 160
holistic health institutions, 136–137
Holistic Institutes of Health, 204
holistic medicine, 111–114, 177, 188
hope. See positive thinking; suggestion/ placebo effect
hougan, 161, 166
Human Possibilities (Krippner), 74
Human Volunteers Research Committee of the FDA, 239
humility, self image in healers, 196
Hunt, Valerie, 82–84
hydrochloric acid, 112
hydrotherapy, 124
hyperactivity, 117
hypertension, 154
hyperthermia, treatment for cancer, 135
hyperventilation in regression exercise, 230–233
hypnosis and hypnotherapy
    attempt to enter state of, 230–231
    in holistic medicine, 182, 186
    power of, 169, 261
    in regression therapy, 266
    in Unity church, 93
hypoactivity, 117
hypochondria, 24

I

illness. See diseases and disorders

immune system, 112, 201
immunoglobulin A, 262
independence, personality trait in healers, 197-198, 268-269
Inevitable Journey (Galloway), 7
infant development and receptivity to healing, 198
infections, risk of, 40-41, 58-60
infrared thermography, 155
injections, spiritual, 53
"intelligent direction," 101
intractable symptoms, 222
intuition, role of in psychic readings, 9
investigations of healers, 101
ion field, changing, 81
iridology, 112

J
Jacobson, Edmond, 179
James, William, 6
jaundice in diagnosis, 157
Johnson, David Kendrick, 211
Johnson, Lyndon, 109
Jolicouer, Aubelin, 165
Judaism as referred to by Oral Roberts, 88
juice
    carrot, 125
    fasting, 114
    machines (juicing), 114
Jung, Carl, 180, 221

K
Kammann, Richard, 43
kapok, 254
karma, 81
Kelly Anti-Cancer Diet, 123
kidneys, preventative medicine for, 254
kinesiology, 112, 199-203
Kirlian photography, 73-74, 83, 141
Krippner, Stanley, 64, 160, 175
Krippner and Villoldo court ruling, 43
Kuhlman, Kathryn, 104

L
labor, difficult, 236
Laryngoscope, 134
laying on of hands
    author's ability, 63-66
    for cancer, 120-121, 129
    Faith of God Foundation, 16
    Olga Worrall, 206
Le Peristyle, 166
lead poisoning, 155

left-brain/right brain, significance of in healing, 93
Leichtman, Robert, 190, 210-215
Leonard, George, 200
LeShan, Lawrence, 194, 196-197, 263, 268
libido, 73, 266
life force, 70, 73
live cell therapy, 202
loas, 163
Long, Coletta, 92-99
Louisiana, 160
Lourdes, 258-259
love
    as a curative agent, 270
    fundamental to healers' abilities, 196
    and healers, 262-263
low density lipids (LDL), 154
Lozanov teaching method, 96
LSD, 215-250. *See also* regression
    author's account of, 244-250
    contraindications for, 241
    Francis Di Leo, 239-242
    genetic mutations from, 240-241
    Human Volunteers Research Committee of the FDA, 239, 242-243
    panic as a common experience, 245
    as a therapeutic tool, 227, 239-250, 266
lymphocytes, 201

M
machinery, diagnostic, 111
Madame C, 162-165
magic and powerlessness, 159
magicians, consultants in psychic surgery studies, 33-43
magnetic polarity in body, 142
magnets, used in diagnosis, 116-120
mail, energy transfer through, 69
mambo, 162
Man Beneath the Gift, The (DiOrio), 103-104
marasmus, 264
massage, 177
    of feet, 143-144
    in healing ceremony, 171
materialization of objects, 44
May, Rollo, 268
medical education, 86-87, 262
medication, prescription of, 120
meditation, 64-65, 181, 186
mediums. *See also* psychic readings
    accuracy in readings, 8-14
    as conduits of God's power, 5

mediums *(Continued)*
   spirits communicating through, 51, 78–79, 101, 162
   spiritualists, 7
memories
   recovery of, 234
   stored in body tissue, 83
mental illness, as "spiritual emergencies," 233
meridians in acupuncture, 73, 130–131
Midwest Research, 135–137
Miller, Robert, 71–72
mind/body connection, 2, 5, 260–261, 266, 269
minerals. *see* vitamins and minerals
money. *See* cost of healing
mood, effects on healing, 75–76
morality, effects on health, 51
mother-child relationship and healing, 198, 267
moxibustion, 256
mushrooms, 255
music
   effects on the unborn, 237
   as tool in LSD regression, 244
mysterious leap concept, 261

N

National Enquirer, 43
Natural Health, Natural Medicine (Weil), 255
Nature-all Formulas, 200
Nature of Reality: Dawning of a New Paradigm, The (Grof), 238
naturopath, 124
nerve blocks, 176
nerves, electrical stimulation of, 176
New Realities (Shealy), 176
Newman, Alan, 204
Ninety Days to Self Health (Shealy), 176
Nolen, William, 31
Novak, Warren, 111–113, 135–136
novelty, significance of the role of in healing, 235
nutrition
   and cancer, 123, 125, 127–128
   for hypertension, 154
   supplements for circulatory problems, 141

O

obel, 253
obesity, related to post-birth deprivation, 223
Occult Medicine Can Save Your Life (Shealy), 175
od, 73
opinions, medical, 153, 158
oral characteristics of healers, 197
Oral Roberts University, Tulsa, OK, 85–91
Orbito, Alex, 45, 47–50
orgone, 70, 73, 266
orthodox medicine
   and alternative medicine, 6, 269–270
   mixed results of, 5, 116–117
   as a tool of God, 89–90
   and voodoo, 161, 165
Out in Inner Space (Applebaum), 9, 127

P

Pain and Rehabilitation Institute, 137, 173–174, 178
pain control
   clinics, 176
   in etheric surgery, 25
   folk remedies for, 253
   with needle electrodes, 174
   in psychic surgery, 30, 37
   in psychic tooth pulling, 58–62
   through laying on of hands, 63
Pain Game, The (Shealy), 176
Palmer Chiropractic School, 140
pancreas, 112
Pangasinan's Spiritualist Center, 52
papillomas, 41
para-electricity, type of spiritual healing, 208
parapsychology, 67
passivity in psychic work, 194
"Peace Song, The," 93–94
peaches. *See* seed pits
Pease, Jean, 123
   healing group meeting, 124–125
   psychic diagnosis, 115–116
   treatments, 129–132, 143–144
perinatal development stage, 219
perinatal matrices, 225–227
personality
   affect of on healers' styles, 97
   effect of patient's, on physical illness, 167–168
   traits of healers, 74, 189–198, 194
perspective, 2
Pfeiffer, Harry L., 116–124, 149–152
   background of, 140
   bedside manner of, 150–151
   diagnosis of author's cancer, 120–123
   examinations of author, 137–138, 147–148
   laying on of hands, 120–121
   use of magnets in diagnosis, 116–120
Philippines. *See also* psychic surgery
   exorcism, 56–57
   travel restrictions imposed by the Federal Trade Commission, 43

Philippines *(Continued)*
   treatments in, 30–62
phlebitis, 141
photography of psychic activity, 74–75
physical examinations, 25–26, 111
physical memory, 219
pichoja, 254
pinpricks, administering psychically, 53
placebo effect. *See* suggestion/placebo effect
plants
   in folk healing, 254
   healer's ability to affect growth of, 69, 72
   used in remedies, 252–256
   in voodoo, 166, 171
plasmapharesis, 135
pleasure scale, 177
plythesmograph, 157
polarity, 117, 141, 200
Port-au-Prince, 165
positive thinking, 257–260. *See also* suggestion/placebo effect
   in holistic medicine, 182
   physiological effects of, 126–127
   in the Unity Movement, 92–97
postoperative symptoms, as evidence of validity, 28
prana, 38, 73, 266
prayer, 86–87, 89
predictions. *See* psychic readings
pregnancy, stress during, 236–237
premenstrual distress, remedy for, 252
preoedipal stages or development, 219
Primal Therapy, 231
problems, perspective on, 2
psychic ability
   atrophy of, 144
   evidence of, 207
psychic diagnosis, anecdotal nature of, 144
psychic gland, 101–102
psychic healing, 117, 120–121, 271
psychic readings, 131–132. *See also* mediums; Tarot readings
   accuracy of, 8–14
   author's readings, 19–20, 55, 131–132
   effect of mood on, 14–15
   generality of, 214
   predictions, 131–132, 185
   role of perception in, 8, 12
   validity of, 213–214
psychic surgery, 30–62
   author's experiences with, 49–50
   Bibles used in, 38, 41, 47, 52

psychic surgery *(Continued)*
   conditions treated, 49
      cancer, 36, 45–46, 54
      curses, 48
      heart problems, 46
      vision problems, 41
   described, 34–39, 53
   discrediting, 54–55
   experiments to authenticate, 32–43
   explained, 51–52
   injections, administering without implements, 53
   pain control in, 30, 37, 40
   payment for, 50–51
   spirituality in, 36
   statistics on, 32
psychic tooth pulling, 58–62
psychic X-ray vision, 52, 80, 129
psychology. *See also* psychotherapy
   of healing, 67, 75, 264–265
   role of in fighting cancer, 127–129
   Unity church's emphasis on, 92–99
psychoneuroimmunology, 271
Psychopharmacological Drugs Advisory Committee, 242
psychosomatic medicine, voodoo as, 159
psychosynthesis, 180
psychotherapy
   compared to psychosynthesis, 180
   contrasted with counseling, 181n
   efficacy of, 76
   as practiced in the Unity church, 94–96
   training in, 265
   voodoo compared to, 161
pulse diagnosis, 164
Purpura, Dominic, 238
pyelogram, 146

R

radiation, treatment for, 155
Randi, James, 43, 105
readings. *See* mediums; psychic readings
reality, concepts of, 55, 220
receptivity
   author's, 79, 213
   encouraged by breathing exercises, 102
   familiarity negating, 108
   as a function of evolution, 67
   as the fundamental requirement of all healing, 198
   in psychic healing, 21
   and resistance to healing, 78
recording devices, failure to work, 27–28

Reed, William Standish, 89
regeneration, 71, 80
regression, 217–250. *See also* LSD
   author's attempts at, 228–233, 244–250
   conditions associated with birth trauma, 222–225
   consciousness concepts, 221–222
   defined, 217–218
   Esalen workshop, 228–233
   resistance to, 231
   screams during exercises, 231
Reich, Wilhelm, 71
reincarnation, 175–176, 184–185, 220
relationships
   of healers (early), 270
   significance of in healing, 263–264
religion
   atheists and healing, 181
   healing ministries emphasizing, 15–17
   role of in healing, 38, 67, 85, 142, 181
remote viewing, 221
research
   critically evaluating methodology, 72
   on healing, 66–77
   importance of, 269–273
   on Olga Worrall, 207
   on Rolfing, 82–84
rheumatism, pain remedy for, 253
Rhine, J. B., 174–175
Roberts, Oral, 85–91
   healing services, authenticity questioned, 90–91
   soliciting donations, 87–88
   theory on healing, 89
Roberts, Richard, 87
Rolfing, 82
Rorschach Test, 190, 195
Rosalita, 252
"royal touch," 3
Rucker, Henry E., 182–185
rutin, 141

S

Sanford, Agnes, 196
Satanic healing, 90
schizophrenia, 80, 226
Scholes, Vernon, 89–90
Schultz, J. H., 179
scientific method
   lack of in alternative healing, 145
   nature of, 4
   shortcomings of, 153

screaming in regression exercises, 231
second opinions, 153
Secret of the Unborn Child, The (Verney), 237, 250
"seed faith," 87
seed pits, in diagnosis, 119, 148
self-healing, 91
Self-Healing, 134
self-responsibility, 98, 177
sensitivity, in lieu of psychic abilities, 15
Serpent and the Rainbow, The (Davis), 167
Seutemann, Sigrun, 32
sexuality in infants, 224
Shealy, C. Norman, 173–188, 204
Shiatsu, 130, 144, 200
shiitake mushrooms, used in folk remedies, 255
sickness. *See* diseases and disorders
Silva Mind Control, 74
Silverman, Lloyd, 197
Simonton, Carl, 127–129
Simonton, Stephanie, 127–129
Singer, Phillip, 32–43
skin, diagnosis through, 71
slaves, 163. *See also* zombies
slaying, 104
Smith, M. Justa, 68–70, 75, 196
Southwestern Missouri State University, 204
speaking in tongues, 104
spirits
   appearances of, 205–206, 208
   communicating through mediums, 78–79, 162, 210, 212–213
   definition of, 99
   guiding surgical procedures, 22–26
   intervention of, 167–168
   role of in healing, 5
Spiritual Emergency Network (S.E.N.), 233–234
spiritualists, 7, 15
spirituality
   enlightenment, as related to schizophrenia, 226
   of healers, 190, 262–263
   healing achieved through, 99
   as the main purpose of healing, 107
spontaneous healing, 2
St. Claire, Magdalen, 16
Stelter, A., 31–32
stomach distress, remedy for, 253
stress, 180, 237
stroke, 155–156
Structural Integration. *See* Rolfing
subconscious, 95–96

suggestion/placebo effect
   as component of psychotherapy, 95
   connection to Freud's "mysterious leap," 261
   connection to need, 262
   connection with healers reputation, 207
   description of, 4, 257
   as explanation for healing by touch, 67
   as tool of healer, 28
   transient nature of, 106
   in Unity movement, 99
   of voodoo potion, 171
suicide, 223
Summa Theologica (Aquinas), 51
surgery. *See* etheric surgery; psychic surgery
Surgery of the Soul (Reed), 89
synchronicity, 181

T
T cells (thymus cells), 201
Talcott, Linden, 120, 126–127
Tarot readings, 164–165, 184–185
technology of healing, 4, 260, 265
teeth. *See* psychic tooth pulling
telepathy, 75, 132
Ten Commandments of Good Health (Shealy), 186–187
tension, effects of on healing, 76
testimonials, 265
   for etheric surgery, 29
   for laying on of hands, 206
   for psychic surgery, 31
Thematic Appercetion Test, 191
throat cancer, symptoms of, 130
Thundercloud, 22
thymus, 201–203
tics, related to birth trauma, 224
touch, healing with, 66–68. *See also* laying on of hands
trances, 51, 168
transcendence, 5, 224
transience of healing results, 182, 197, 202
transpersonal experiences, 217
transpersonal mind, 220
Treadway, George, 89–90
treatments, 176
tremors, related to birth trauma, 224
tukis Mayan, 254
turtles, used in folk remedies, 254

U
Unity Movement, 91–99, 109

universal consciousness, 234
University of Arizona Program in Integrative Medicine, 134

V
Vagina dentata, 224
Valentine, Tom, 53
validity
   questions of, 47, 125, 212–213
   return customers as evidence of, 28–29
Vanderbilt Divinity School, 140
varicosities, 141
vascular diagnosis, 157
Verney, Thomas, 237
vibrations of spirits, 208
visions, as guidance in diagnosis, 131
vitamins and minerals, 112, 149
voodoo, 159–172
   compared to Western health care, 161–162
   diagnoses, 164
   healing ceremony, 168–171
   as a psychosomatic medicine, 159
   as quasi-legal system, 161–162, 163, 167
   as self-defense measure, 163
"voodoo death," 259

W
Watson, Lyall, 53
weight loss, from treatment, 139–140
Weil, Andrew, 134, 255
Western medicine. *See* orthodox medicine
white blood cells, 201
white crow, search for, 6, 270–273
wormwood for colonic irrigation, 25
Worrall, Olga
   accounts of the paranormal involving, 71–72, 205–210
   brain waves experiments on, 93
   views on love in healing, 196
Worrell, Ambrose, 196, 205–210

X
X-ray vision in healers, 52, 80, 129
Xuehin, Gong, 61

Y
Yoga, 179
yogis, 259

Z
Zen, 179
zombies, 163, 167

About the Author

After many years on the staff of the Menninger Clinic in Topeka, Kansas, Dr. Stephen A. Appelbaum was in private practice of psychoanalysis and clinical psychology in Kansas City and Professor at the University of Missouri–Kansas City. He then became the Erik H. Erikson Scholar in Residence at the Austen Riggs Center in Stockbridge, Massachusetts. He is now Visiting Professor in the Department of Psychiatry, Harvard Medical School. Author of over 100 professional journal articles, his previous books include *The Anatomy of Change* (Plenum Press), *Effecting Change in Psychotherapy* (Jason Aronson Publishing Co./Jason Aronson Masterworks Series), and *Out in Inner Space: A Psychoanalyst Explores the New Therapies* (Doubleday/Anchor).